D1568736

Gastrointestinal Motility Disorders

Diagnosis and Treatment

Gastrointestinal Motility Disorders

Diagnosis and Treatment

Edited by

Richard W McCallum, MD

Professor of Internal Medicine
Chief, Division of Gastroenterology
University of Virginia School of
Medicine
Charlottesville, Virginia

Malcolm C Champion, MB

Associate Professor of Medicine
Division of Gastroenterology
University of Ottawa
Ottawa Civic Hospital
Ottawa, Ontario, Canada

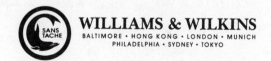
WILLIAMS & WILKINS
BALTIMORE · HONG KONG · LONDON · MUNICH
PHILADELPHIA · SYDNEY · TOKYO

Editor: Michael G. Fisher
Associate Editor: Carol Eckhart
Production: Barbara J. Felton

Copyright © 1990
Williams & Wilkins
428 East Preston Street
Baltimore, MD 21202, U.S.A.

Accurate indications, adverse reactions, and dosage schedules for drugs are provided in this book, but it is possible that they may change. The reader is urged to review the package information data of the manufacturers of the medications mentioned.

Printed in Canada
To be sold in the United States of America only

Library of Congress Cataloging-in-Publication Data

Gastrointestinal motility disorders : diagnosis and treatment / edited by Richard W. McCallum, Malcolm C. Champion.
     p. cm.
  Based on a symposium held in Chicago on May 8, 1987.
  Includes index.
  ISBN 0-683-05748-0
  1. Gastrointestinal system — Motility — Disorders — Congresses.
I. McCallum, Richard W. II. Champion, Malcolm C. III. Title: Gastrointestinal motility disorders: diagnosis & treatment. [DNLM: 1. Gastrointestinal Diseases — diagnosis — congresses. 2. Gastrointestinal Diseases —therapy — congresses. 3. Gastrointestinal Motility — congresses. WI 102 P5777 1987]
RC811.G37   1989   616.3'3—dc19   88-38740

92 93 94
10 9 8 7 6 5 4 3 2

Contents

Preface

What, another book on motility! Why? Because new discoveries have been made concerning the motor action of the alimentary canal, providing new insights into the problems that afflict our patients and novel therapies for their disordered motility.

These advances come from the generation next to mine. There has been a dry spell in between, but renewed life is now spreading through the field and the fertile areas are well represented in this book.

It is easy reading. You can pick up or put it down, for there is no continuity except in time. Each piece is presented by an expert. Each piece stands alone. The chapters are good to read, not only for the knowledge they present, but also for the glimpse into the future they provide.

New drugs, new regulators with wonderful names and actions are here to stay. Drugs like domperidone to turn things on and hormones like somatostatin to turn them off.

There is improvement, too, in the tools at hand. This applies also to the recognition of disordered segments whose removal may cure or greatly improve disorganized motor action.

It is clear from this book that the most accurate information and the greatest quantity of data available relate to the two ends of the alimentary canal. The deeper the penetration from either end, the thinner the knowledge. This is particularly true in the large bowel where the relationship between electrical activity and contraction, so firm in the stomach and small bowel, appears to have broken down. We still do not understand it. The contrast is at a stand off. Is it that some features of the mechanical or electrical changes in the bowel are absent from our recordings? The modus operandi of the system still eludes us.

I have enjoyed the book. I think you will, too. The editors and the contributors have my gratitude and my admiration. I hope they will have yours.

Charles F Code MD PhD
University of California
San Diego, LA

Foreword

The importance of motility as a major cause of gastrointestinal problems has become increasingly recognized in recent years. There has been a realization that while acid does play a role in the pathophysiology of some symptom states in the esophagus and stomach, inhibiting acid secretion is not appropriate therapy for those disorders resulting from impaired smooth muscle function. This need to reassess the role of acid begins in the esophagus and stomach with realization that the entity of non-ulcer dyspepsia is often explained by delayed gastric emptying. In addition there are motor abnormalities of the small intestine such as pseudo-obstruction and the spectrum of constipation and irritable bowel syndrome, including colonic motility problems. Indeed, it has been estimated that disorders of gastrointestinal (GI) motility account for 50–60% of complaints seen by primary care physicians and 40–60% of patients referred to a gastroenterologist.

Many of the underlying mechanisms controlling the motility of the gut are not yet fully understood. However, recent advances in diagnostic methodology have enhanced our ability to perform manometric, scintigraphic and electrophysiologic measurement of the gut's activities, and have provided many new insights into the pathophysiology of some of these entities. In addition, novel pharmacologic approaches have evolved to treat the disorders. A new class of agent has appeared in the 1980s — prokinetic agents. The definition of this new class is that they restore and normalize impaired or abnormal smooth muscle function resulting in improved aboral transit of digested nutrients through the GI tract.

The founding father of this class of agents was metoclopramide (Reglan® in the USA, Maxalon® in Britain, Primperan® in France). Since then domperidone (Motilium®) has been cloned as a more refined model. It is interesting that there is a perception that motility disorders of the GI tract may still be addressed by empiric therapy with acid-inhibiting drugs (specifically H_2 blockers) and this will require time and education to change.

Currently, new agents are being developed where promotility effects are not limited to the upper GI tract as is the situation with metoclopramide and domperidone. Rather promotility benefits may also extend to the distal small bowel, establishing the concept of a 'pan-prokinetic' agent. Cisapride (Prepulsid®) is the drug which represents the evolution of pharmacologic development. When new pharmacology is on the horizon, better methodology for objective quantitation of results seems to emerge and we are motivated into more creative techniques. We believe this will also occur in the colon, enabling major strides to be accomplished in this poorly understood area. This is because new therapeutic agents offer so much hope for symptom relief for our patients and it is crucial that at the same time we objectively document their benefits.

To provide a timely, in-depth review of the current state of knowledge in the field of motility and also predict future developments, a major symposium entitled *Physiology, Diagnosis & Therapy in GI Motility Disorders* was held in Chicago on May 8, 1987. Nineteen of the world's experts in GI motility disturbances took part in this symposium, which was attended by over 400 physicians and surgeons. Presentations reflected state-of-the-art knowledge on motor disorders of the esophagus, stomach, small intestine and colon, with presentation of the latest theories, diagnostic tests, therapies (both surgical and nonsurgical) and research results. The symposium thus represented a major landmark in announcing the arrival of motility disorders as a clinically prominent entity as well as advancing our full understanding of the area.

The faculty who contributed to this scientific gathering are the authors of the chapters in this text book entitled *Gastrointestinal Motility Disorders: Diagnosis and Treatment*. We, the editors of this publication, believe this text provides a timely summary of current concepts in an exciting and evolving major field of gastroenterology. The contents attempt to relate basic research to diagnostic findings in patients and provide an up-to-date assessment and preview of therapeutic approaches to motility problems from the esophagus to the rectum.

Malcolm C Champion BSc MB ChB
MRCS MRCP(UK) FRCPC

Richard W McCallum MB BS MD
FACP FRACP(Aust) FACG

®Registered trademark

Contributors

Donald O Castell MD
Professor of Medicine
Chief of Gastroenterology
Bowman Gray School of
  Medicine
Winston-Salem, North Carolina

Malcolm C Champion BSc MB ChB
  MRCS MRCP(UK) FRCPC
Associate Professor of Medicine
Division of Gastroenterology
University of Ottawa
Ottawa Civic Hospital
Ottawa, Canada

Nicholas E Diamant MD FRCPC
Professor of Medicine and Physiology
University of Toronto
Head, Division of Gastroenterology
Toronto Western Hospital
Toronto, Canada

Michael RB Keighley MRCS LRCP
  MB BS FRCS
Professor of Surgery
General and Dental Hospital
University of Birmingham
Birmingham, England

Keith A Kelly MD
Professor, Chairman
Department of Surgery
Mayo Medical Center
Rochester, New York

Richard W McCallum MB BS MD
  FACP FRACP(Aust) FACG
Professor of Internal Medicine
Chief, Division of Gastroenterology
University of Virginia School of Medicine
Charlottesville, Virginia

Juan-Ramon Malagelada MD
Chief of Gastroenterology
Hospital 'Valle de Hebron'
Autonomous University of Barcelona
Barcelona, Spain

John R Mathias MD
Professor of Internal Medicine
University of Texas Medical Branch
Galveston, Texas

James H Meyer MD
Professor of Medicine
University of California, Los Angeles
Chief, Division of Gastroenterology
Veterans Administration Medical Center,
  Sepulveda
Los Angeles, California

Sidney F Phillips MD FRACP FACP
Director, Gastroenterology Unit
Mayo Clinic
Rochester, New York

Nicholas W Read MB MD MRCP FRCP
Honorary Consultant Physician
Royal Hallamshire Hospital
Reader in Physiology and Honorary
    Lecturer in Medicine
University of Sheffield
Sheffield, England

Michael D Schuffler MD
Professor, Department of Medicine
University of Washington School
    of Medicine
Chief of Gastroenterology
Pacific Medical Center
Seattle, Washington

William J Snape Jr MD
Professor of Medicine
University of California, Los Angeles
Director of Inflammatory Bowel Disease
    Center
Harbor-UCLA Medical Center
Los Angeles, California

Grant Thompson MD FACP FRCPC
Assistant Dean, Professor of Medicine
University of Ottawa
Chief, Division of Gastroenterology
Ottawa Civic Hospital
Ottawa, Canada

Gaston Vantrappen MD PhD
Professor and Chairman of Medicine
Head, Division of Gastroenterology
University Hospital of Leuven
Leuven, Belgium

William E Whitehead PhD
Johns Hopkins University School
    of Medicine
Francis Scott Key Medical Center
Baltimore, Maryland

I
Physiology

Physiology of the esophagus

N E Diamant

Current knowledge of the more basic physiology of the esophagus is derived primarily from studies in animal species and to a lesser extent from humans and non-human primates. Unfortunately, there are marked species differences that invite some caution when applying findings from animal studies to normal human esophageal physiology.

Nevertheless, normal control of the human esophagus can be viewed with some general functional characteristics in mind.

• Functionally, the esophagus can be divided into three zones: the upper esophageal sphincter (UES), the esophageal body and the lower esophageal sphincter (LES).

• There are a number of control mechanisms for esophageal motor activity, harboured within the central nervous system, as well as peripherally within the intramural neural and muscle properties.

• Deglutition, or the act of swallowing, is the primary initiator of integrated esophageal activity.

• In the human, normal activity of the esophagus is programmed to proceed in the aboral direction.

Several recent reviews cover the topic in detail.[1-4]

Anatomy of the esophagus

The esophageal length is about 20 cm (*Figure 1*). Five percent of the upper esophageal body, including the UES, along with the muscles involved in the buccopharyngeal phase of swallowing, are entirely striated. Approximately 50–60% of the distal esophagus, including the LES, is entirely smooth muscle, the circular muscle layer extending more proximally than the longitudinal layer. The transition zone of striated and smooth muscle includes up to 35–40% of the esophageal length in between. The area where muscle is equally striated and smooth is found about 5 cm below the proximal portion of the cricopharyngeus muscle.[5]

Striated muscle

Pharynx: the oropharynx and hypopharynx form a contractile funnel which leads to the upper end of the esophagus at the UES. There is a good deal of structural complexity and associated functional complexity which provides ample scope for difficulty in swallowing during the buccopharyngeal stage of swallowing.[6]

Upper esophageal sphincter: the UES (2–4.5 cm by manometry) is formed primarily by the horizontal fibres of the cricopharyngeus muscle which forms a loop posteriorly. The anterior wall of the UES is rigid because of the cricoid cartilage and other

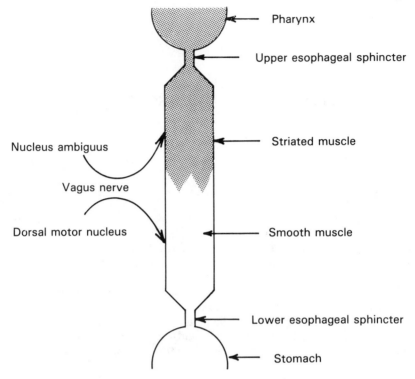

Figure 1   Muscle composition of the esophagus and its vagal innervation.

structures that form the posterior wall of the larynx.[2-4,6] Because of the anatomical features, the UES forms a transverse slit-like structure when closed.

Esophageal body: the striated muscle portion of the esophageal body begins at the inferior border of the cricopharyngeus muscle. Generally, there is a longitudinal outer layer and a circular inner layer. The longitudinal layer extends more distally than the circular layer.

Smooth muscle

Esophageal body: the smooth muscle in the human esophageal body also has an outer longitudinal and a thicker inner circular layer, the latter extending more proximally. Cell-to-cell contact is common particularly in the circular layer.[7]

Lower esophageal sphincter: at the gastroesophageal junction, which is characterized by a higher pressure zone of 2-4 cm in length and functional and radiological features of a sphincter, there is a thicker ring of the circular smooth muscle. This ring is intimately connected with some smooth muscle fibres of the stomach.[8] Many smooth muscle cells in the region of the LES show numerous branches and increased cell-to-cell contacts, which probably relate to the ability of this zone to maintain tone.[7]

Innervation of the esophagus
The esophageal innervation provides the mechanism for excitation of the muscle at all levels and serves as the coordinating mechanism for the swallowing sequence in the buccopharyngeal region and the striated muscle portion of the esophagus. In addition, innervation affords at least three potential control mechanisms for coordina-

tion of peristalsis within the smooth muscle esophagus. Finally, it serves as the major control mechanism for normal function of both the UES and LES, and includes the network for sensory and reflex modulation of the esophageal body and sphincter motor activities.

Extrinsic innervation

Extrinsic control for esophageal motor function resides in a brainstem swallowing centre (*Figure 2*)[1,4,9,10] that has three functional components: an afferent reception system, an efferent system of motor neurons, and a complex organizing or internuncial system of neurons. These components can also be conveniently subdivided topographically into buccopharyngeal (to include the UES), esophageal and LES control functions.

Afferent reception system: afferent information from the periphery ultimately enters into the solitary tract, the afferent reception portion of the swallowing centre. This sensory information can serve to initiate deglutition and the swallowing sequence, alter previously initiated activity in the swallowing centre and therefore modify ongoing motor activity, or function within reflexes affecting the esophageal body and its sphincters independent of swallowing. Sensory information from the entire esophagus, including the sphincters, is carried in the vagus, with the cell bodies in the nodose ganglion, while some sensory information also passes via the sympathetics to the spinal cord segments T3–T12.[11]

Sensory information from the buccopharyngeal area enters through the extravagal cranial nerve (trigeminal, facial, hypoglossal and glossopharyngeal) and vagal nerve pathways.[6,9]

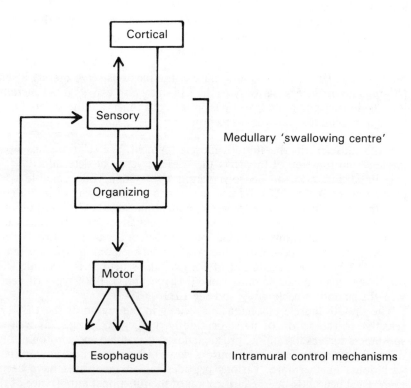

Figure 2 Diagram representing the central organization of swallowing.

Coordinating region: the portion of the swallowing centre that programs the entire swallowing sequence is probably located in the solitary tract nucleus (STN) and the neighbouring reticular substance.[10] It has two levels of integration, one for the initiation of swallowing and organizing of the entire swallowing sequence, and the other serving as a connecting pathway to the various motor neuron pools involved in the swallowing sequence.

Efferent output: motor neurons involved in the swallowing sequence lie mainly in the trigeminal, facial and hypoglossal nuclei, the nucleus ambiguus (for esophageal striated muscle) and the dorsal motor nucleus of the vagus (for esophageal smooth muscle).[1,6,9] The vagus nerve receiving fibres both from the nucleus ambiguus and the dorsal motor nucleus innervates the striated and smooth muscle esophagus respectively, including the sphincters (*Figure 1*). The cervical esophagus is innervated by the recurrent laryngeal nerves and the esophagus distally by the branches from the thoracic vagal trunks. In the region of the cricopharynx, fibres from the pharyngeal branches of the vagus and the superior laryngeal nerves intersect with fibres from the recurrent laryngeal nerves.

Sympathetic: the efferent sympathetic connections to the esophagus arise in the cervical ganglia and ganglia of the paravertebral chains and reach the esophagus via the vascular supply and, to a lesser extent, through connections to the vagus nerves. The pre-ganglionic cell bodies are said to lie in spinal segments T5 and T6.[12] It is likely that, in humans, sympathetic innervation to the LES also occurs via the splanchnic nerves.

Intramural innervation
There is a myenteric nerve plexus in both the striated and smooth muscle segments of the esophagus; this is less well developed in the striated muscle portion. The submucosal plexus is present but also sparse.[3]

Striated muscle: in the striated muscle, the plexuses serve mainly a sensory role, although an inhibitory pathway to the LES may also exist.[13] It is generally held that the vagal post-ganglionic fibres pass directly to innervate the striated muscle fibres through cholinergic, nicotinic receptors.[1,3,4]

Smooth muscle: in the smooth muscle segment, the relationships between morphology and function of the nerve plexuses are yet to be determined.[3,14,15] There are two important effector neurons within the system, one capable of mediating cholinergic excitation of both longitudinal and circular layers of smooth muscle, and the other of mediating nonadrenergic, noncholinergic (NANC) inhibition mainly of the circular muscle layer (*Figure 3*).[1-4,16-21] The neurotransmitter released by the latter neuron(s) is unknown although purine nucleotides and peptide hormones, such as vasoactive intestinal polypeptide (VIP), have been among the substances proposed.[1-4,22,23] Cholinergic excitation of the excitatory neuron is nicotinic while that of the NANC neuron can be muscarinic (M1 receptors). Both types of neurons innervate the smooth muscle body and the LES.

   The smooth muscle esophagus, especially in the region of the LES (*Table 1*), is sensitive to the action of most peptide hormones and drugs, as well as to other substances such as histamine, prostaglandins, dopamine and serotonin.[1-4,22] The majority of these agents can act on muscle, nerve or both and there are significant species variations. Furthermore, various peptides including opiates have been found in esophageal neural tissue.[2-4] Clarification of the functional importance of these agents awaits further study.

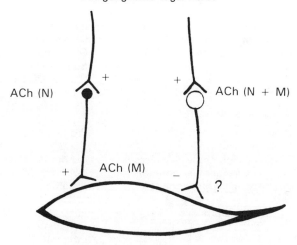

Figure 3   Major known motor innervation of the smooth muscle esophagus. Interneurons, adrenergic innervation and other possible neurotransmitters are not shown since the circuitry is not known (other than a modulatory role is not established for adrenergic supply) and the functional role of other putative neurotransmitters is unclear. • = excitatory neuron; O = inhibitory neuron; ACh = acetylcholine; N = nicotinic; M = muscarinic.

Sympathetic: sympathetic nerves are also present within the myenteric plexus of the striated and smooth muscle esophagus. Sympathetic nerves appear to modulate the activity of other neurons and the release of their respective neurotransmitters, and act to modify features such as contraction amplitude and velocity, and LES tone.[25,26] Beta-adrenergic effect is inhibitory and alpha-adrenergic effect is excitatory.

Coordinated esophageal motor activity

Accurate and reliable measurement techniques are of particular importance in assessing coordinated esophageal motility.[27-29] Furthermore, structural and functional factors affect measurements such as pressure, especially in the area of the sphincters.[30-32]

At rest, the esophageal body is usually quiet and without motor activity, while the sphincters at either end maintain a contraction which can be manometrically measured as a high pressure zone and characterized as resting tone. Between swallows, neither the resting tone of the sphincters nor the quiescence of the esophageal body are static and unchanging. Within the esophageal body, peristaltic or nonperistaltic esophageal contractions can arise independent of swallowing with such events as gastroesophageal reflux and stress.[33,34] In the sphincter regions, continuous change is the rule. The classical coordinated motor pattern of the esophagus is initiated by the act of swallowing, and is called 'primary' peristalsis (*Figure 4*). A rapidly progressing pharyngeal contraction transfers the bolus through a relaxed UES into the esophagus, and as the UES closes, a progressive circular contraction begins in the upper esophagus and proceeds distally along the esophageal body to propel the bolus through a relaxed LES. Once the bolus is moved voluntarily into the pharynx and the pharyngeal contractions are initiated, the process becomes involuntary.

'Secondary' peristalsis is a progressive contraction in the esophageal body that is not induced by a swallow, but rather by stimulation of sensory receptors in the

	Increase in pressure	Decrease in pressure
Hormones	Gastrin	Secretin
	Motilin	Cholecystokinin
	Substance P	Glucagon
		Somatostatin
		Gastric inhibitory polypeptide
		Vasoactive intestinal polypeptide
		Progesterone
Neural agents	α-Adrenergic agonists	ß-Adrenergic agonists
	ß-Adrenergic antagonists	α-Adrenergic antagonists
	Cholinergic agonists	Anticholinergic agents
Foods	Protein meals	Fat
		Chocolate
		Ethanol
		Peppermint
Other	Histamine	Theophylline
	Antacids	Caffeine
	Metoclopramide	Gastric acidification
	Domperidone	Smoking
	Cisapride	Pregnancy
	Prostaglandin ($F_{2\alpha}$)	Prostaglandins (E2, I2)
	Coffee	Serotonin
	Migrating motor complex	Meperidine, morphine
	Raised intra-abdominal pressure	Dopamine
		Calcium blocking agents
		Diazepam
		Barbiturates

Table 1   Factors influencing LES pressure.

esophageal body. Secondary peristalsis is usually caused by distension with refluxed gastric content, or following incomplete clearing of the esophageal content by a primary swallow. Secondary peristalsis occurs only in the esophagus, usually begins at or above a level corresponding to the location of the stimulus, closely resembles the peristalsis induced by a swallow, and is also swallowing centre mediated.

In the absence of connections to the swallowing centre, a local intramural mechanism can at times produce peristalsis in the smooth muscle esophagus. This has been called 'tertiary' peristalsis,[36,37] and should not be confused with tertiary contractions, incoordinate or simultaneous contractions in the esophageal body.[38]

Upper esophageal sphincter
At rest the UES is tonically closed with marked radial asymmetry to the profile of the intraluminal pressure.[30] Pressures are higher anteriorly and posteriorly (*Table 2*). UES pressure increases when necessary to provide extra protection for the airway, such as with acid in the upper esophagus.[4,32] On the other hand, a belch, vomiting

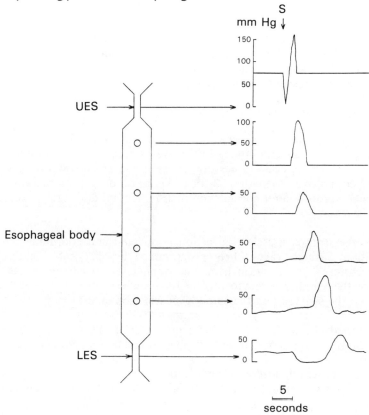

Figure 4 Manometric pressure changes with a swallow (S). Proximal and distal tracings are from the upper (UES) and lower (LES) esophageal sphincters respectively. Immediately after a swallow UES pressure falls transiently. Shortly thereafter, LES pressure falls and remains low until the peristaltic contraction passing aborally through the UES and then the esophageal body closes the LES.

	Mean (mmHg)	Range (mmHg)
Resting UES pressure[32]		
— posterior axis	101	60–142
— anterior axis	84	55–123
— lateral axis	48	30–65
Resting LES pressure[72]		10–65
Esophageal contraction amplitude[72]		
— distal esophagus		50–110

Table 2 Typical esophageal manometric pressures. UES = upper esophageal sphincter; LES = lower esophageal sphincter.

and abrupt esophageal distension are associated with a fall in UES pressure to permit release of esophageal contents or decompression of the esophagus.[39]

After a swallow (within 0.2–0.9 seconds) both cessation of neural excitation to the UES and elevation and forward movement of the cricoid cartilage act together to decrease the UES resting pressure and to open the sphincter.

Esophageal body

It takes 6–8 seconds for peristalsis to proceed through the esophagus with an average velocity of 3–4 cm/second. The amplitude of the waves is highest in the distal 5 cm of the esophagus, and waves of low pressure are seen 4–6 cm below the upper esophageal sphincter and over a length of 2–3 cm. Duration of the contractions is usually less than 7 seconds and normal contraction amplitudes rarely exceed 150 mmHg.[1-4,38]

Striated muscle: the striated muscle contraction is directed and coordinated by sequential excitation through vagal fibres programmed by the central control mechanism.[1-4,9,40] Afferent information from the esophagus and elsewhere has a significant effect on the central program to alter the force and velocity of the peristaltic contraction in both the striated and the smooth muscle esophagus.

Smooth muscle: there are at least four different potential mechanisms for the production of peristalsis in the smooth muscle esophagus, and these reside at different levels of control.
• Arising in the central program, different efferent motor fibres fire sequentially during both primary or secondary peristalsis in the smooth as well as the striated muscle esophagus.[40,41]
• There is an intramural neural mechanism that can be excited to produce peristalsis near the onset of vagal stimulation or intraluminal balloon distension — the 'on-contraction'.[17-21,42]
• There is an intramural neural mechanism that can be excited to produce peristalsis onsetting after the vagal or balloon stimulus is terminated — the 'off-response' or 'off-contraction'.[17,18,20,21]
• There is some type of mechanism for myogenic propagation of a contraction, and therefore an indication that muscle properties contribute to the nature of peristalsis.[43,44]

In the human, cat and monkey, direct smooth muscle excitation by the intramural cholinergic neurons is the predominant mechanism for muscle contraction during normal peristalsis.[45-47] This would dictate that coordination of the excitation, and therefore of the peristaltic contraction, is primarily due to sequencing and activation of the intramural excitatory neurons. Yet to be determined is how the centrally programmed sequential vagal discharge interacts with the local control mechanisms to produce normal primary and secondary peristalsis.

Two main hypotheses for control of peristalsis in the smooth muscle have arisen. The first hypothesis proposes that the central program directs the cholinergic excitatory neurons as the final common pathway, with the intramural mechanism normally serving to modulate activity and to provide a local mechanism for distal inhibition.

The second hypothesis proposes that the swallowing centre triggers the peripheral intramural mechanism which then is primarily responsible for coordinating the peristaltic contraction, but modulated by the central mechanism through temporal and frequency differences in vagal discharge. In some species, such as the opossum and cat, the intramural mechanism can produce neurally mediated peristalsis in the absence of extrinsic vagal innervation, or with experimental vagal stimulation that does not incorporate sequential excitation.[17,18,21,22,40–42] How muscle properties contribute to peristalsis directed by either central or intramural neural mechanisms is not clear.

Intramural control mechanisms: Dodds and his co-workers have characterized the two intramural neural mechanisms for control of peristalsis in the opossum and cat.[17,18,21] The 'on-contraction' (A wave) has an apparent propagation velocity that resembles that of swallow-induced peristalsis, is atropine-sensitive and is induced by low frequency stimulation. On the other hand, the 'off-contraction' (B wave) has a much more rapid propagation similar to the 'off-response' delays of serial muscle strips *in vitro*, is atropine-resistant and occurs at higher stimulation frequencies. The former mechanism is attributed to the activation of the excitatory cholinergic neurons, although the nature of the circuitry dictating the progressive distal delays is not known.[16] The latter mechanism of contraction has been attributed to a muscle response that follows muscle hyperpolarization through activation of the NANC inhibitory neurons, membrane depolarization and contraction due both to passive rebound as well as to some type of active excitation.[4,48,49]

In the opossum the cholinergic 'on-response' mechanism is more prominent proximally and decreases distally,[20,21] while the noncholinergic, 'off-contraction' is more prominent distally. Therefore, in the opossum, both intramural mechanisms appear to contribute to peristalsis. In this species, different frequencies of vagal stimulation can alter and shift the mechanism from one to the other and therefore change either the propagation velocity or even the direction of peristalsis.[20] In humans, if an intramural mechanism is responsible for producing peristalsis, the predominant mechanism would normally be the cholinergic 'on-contraction' mechanism *(Figure 5)*. However, it is possible that under circumstances not yet defined, the 'off-response' contraction mechanism is also called into play in humans, especially distally.

Central control mechanisms: there is a well defined set of programmed neurons in the swallowing centre responsible for striated muscle peristalsis.[9,10] Presumably similar neurons are also present for the smooth muscle portion, but this has not yet been demonstrated. However, in both the baboon and the opossum, different vagal fibres discharge with a timing corresponding to the peristaltic contractions in both striated and smooth muscle sections.[40,41] Furthermore, in a number of animal species with intrinsic nerves intact, continuity of the intramural mechanism is not necessary for primary or secondary peristalsis to cross a level of transection regardless of whether the ends are reanastomosed, or are separated with deviation of the bolus.[51] In the cat, neither primary nor secondary peristalsis occurs in the smooth muscle esophagus when the vagi are temporarily blocked in the neck.[52] Afferent stimulation acting centrally has a major effect on peristalsis.[40,53,54]

Integration of central and peripheral mechanisms: regardless of which control mechanism is primary, it is clear that both central and peripheral levels of control are highly integrated, and the focus of this integration is likely to be the excitatory cholinergic neuron. Whether this neuron reaches threshold and induces a contraction would be determined by both excitatory and inhibitory influences, and may depend on more than one excitatory input. For example, in addition to the excitatory vagal fibres impinging on this neuron, other excitatory influences include central or local sensory reinforcement from an intraesophageal bolus, activity within the intramural peristaltic mechanism itself, and sensory information from a contraction.[55] Inhibitory influences that might act on this neuron have not yet been elucidated. In

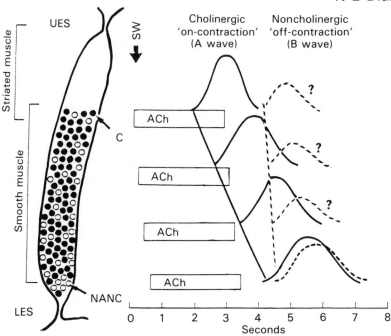

Figure 5   Schematic drawing of possible cholinergic (C, ●) and noncholinergic
(NANC, ○) influences in the human smooth muscle esophagus, and the
potential interplay of two intramural neural mechanisms for the production of
peristalsis. Cholinergic influence is shown as most prominent except for very
distal esophagus and LES. Where the cholinergic influence is dominant, the
'on-contraction' (A wave) will occur; where the noncholinergic influence is
dominant, or with cholinergic blockade, contraction will occur predominantly
as an 'off-response' (B wave). Release of acetylcholine (ACh) and the
noncholinergic inhibitory neurotransmitter could potentially occur through
either activity of the intramural nerve plexus itself or activation of the
intramural neurons by pre-ganglionic vagal fibres. Adapted with permission
from: Crist J, Gidda JS, Goyal RK. Intramural mechanism of esophageal
peristalsis: roles of cholinergic and noncholinergic nerves. *Proc Natl Acad Sci*
1984; **81**: 3593–9; and Gilbert RJ, Dodds WJ. Effect of selected muscarinic
antagonists on peristaltic contractions in opossum smooth muscle. *Am J
Physiol* 1986; **250**: G50–4.

those species and circumstances where the NANC inhibitory neuron is also present
and active, the mechanism for induction of the contraction will depend on the balance
between release of acetylcholine and the inhibitory neurotransmitter.[21]

Deglutitive inhibition: deglutitive inhibition in the esophagus is primarily a function
of the swallowing centre. A second swallow, initiated when a previous swallow is
in the striated muscle esophagus, causes rapid and complete inhibition of contractile
activity induced by the first swallow.[56,57] Once the first swallow wave has reached
the smooth muscle esophagus, it can proceed distally for at least 3 seconds after a
second swallow,[56,58] its amplitude diminishing progressively until it disappears. In
addition to the effect of a second swallow on a previous swallow, that is 'deglutitive
inhibition', the recent occurrence of a swallow or the presence of a swallow wave
within the esophagus can alter dramatically the nature of a subsequent swallow wave,
decreasing its amplitude, either increasing or decreasing its velocity and at times
rendering it nonperistaltic.[58-60] These effects can last for 20–30 seconds.

Lower esophageal sphincter

The LES is tonically closed at rest owing to a combination of myogenic properties and active tonic neural excitation, modulated by a complex interaction of numerous other neural and hormonal factors. Radial asymmetry in the recorded pressures is less marked than in the UES. The myogenic component of tone is calcium dependent and calcium blocking agents reduce LES pressure, a potentially useful therapeutic effect in patients with achalasia.[61]

In the human, as well as the cat, dog and monkey, the majority of this tone is due to the release of acetylcholine from excitatory neurons.[45,62] Some of this release is likely to be a result of tonically firing vagal fibres as in the dog,[50] and perhaps there is some adrenergic release of acetylcholine, as in the cat.[26,63] Beta-adrenergic antagonists also increase LES tone in the human.[64] Therefore, resting tone is regulated by a balance between excitatory and inhibitory neural influences. Both are highly centrally mediated.

A number of reflex mechanisms, physiologic alterations and ingested substances can markedly alter resting LES tone. LES pressure fluctuates with the migrating motor complex (MMC),[65] and increases after a meal and with raised intra-abdominal pressure.[66] On the other hand, the LES relaxes transiently independent of swallowing (TLESR) and this relaxation is frequently associated with gastroesophageal reflux.[33,67] The mechanism for this TLESR is unknown but presumably it is neurally mediated and can occur at least in response to intraesophageal stimuli.[68]

The large number of factors that may influence LES pressure are summarized in *Table 1*. Many of these have obvious clinical and therapeutic implications.

On swallowing, LES pressure falls within 1.5–2.5 seconds and remains low for 6–8 seconds as the peristaltic contraction traverses the esophageal body. The LES relaxes with virtually 100% of swallows, even though the swallow may not induce esophageal body motor activity. In humans, as in other species, the swallow-induced inhibition likely includes both active inhibition of the muscle and cessation of tonic neural excitation to the sphincter.[50] There is provision for central participation in control of this LES relaxation. However, intramural pathways within at least the smooth muscle esophageal body can also serve to inhibit the LES.[42,68] There is reason to believe that efferent vagal fibres serving both LES excitation and relaxation enter the esophagus at some point above the LES.[70,71]

References

1 Roman C, Gonella J. Extrinsic control of digestive tract motility. In: Johnson LR, ed. *Physiology of the Gastrointestinal Tract* 2nd ed. New York: Raven Press 1986; 507–54.

2 Christensen J. Motor functions of the pharynx and esophagus. In: Johnson LR, ed. *Physiology of the Gastrointestinal Tract* 2nd ed. New York: Raven Press 1986; 595–612.

3 Christensen J. The esophagus. In: Christensen J, Wingate D, eds. *A Guide to Gastrointestinal Motility*. Bristol: Wright. PSG 1983; 75–100.

4 Diamant NE. Normal esophageal physiology. In: Cohen S, Soloway RD, eds. *Diseases of the Esophagus*. New York: Churchill Livingstone 1982; 1–33.

5 Meyer GW, Austin RM, Brady CE III, Castell DO. Muscle anatomy of the human esophagus. *J Clin Gastroenterol* 1986; **8**: 131–4.

6 Bosma JF, Donner MW, Tanaka E, Robertson D. Anatomy of the pharynx, pertinent to swallowing. *Dysphagia* 1986; **1**: 23–33.

7 Daniel EE, Bowes KL, Duchon G. The structural basis for control of gastrointestinal motility in man. In: Vantrappen G, ed. *Proceedings of the Fifth International Symposium on Gastrointestinal Motility*. Herentals: Typoff-Press 1975; 142–51.

8 Liebermann-Meffert D, Allgower M, Schmid P, Blum AL. Muscular equivalent of the lower esophageal sphincter. *Gastroenterology* 1979; **76**: 31–8.

9 Doty TW. Neural organization of deglutition. In: Code CF, ed. *Handbook of Physiology*. Vol 4. Washington DC: American Physiological Society 1968; 1861–902.

10 Jean A. Brainstem organization of the swallowing network. *Brain Behav Evol* 1984; **25**: 109–16.

11 Christensen J. Origin of sensation in the esophagus. *Am J Physiol* 1984; **246**: G221–5.

12 Weisbrodt NW. Neuromuscular organization of esophageal and pharyngeal motility. *Arch Intern Med* 1976; **136**: 524–31.

13 Mann CV, Code CF, Schlegel JF, Ellis FH Jr. Intrinsic mechanisms controlling the mammalian gastro-oesophageal sphincter deprived of extrinsic nerve supply. *Thorax* 1968; **23**: 634–9.

14 Yamamoto T. Histologic studies on the innervation of the esophagus in Formosan macaque. *Arch Hist Jap* 1960; **18**: 545-64.

15 Seelig LL Jr, Goyal RK. Morphological evaluation of opossum lower esophageal sphincter. *Gastroenterology* 1978; **75**: 51–8.

16 Diamant NE, El-Sharkawy TY. Neural control of esophageal peristalsis. A conceptual analysis. *Gastroenterology* 1977; **72**: 546–56.

17 Dodds WJ, Steff JJ, Stewart ET, Hogan WT, Arndorfer RC, Cohen EB. Responses of feline esophagus to cervical vagal stimulation. *Am J Physiol* 1978; **235**: E63–73.

18 Dodds WJ, Christensen J, Dent J, Wood JD, Arndorfer RC. Esophageal contractions induced by vagal stimulation in the opossum. *Am J Physiol* 1978; **235**: E392–401.

19 Gilbert R, Rattan S, Goyal RK. Pharmacologic identification, activation and antagonism of two muscarinic receptor subtypes on the lower esophageal sphincter. *J Pharmacol Exp Ther* 1984; **230**: 284–91.

20 Crist J, Gidda JS, Goyal RK. Intramural mechanism of esophageal peristalsis: roles of cholinergic and noncholinergic nerves. *Proc Natl Acad Sci* 1984; **81**: 3595–9.

21 Gilbert RJ, Dodds WJ. Effect of selective muscarinic antagonists on peristaltic contractions in opossum smooth muscle. *Am J Physiol* 1986; **250**: G50–4.

22 Goyal RK, Rattan S. Neurohumoral, hormonal and drug receptors for the lower esophageal sphincter. *Gastroenterology* 1978; **74**: 598–619.

23 Goyal RK, Rattan S, Said SI. VIP as a possible neurotransmitter of non-cholinergic non-adrenergic inhibitory neurones. *Nature* 1980; **288**: 378.

24 Aggestrup S, Uddman R, Jensen SL *et al*. Regulatory peptides in the lower esophageal sphincter of man. *Regulatory Peptides* 1985; **10**: 167–78.

25 Lyrenas E, Abrahamsson H. Beta adrenergic influence on oesophageal peristalsis in man. *Gut* 1986; **27**: 260–6.

26 Gonella J, Niel JP, Roman C. Sympathetic control of lower esophageal sphincter motility in the cat. *J Physiol (Lond)* 1979; **287**: 177–90.

27 Dodds WJ, Stef JJ, Hogan WJ. Factors determining pressure measurement accuracy by intraluminal manometry. *Gastroenterology* 1976; **70**: 117–23.

28 Hollis JB, Castell DO. Amplitude of perstalsis as determined by rapid infusion. *Gastroenterology* 1972; **63**: 417–22.

29 Dent J. A new technique for continuous sphincter pressure measurement. *Gastroenterology* 1976; **71**: 263–7.

30 Winans CS. The pharyngoesophageal closure mechanism: a manometric study. *Gastroenterology* 1972; **63**: 768–77.

31 Winans CS. Manometric asymmetry of the lower esophageal high-pressure zone. *Am J Dig Dis* 1977; **22**: 348–54.

32 Gerhardt DG, Castell DO. Anatomy and physiology of the esophageal sphincters. In: Castell DO, Johnson LF, eds. *Esophageal Function in Health and Disease*. New York: Elsevier Biomedical 1983; 17–29.

33 Dent J, Dodds WJ, Friedman RH *et al*. Mechanism of gastroesophageal reflux in recumbent asymptomatic human subjects. *J Clin Invest* 1980; **65**: 256–67.

34 Stacher G, Schmierer G, Landgraf M. Tertiary esophageal contractions evoked by acoustic stimuli. *Gastroenterology* 1979; **77**: 49–54.

35 Dodds WJ, Stewart ET, Hodges D, Aboralske FF. Movement of the feline esophagus associated with respiration and peristalsis. An evaluation using tantalum markers. *J Clin Invest* 1973; **52**: 1–13.

36 Jurica EJ. Studies on the motility of the denervated mammalian oesophagus. *Am J Physiol* 1926; **77**: 371–84.

37 Roman C, Tieffenbach L. Electrical activity of esophageal smooth muscle in vagotomized and anesthetized cats. *J Physiol (Paris)* 1971; **63**: 733–62.

38 Meyer GW, Castell DO. Anatomy and physiology of the esophageal body. In: Castell DO,

Johnson LF, eds. *Esophageal Function in Health and Disease.* New York: Elsevier Biomedical 1983; 1–15.

39 Kahrilas PJ, Dodds WJ, Dent J, Wyman JB, Hogan WJ, Arndorfer RC. Upper esophageal sphincter function during belching. *Gastroenterology* 1986; **91**: 133–40.

40 Roman C, Tieffenbach L. Activity of vagal efferent fibres innervating the baboon's esophagus. *J Physiol (Paris)* 1972; **64**: 479–506.

41 Gidda JS, Goyal RK. Swallow-evoked action potentials in vagal preganglionic efferents. *J Neurophysiol* 1984; **52**: 1169–80.

42 Tieffenbach L, Roman C. The role of extrinsic vagal innervation in the motility of the smooth-muscled portion of the esophagus: electromyographic study in the cat and the baboon. *J Physiol (Paris)* 1972; **64**: 193–226.

43 Bartlet AL. Myogenic peristalsis in isolated preparations of chicken esophagus. *Br J Pharmacol* 1973; **48**: 36–47.

44 Sarna SK, Daniel EE, Waterfall WE. Myogenic and neural control systems for esophageal motility. *Gastroenterology* 1977; **73**: 1345–52.

45 Dodds WJ, Dent J, Hogan WJ, Arndorfer RC. Effect of atropine on esophageal motor function in humans. *Am J Physiol* 1981; **240**: G290–6.

46 Hollis JB, Castell DO. Effects of cholinergic stimulation on human esophageal peristalsis. *J Appl Physiol* 1976; **40**: 40–3.

47 Humphries TJ, Castell DO. Effect of oral bethanecol on parameters of esophageal peristalsis. *Dig Dis Sci* 1981; **26**: 129–32.

48 Chan WW-L, Diamant NE. Electrical off-response of cat esophageal smooth muscle: an analogue simulation. *Am J Physiol* 1976; **230**: 233–8.

49 McKirdy HC, Marshall RW. Effect of drugs and electrical field stimulation on circular muscle strips from human lower oesophagus. *Quart J Exp Physiol* 1985; **70**: 591–601.

50 Miolan JP, Roman C. Activité des fibres vagales efferentes destinées à la musculature lisse du cardia du chien. *J Physiol (Paris)* 1978; **74**: 709–23.

51 Janssens J. *The Peristaltic Mechanism of the Esophagus.* Leuven: Acco 1978.

52 Reynolds RPE, El-Sharkawy TY, Diamant NE. Esophageal peristalsis in the cat: the role of central innervation assessed by transient vagal blockade. *Can J Physiol Pharmacol* 1985; **63**: 122–30.

53 Dodds WJ, Hogan WJ, Reid DP, Steward ET, Arndorfer RC. A comparison between primary esophageal peristalsis following wet and dry swallows. *J Appl Physiol* 1973; **35**: 851–7.

54 Dodds WJ, Hogan WJ, Stewart ET, Stef JJ, Arndorfer RC. Effects of intra-abdominal pressure on esophageal peristalsis. *J Appl Physiol* 1974; **37**: 378–83.

55 Mei N. Anatomical arrangement and electrophysiological properties of sensitive vagalneurones in the cat. *Exp Brain Res* 1970; **11**: 465–79.

56 Vantrappen G, Hellemans J, Pelemans W, Janssens J. Electromyographic and manometric studies of the deglutitive inhibition of the esophagus. *Rendic R Gastroenterol* 1971; **3**: 139 (abstr).

57 Hellemans J, Vantrappen G, Janssens J. In: Vantrappen G, Hellemans J, eds. *Diseases of the Esophagus.* New York: Springer-Verlag 1974; 280–4.

58 Meyer GW, Gerhardt DC, Castell DO. Human esophageal response to rapid swallowing: muscle refractory period or neural inhibition? *Am J Physiol* 1980; **241**: G129–36.

59 Ask P, Tibling L. Effect of time interval between swallows on esophageal peristalsis. *Am J Physiol* 1980; **238**: G485–90.

60 Vanek AW, Diamant NE. Responses of the human esophagus to paired swallows. *Gastroenterology* (In press).

61 Bortolotti M, Labo G. Clinical and manometric effects of nifedipine in patients with esophageal achalasia. *Gastroenterology* 1981; **80**: 39–44.

62 Price LM, El-Sharkawy TY, Mui HY, Diamant NE. Effect of bilateral cervical vagotomy on balloon-induced lower esophageal sphincter relaxation in the dog. *Gastroenterology* 1979; **77**: 324–9.

63 Reynolds RPE, El-Sharkawy TY, Diamant NE. Lower esophageal sphincter function in the cat. The role of central innervation assessed by transient vagal blockade. *Am J Physiol* 1984; **246**: G666–74.

64 Thorpe JAC. Effect of propranolol on the lower esophageal sphincter in man. *Curr Med Res Opin* 1980; **7**: 91–5.

65 Dent J, Dodds WJ, Sekiguchi T, Hogan WJ, Arndorfer RC. Interdigestive phasic control of the human lower esophageal sphincter. *Gastroenterology* 1983; **3**: 453–60.

66 Crispin JS, McIver DK, Lind JF. Manometric study of the effect of vagotomy on the gastro-oesophageal sphincter. *Can J Surg* 1967; **10**: 299–303.

67 Dodds WJ, Dent J, Hogan WJ *et al*. Mechanisms of gastroesophageal reflux in patients with reflux esophagitis. *N Engl J Med* 1982; **307**: 1547–52.

68 Patterson WG, Rattan S, Goyal RK. Experimental induction of isolated lower esophageal sphincter relaxation in anesthetized opossum. *J Clin Invest* 1986; **77**: 1187–93.

69 Mann CV, Code CF, Schlegel JF, Ellis FH Jr. Intrinsic mechanisms controlling the mammalian gastro-oesophageal sphincter deprived of extrinsic nerve supply. *Thorax* 1986; **23**: 634–9.

70 Higgs RH, Castell DO. The effect of truncal vagotomy on lower esophageal sphincter pressure and response to cholinergic stimulation. *Proc Soc Exp Biol Med* 1976; **153**: 379–82.

71 Temple JG, Goodall RJR, Hay DJ, Miller D. Effect of highly selective vagotomy upon the lower oesophageal sphincter. *Gut* 1981; **22**: 368–70.

Physiology of the stomach

J H Meyer

The stomach plays two important roles in digestion:
• It stores food and controls gastric emptying so that the food enters the intestine at rates which can be easily assimilated;
• It breaks up solid food and fats into tiny particles with large surfaces that are easily attacked by pancreatic enzymes.

In the first half of this century, physiologists studied these motor functions of the stomach primarily by fluoroscopy or by examining gastroduodenal transit in animals with gastrointestinal fistulas. Observations were qualitative rather than quantitative. The visible peristaltic contractions which periodically swept the gastric antrum were assumed to pump food out of the stomach.[1] This impression was reinforced by the observation in dogs with duodenal fistulas that chyme left the stomach in interrupted spurts.[2] The finding that fat in the intestine inhibited antral peristalsis and slowed gastric emptying was entirely consistent with the theory of the antral pump.[3]

Beginning in the 1960s, a number of simultaneous developments led to changes in the understanding of how the stomach works. Rapid advances in physiology of smooth muscle, in chemistry of GI hormones and in instrumentation for measuring muscle contractions or GI transit allowed new insights into the function of the stomach. Also important during this period were trials of various kinds of gastric operations for peptic ulcer and the observations on how these various operations affected gastric emptying. Out of this period of advancement the hypothesis of the two-component stomach was born.[4]

The two-component stomach

To the smooth muscle physiologist, the stomach is two organs. The proximal one-third, which contains the fundus, is an electrically stable muscle which does not rapidly contract but instead exhibits mostly tonic alterations in volume. Relaxation of tone in the region is regulated by nonadrenergic, noncholinergic fibres in the vagi during distension of the esophagus, stomach or duodenum. By contrast, smooth muscle in the distal two-thirds of the stomach exhibits a decaying and thus fluctuating electrical membrane potential. This potential change is propagated in waves, spreading circumferentially and downward, in cycles of 3/minute in man. Unlike the fundus, the distal stomach undergoes periodic contractions over 10–20 seconds which move distally in a peristaltic fashion as ring-like indentations of the stomach wall. As it passes over the muscle cells, the fluctuating, pacesetter potential alters calcium channels and thus sensitizes the cell to contract. Thus, the orderly propagation of the pacesetter potential organizes peristaltic contractions.

Of course, not every pacesetter potential results in a contraction. Both neural and hormonal mediators act at the muscle cell to enhance or diminish the cell's contractility. Thus, depending on incoming messages, antral muscle may contract at a rate from 0 up to a maximum of 3/minute and the advancing peristaltic wave may spread along the entire distal two thirds of the stomach or may die out.[5] The sequence of contractions of the terminal antrum is always the same. Therefore, this cycle of events may be important in both regulating the rate of gastric outflow and in sieving and grinding solid foods. As the peristaltic wave advances into the distal antrum, the pylorus closes just before the terminal antrum is obliterated by advancing contraction. Residual content in the terminal antrum is then retropelled backward as the terminal antrum closes down.[6]

At times the two regions of the stomach also differ in how they are affected by GI hormones or by nervous reflexes. All known GI hormones, except motilin, relax the fundus, but some of these same hormones, like gastrin or cholecystokinin, excite antral contractions. While nutrients in the small intestine both relax fundic tone and inhibit antral contractions, gastric distension has the opposite effects on the proximal and distal stomach. Vasovagal reflexes inhibit fundic tone but increase antral contractility when the stomach is distended (*Table 1*).

These observations suggest that truncal or complete gastric vagotomy might: (a) impair relaxation of the fundus; and (b) reduce antral peristalsis as the stomach is filled with food. In fact, truncal vagotomy has both of these effects in man.[7] Intragastric pressure rises much more rapidly with distending volume after truncal vagotomy than before this operation; and phasic pressure waves generated by antral contractions in response to gastric distension are diminished by the vagotomy. Sometimes, patients who have undergone truncal vagotomy exhibit both rapid emptying of fluids and impaired emptying of solid foods.[8,9] In view of the dissociation between electrical and mechanical behaviour of the two regions, opposite responses to some GI hormones and to vagal denervation, and, especially, this clinical dissociation in gastric emptying of liquids vs. solids, the hypothesis that tonic pressures in the proximal stomach regulate gastric emptying of liquids, while gastric transit of solid foods is controlled by antral peristalsis, seems a reasonable one.

More recent observations, both clinical and experimental, cannot be accounted for by this simple two-component model of gastric emptying. Instead, it appears that gastric emptying of both liquids and solids is controlled by concerted and complex actions of fundus, antrum, pylorus and duodenum.

The stomach as a storage organ
Fat, sugars, certain amino acids (especially tryptophan) and titrateable acid of high osmolality trigger sensory mechanisms from the intestine which inhibit gastric emptying. Of these nutrients, the most potent inhibitor of gastric emptying is fat. Fat in the intestine has a number of effects on the stomach (*Table 2*). It:

Region	Effect	Stimulus	Pathway
Fundus	Relaxation	Esophageal distension	Vagus
Fundus	Relaxation	Gastric distension	Vagus
Fundus	Relaxation	Duodenal distension	Vagus
Antrum	Contraction	Gastric distension	Vagus
Antrum	Relaxation	Gut nutrients	Vagus
Antrum	Relaxation	Gut distension	Vagus and splanchnic
Antrum	Contraction	Muscle stretch	Myogenic

Table 1 Reflexes affecting the stomach.

	Inhibitor			
	Fat	Sugar	AA/protein	Acid
Fundus	– –	0	–	?
Antrum	– –	–	– –	– –
Pylorus	+ +	+	+	+ +
Proximal gut*	– –	–	–	–

Table 2 Effects of gut inhibitors on the function of the stomach. AA = amino acid; + = stimulate; – = inhibit; 0 = no effect.
*In proximal gut, inhibition is conversion of propagated to segmenting contractions and/or decreased flow at constant pressures.

- relaxes or dilates the fundus which reduces pressures that might expel liquids or push contents into the antrum;[10]
- inhibits antral peristalsis, reducing the tendency for the antrum to pump material from the stomach;[3,11,12]
- narrows the calibre of the antrum, pyloric canal and duodenum, increasing resistance to outflow;[12]
- stimulates phasic contractions and tonic narrowing of the pylorus;[12-14]
- reduces coordination of contractions between antrum and duodenum, further impeding outflow;
- reduces the frequency and length of spread of peristaltic activity in the duodenum while increasing the frequency of segmenting contractions[13] — the former is associated with propulsion, the latter with reduction of transit.[15]

The effect of fat at every site seems to be directed toward limiting outflow. The other inhibitors of gastric emptying act similarly but somewhat less dramatically.

Experimental evidence

Several experiments have been conducted to ascertain the roles of the various sites in the stomach on controlling gastric emptying. In one experiment the stomachs of dogs were filled with saline, 600 mM glucose or 40 mM fatty acid from a barostat. The barostat set the pressures in the stomach. With all three solutions gastric outflow increased as pressure was raised, but the rate of increase was much less with the nutrients than with the saline (*Figure 1*). Thus, whatever forward pressure the fundus or barostat could provide was modified by the antrum, pylorus and/or small intestine. Following truncal vagotomy and pyloroplasty, there was no change. Therefore, the *pyloric* integrity was not necessary for this regulation of nutrient outflow. Similar regulation also persisted in other experiments after antropyloric resection, indicating that at least some of this resistance to outflow was generated by the small intestine.[16,17] In other experiments, it was found that the gastric emptying rate of liquids was increased by myotomy of duodenal circular muscle,[18] lending further support to the role of the duodenum in the regulation of outflow.

In another canine experiment, gastroduodenal pressure gradients were controlled by barostats in continuity with the stomach and the duodenum (*Figure 2*).[6] In con-

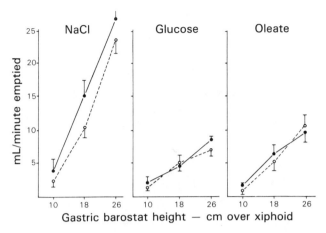

Figure 1 Rate of canine gastric emptying (vertical axes) of liquid meals of saline, oleate or glucose when meals were held in the fundus by a barostat at pressures (cm of water over the xiphoid) indicated on the horizontal axes. Experiments were performed before (solid lines) and after (dotted lines) truncal vagotomy and pyloroplasty. With each meal, gastric outflow increased linearly with gastric pressure, but the magnitude of increase was significantly smaller with meals of oleate or glucose than with saline meals. This finding indicates that while rates of outflow may depend on pressures generated in the fundus, outflow is modified by structures beyond the fundus so that rates vary according to nutrient concentrations, despite similar fundic pressures with the different meals. Reproduced with permission from Miller J, Kauffman G, Elashoff J *et al*. Search for resistances controlling gastric emptying of liquid meals. *Am J Physiol* 1981; **241**: G403–25.

trol experiments with solutions of taurocholate in saline or saline alone, transpyloric flow increased as the gastroduodenal pressure gradient increased.

Outflow continued even when gastroduodenal pressure was zero or − 2 cm of water, indicating that the antrum was capable of pumping out fluid against a small pressure gradient. When the intestine was perfused with increasing concentrations of oleic acid emulsified in taurocholate or increasing concentrations of glucose with gastroduodenal pressure set at zero, transpyloric flow diminished. This verifies the concept of the antral pump for liquids and shows that inhibitors of antral contractions may slow outflow.

In addition, at each gastroduodenal pressure gradient intestinal oleate inhibited outflow in a dose-related fashion. This inhibiting effect of intestinal fat was abolished by pyloroplasty (*Figure 2*). The findings of this experiment are consistent with the theory that the pylorus can regulate fluid outflow. Using an *ex vivo* stomach in an organ bath, Schulze-Delrieu observed that gastric outflow early after the stomach was filled with liquid was slower when the pylorus was intact than when it was stented open.[19] Clinical observations in humans indicate that a pyloroplasty accelerates early gastric emptying of liquids, especially after proximal gastric vagotomy which enhances fundic tone.[20,21]

All of these experiments support the hypothesis that the antrum, pylorus and duodenum work in a coordinated fashion to augment or modulate input from the fundus. Because the fundus is in linear series with the antrum and duodenum, increased fundic tone and intragastric pressure following vagotomy may force the rapid evacuation of liquids by overwhelming antropyloric and duodenal mechanisms. Such pathology after vagotomy does not necessarily mean that fluid outflow is normally controlled by fundic tone alone.

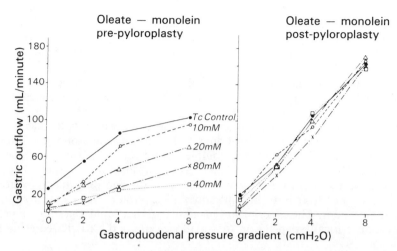

Figure 2 Rates of canine gastroduodenal outflow (vertical axes) of saline solutions during small bowel perfusion with different concentrations of oleate in taurocholate as gastroduodenal pressure gradients (cm of water, horizontal axes) were modified by a system of gastric and duodenal barostats. Gastroduodenal outflow was noted even at zero gastroduodenal pressure gradients and increased with increasing gastroduodenal pressures. Oleate in the proximal small intestine inhibited these outflows (left panel) in a dose-related fashion before pyloroplasty, but this inhibition was abolished (right panel) by pyloroplasty (pyloric myotomy). The observations indicate that the pylorus may function as a variable resistance to gastroduodenal flow. Reproduced with permission from Miller J, Kauffman G, Elashoff J *et al*. Search for resistances controlling gastric emptying of liquid meals. *Am J Physiol* 1981; **241**: G403–25.

Scintigraphy: scintigraphic and radiographic studies indicate that both liquids and solids are normally stored in the relaxed fundus and are slowly pressed into the antrum, where peristalsis forces the contents out of the stomach.[22] Scintigraphic studies have shown that the rate of gastric emptying parallels the rate of loss of fundic counts, while antral radioactivity (the volume of food in the antrum) remains fairly constant throughout most of the emptying time-course. Liquids appear to make their way into the antrum more quickly than solids. Moreover, there is a gradient of particle size between fundus and antrum such that large masses of solid food are retained in the fundus, while smaller particles drain into the antral area.[3] Exactly how this gradient is maintained is uncertain, but it is probably actively controlled. For example, Collins and co-workers recently observed that infusing fat into the intestine not only slowed gastric emptying but also redistributed radiolabelled, solid food from the antrum into the fundus.[23]

The stomach as a digestive organ
In addition to its ability to store and slowly meter out nutrients at rates which can be easily assimilated into the body, the stomach also has a second major function as a digestive organ. It breaks food up into tiny particles which have a large surface to volume ratio so that they can be easily digested by pancreatic enzymes at the particle surfaces. Furthermore, the stomach retains food until it has been broken down into small particles.[24-26] In dogs, both the pylorus and the terminal antrum have to be resected to impair these processes and induce the gastric emptying of large pieces of food. Similarly, food particles empty from the stomach in the normal range (below

1 mm) in human patients who have undergone a proximal gastric vagotomy or a vagotomy and pyloroplasty for duodenal ulcers; but in those patients who have had a vagotomy and antrectomy (removal of both the terminal antrum and pylorus), about 30% of ingested meat is emptied into the duodenum as particles much larger than 1 mm.[26]

The importance of this grinding and sieving of food was illustrated by a canine experiment in which the percentage of radiolabelled triolein which remained unabsorbed by the time it reached midintestine was measured.[27] The radiotriolein was fed in margarine, a liquid fat, or was fed as a solid fat which was intracellular within pieces of chicken liver. In both control dogs and dogs with vagotomy and antrectomy, the absorption of fat was nearly complete from the margarine as it reached the midintestine. However, only in normal dogs was absorption of fat nearly complete from tiny particles of liver. By contrast, dogs with vagotomy and antrectomy passed large pieces of liver into their intestine; absorption of fat from these large particles was very poor. The experiment thus indicates that rapid digestion and efficient absorption critically depend on the small size of food particles entering the duodenum.

In a parallel experiment in humans,[28] radioiron was absorbed equally well in normal subjects from hemoglobin in solution as it was from myoglobin in pieces of lamb. However, in patients with vagotomy and antrectomy, absorption of the iron from the pieces of lamb was only half that from the hemoglobin solution. Presumably, the passage of large, poorly digestible pieces of lamb into the duodenums of the patients accounted for the abnormally low efficiency of absorption of the myoglobin iron.

Figure 3 depicts one possible mechanism by which the stomach normally grinds and sieves food into small particles.[29] As peristaltic contractions sweep over the antrum, smaller particles with little inertia are quickly accelerated and distributed in the central, more fast moving stream, while larger particles with more inertia are less rapidly accelerated and are thus distributed toward the sides of the stomach, where fluid velocity is slower. Peristaltic contraction progresses into the terminal antrum,

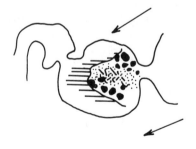   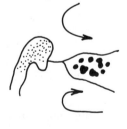

1. Large particles at side, small particles in centre of velocity parabola with contractions.

2. Small particles empty just before pyloric closure. Slower moving, large particles retained and retropulsed.

Figure 3 Keller's hydrodynamic hypothesis of sieving. Reproduced with permission from Meyer JH. Motility of the stomach and gastroduodenal junction. In: Johnson LR, Christensen J, Jacobsen ED, Schultz SG, eds. *Physiology of the Digestive Tract.* New York: Raven Press 1987; 613–30.

first closing the pylorus and then reversing fluid flow as the terminal antrum obliterates against a closed pylorus. The slower moving, large food particles are thus suddenly reversed in direction, and are tumbled as they assume a backwards motion. The shear generated by rapidly changing to-and-fro motions breaks the particles apart.

This theory emphasizes relations between peristaltic contractions, intermittent fluid flow and particle movement. If this entire hypothesis were correct, pyloroplasty itself would greatly alter grinding and sieving, but it does not.[24,25] On the other hand, if intermittent, to-and-fro fluid flows are created by complex coordination between antral and duodenal contractions rather than simply by pyloric closure,[30,31] then resection of the antrum in addition to the pylorus would be required to upset normal grinding and sieving, as has been observed.

Another similar hydrodynamic hypothesis is that transit of particles relative to suspending fluid is determined by how fast food particles sink or float out of the fast-moving central stream. In this hypothesis, particle transit will vary inversely with particle diameter and particle density, but will vary directly with fluid viscosity and fluid velocity. This theory focuses on how particles move in a constantly moving stream of laminar flow, a condition that does not well characterize the intermittent flow in the antral region. Nevertheless, this theory, like the other, stresses that particle diameter and particle density, as well as the viscosity and the linear velocity of suspending, luminal fluid, govern particle transit. Recent canine experiments have confirmed that all four parameters influence gastric emptying of particles.[32,33] In humans, both particle diameter and particle density have been shown to affect rates of particle emptying.[34] Thus, both human and canine experiments support the theory that sieving and emptying of food particles depends in some way on hydrodynamic flow patterns.

It is believed that the antropyloric segment normally extends downward as the food-filled stomach relaxes. The segment forms a U-shaped trap. This configuration, along with intermittent, to-and-fro flows generated by antroduodenal coordination, facilitate hydrodynamic sieving. Thus, resection of the terminal antrum destroys these actions and breaks down the sieving process.

In summary, the stomach is a complicated organ capable of high degrees of discrimination. It can distinguish and selectively retain liquid nutrients. It can sort out particles which vary subtly in physical properties. The intricate systems which permit this discriminating behaviour are only just being recognized.

References

1 Cannon WB. The movements of the stomach studied by means of Roentgen rays. *Am J Physiol* 1898; **1**: 359–82.

2 Stemper TJ, Cooke AR. Gastric emptying and relationship to antral contractile activity. *Gastroenterology* 1975; **69**: 649–53.

3 Thomas JE. Mechanics and regulation of gastric emptying. *Physiol Rev* 1957; **37**: 453–74.

4 Kelly KA. Gastric emptying of liquids and solids: roles of proximal and distal stomach. *Am J Physiol* 1980; **239**: G71–6.

5 Code CF, Carlson HC. Motor activity of the stomach. In: Code CF, Heidel W, eds. *Handbook of Physiology*, Section 6, Volume 4: Alimentary Canal. American Physiological Society: Washington, DC 1968.

6 Szurszewski JH. Electrical basis of gastrointestinal motility. In: Johnson LR, ed. *Physiology of the Gastrointestinal Tract*. Raven Press: New York 1981; 1435–66.

7 Staadas J, Aune S. Intragastric pressure/volume relationship before and after vagotomy. *Acta Chir Scand* 1970; **136**: 611–5.

8 Gulsrud PO, Taylor IL, Watts HD, Dohen MB, Meyer JH. How gastric emptying of carbohydrate affects glucose tolerance and symptoms after truncal vagotomy with pyloroplasty. *Gastroenterology* 1980; **78**: 1463–71.

9 Malagelada J-R, Rees WDW, Mazzotta LJ, Go VLW. Gastric motor abnormalities in diabetic

and postvagotomy gastroparesis: effect of metoclopramide and bethanechol. *Gastroenterology* 1980; **78**: 286–93.

10 Azpiros F, Malagelada J-R. Intestinal control of gastric tone. *Am J Physiol* 1986; **249**: G501–9.

11 Dooley CP, Reznick JB, Valenzuella JE. Variations in gastric and duodenal motility during gastric emptying of liquid meals in humans. *Gastroenterology* 1984; **87**: 1114–9.

12 Keinke O, Ehrlein HJ. Effect of oleic acid on canine gastroduodenal motility, pyloric diameter and gastric emptying. *Quart J Exp Physiol* 1983; **68**: 675–86.

13 Fisher RS, Lipshutz W, Cohen S. The hormonal regulation of pyloric sphincter function. *J Clin Invest* 1973; **52**: 1289–96.

14 Brink BM, Schlegel JF, Code CF. The pressure profile of the gastroduodenal junctional zone in dogs. *Gut* 1965; **6**: 163–71.

15 Schemann M, Ehrlein HJ. Postprandial patterns of canine jejunal motility and transit of luminal content. *Gastroenterology* 1986; **90**: 991–1000.

16 Miller J, Kauffman G, Elashoff J, Ohashi H, Carter D, Meyer JH. Search for resistances controlling gastric emptying of liquid meals. *Am J Physiol* 1981; **241**: G403–25.

17 Williams NS, Miller J, Elashoff J, Meyer JH. Canine resistances to gastric emptying of liquids after ulcer surgery. *Dig Dis Sci* 1986; **31**: 273–80.

18 Bortolotti M, Pandolfo N, Bebiacolombo C, Labo G, Mattioli F. Modifications in gastroduodenal motility induced by the extramucosal section of circular duodenal musculature in dogs. *Gastroenterology* 1981; **81**: 910–4.

19 Schulze-Delrieu K, Wall JP. Determinants of flow across isolated gastroduodenal junctions of cats and rabbits. *Am J Physiol* 1983; **245**: G257–64.

20 Aeberhard P, Walther M. Results of a controlled randomized trial of proximal gastric vagotomy with and without pyloroplasty. *Br J Surg* 1978; **65**: 634–6.

21 Clarke RJ, Alexander-Williams J. The effect of preserving antral innervation and of a pyloroplasty on gastric emptying after vagotomy in man. *Gut* 1973; **14**: 300–7.

22 Collins PJ, Horowitz M, Cook DJ, Harding PE, Shearman DJC. Gastric emptying in normal subjects — a reproduceable technique using a single scintillation camera and a computer system. *Gut* 1983; **24**: 1117–25.

23 Collins PJ, Heddle R, Horowitz M *et al*. The effect of intraduodenal lipid on gastric emptying and intragastric distribution of a solid meal. *Gastroenterology* 1986; **90**: 1377 (abstr).

24 Meyer JH, Thomson JB, Cohen MB *et al*. Sieving of solid food by the normal and ulcer-operated canine stomach. *Gastroenterology* 1976; **76**: 804.

25 Hinder RA, San-Garde BA. Individual and combined roles of the pylorus and antrum in the canine gastric emptying of a liquid and a digestible solid. *Gastroenterology* 1983; **84**: 281.

26 Mayer EA, Thomson JB, Jehn D *et al*. Gastric emptying and sieving of solid food and pancreatic and biliary secretions after solid meals in patients with nonresective ulcer surgery. *Gastroenterology* 1984; **87**: 1264.

27 Doty JE, Meyer JH. Vagotomy and antrectomy impairs absorption of fat from solid, but not liquid dietary sources. *Gastroenterology* 1987; **92**: 1374.

28 Meyer JH, Porter-Fink V, Crott R, Figeuroa W. Absorption of heme iron after truncal vagotomy with antrectomy. *Gastroenterology* 1987; **92**: 1534.

29 Meyer JH. Motility of the stomach and gastroduodenal junction. In: Johnson LR, Christensen J, Jacobsen ED, Schulz SG, eds. *Physiology of the Digestive Tract*. New York: Raven Press 1987; 613–30.

30 Gastroduodenal coordination. In: Schuurkes JAJ, van Neuten JM, Akkermans LMA, Johnson AG, Read NW, eds. *Gastric and Gastroduodenal Motility*. New York: Praeger Scientific 1986.

31 King PM, Adam RD, Pryde A, McDicken WN, Heading RC. Relationships of human antroduodenal motility and transpyloric fluid movement: non-invasive observations with real-time ultrasound. *Gut* 1984; **25**: 1384–91.

32 Meyer JH, Dressman J, Fink AS, Amidon G. Effect of size and density on canine gastric emptying of non-digestible solids. *Gastroenterology* 1985; **89**: 805–13.

33 Meyer JH, Gu YG, Dressman J, Amidon G. Effect of viscosity and flow rate on gastric emptying of solids. *Am J Physiol* 1986; **250**: G161–4.

34 Meyer JH, Elashoff J, Porter-Fink V, Dressman J, Amidon G. What should be the size of pancreatin microspheres? *Gastroenterology* 1987; **92**: 1533 (abstr).

Small intestinal motility physiology

N W Read

Anatomy of the small intestine

The small intestine is a long muscular tube that extends from the stomach to the cecum. It consists of the duodenum, which is retroperitoneal and occupies the first 25 cm, the jejunum, which occupies approximately 50% of the small intestine, and the ileum. There is no obvious anatomical distinction between the jejunum and ileum, although the latter is said to have a smaller diameter. The muscular wall of the small intestine is organized into an outer layer, in which the smooth muscle cells are orientated longitudinally, an inner layer, in which the cells are orientated circumferentially, and a thin layer of muscularis mucosa which lies underneath the mucosa and sends strands up into the villi. The longitudinal and circular layers of smooth muscle are mainly responsible for the movement of intestinal contents. Phasic contraction of the muscularis mucosae may shorten the villi and stir the microclimate adjacent to the mucosa; tonic contraction of this layer may act as a barrier to fluid absorption.[1]

The muscle layers consist of spindle-shaped, tightly-packed smooth muscle cells, approximately 2–8 mm in diameter and 40–100 mm in length. These cells are connected to one another by nexuses or gap junctions. The cells in the circular muscle layer are considered to be linked electrically to those in the longitudinal layer via the interstitial cells of Cajal.[2]

An extensive network of nerve fibres, connected with ganglion cells, lies between the circular and longitudinal layers of smooth muscle. Another nerve plexus lies in the submucosa. These enteric nerve nets are linked to sensory receptors in the epithelium, the submucosa and muscular layers, and supply motor nerve fibres to the smooth muscle. The enteric nervous system or 'gut brain' coordinates the patterns of small intestinal contractile activity in response to luminal stimuli. The small intestine receives an extrinsic nerve supply from the vagus nerve and from the sympathetic nervous system. These nerves modulate the activity of the enteric nervous system according to environmental changes or alterations in the activity of organs at distant sites. The role of extrinsic nerves as modulators of gut motor activity is supported by the fact that there are approximately 10^8 ganglion cells in the enteric nervous system[3] and only 10^4–10^5 efferent fibres in the vagus or splanchnic nerves.

Electrical basis of small intestinal contraction

The timing, maximum frequency and rate of propagation of contractions in the small intestine are all determined by the regular oscillations in the membrane potential of the smooth muscle cells. These fluctuations have been termed slow waves, pacesetter potentials or electric control activity (ECA). The ionic mechanism for these oscillations has not been resolved. One hypothesis states they are caused by regular changes in activity of a membrane-bound sodium pump; the other ascribes them to cyclic changes in the permeability to sodium and chloride across the smooth muscle membrane.

Although regular slow waves can be recorded from both longitudinal and circular smooth muscle layers in intact preparations, they cannot be recorded from isolated preparations of longitudinal smooth muscle unless these contain a thin layer of circular muscle. Also, isolated preparations of the outer layer of circular muscle are electrically silent unless they include a thin strip of longitudinal muscle.[4] These recent observations are compatible with the concept that slow waves arise from the interstitial cells of Cajal, which lie between the two muscle layers and act as pacemakers entraining adjacent smooth muscle cells to the same frequency.[5] These pacemaker cells do not only coordinate the slow waves in the circular and longitudinal layers, they also determine the slow wave frequency along the length of the intestine.

In humans, the frequency of the slow waves declines in a series of frequency plateaux from the duodenum (12/minute) to the ileum (8/minute), each plateau being dominated by a pacemaker situated at its orad aspect. These frequency plateaux vary in length and position, even in the same individual, and it appears as if the function of the dominant pacemaker can be assumed by different cells at different times.

The slow wave is propagated rapidly in a circumferential direction, creating the conditions for the development of a ring constriction. Propagation in a longitudinal direction is directed aborally and is slower (60–100 cm/minute).

Contractions of intestinal smooth muscle only occur during maximum depolarization of the smooth muscle membrane. Unlike cardiac muscle, these contractions do not occur in association with every electrical depolarization, only when the depolarization exceeds a given threshold. Contractions are accompanied in the inner circular and longitudinal layers of smooth muscle by a burst of spike potentials.[6] These

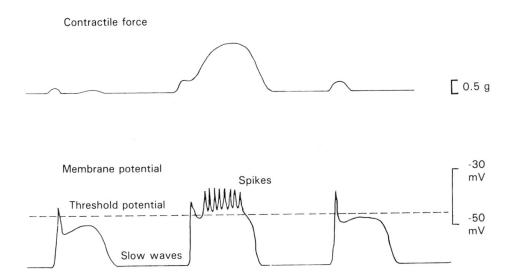

Figure 1   Diagram of the electrical and mechanical activity of smooth muscle showing the relationship between fluctuations in membrane potential and contractile force.

spikes are rapid depolarizations and repolarizations of smooth muscle membrane and are thought to be caused by the entry of calcium into the smooth muscle cells. Thus, although the slow waves determine the potential timing, frequency and rate of propagation of contractions, the actual occurrence of contractions in inner circular and longitudinal layers depends on the presence or absence of spikes (*Figure 1*) and the strength of the contractions is determined by the number of spikes associated with the slow wave. Spike potentials are caused by the opening of voltage-dependent calcium channels and occur when the membrane potential exceeds a certain threshold. Neurotransmitters, released from the enteric nervous system, alter the membrane potential by changing its permeability to small ions, and this influences the coupling of membrane oscillations to spike potentials and contractions. Acetylcholine increases the depolarization of smooth muscle and increases the frequency of spike potentials and contractions, while noradrenaline reduces the depolarization of the muscle membrane and inhibits spike potentials and contractions.

Contraction in the outer layers of circular smooth muscle of canine small intestine is not associated with the presence of spike potentials, but depends solely on the degree of depolarization of the slow wave.[6] Moreover, the resting potential of the cells in the outer circular layer is further from the threshold required to initiate contraction than it is in the inner circular and longitudinal layers. These arrangements would make it possible for the propulsion of fluid to occur when the intestine was tonically contracted; the release of large amounts of acetylcholine could depolarize the inner circular and longitudinal layers sufficiently to cause continuous spikes and tonic contractions, while at the same time generating phasic contractions in the outer longitudinal layers.

Control of motor patterns

Intrinsic nerves: the occurrence of patterns of contractions are caused by neurohumoral influences that work through the normal relationships between slow waves and contractions. Any contraction will potentially migrate at the rate of propagation of the slow wave for long distances if the activity in the enteric nervous system causes sequential release of an excitatory neurotransmitter.

Not all patterns of contractile or myoelectrical spiking activity in the small intestine are associated with propagated slow waves. The large retroperistaltic contractions that occur during emesis and the large propagating contractions and spike burst that can be observed in the distal small intestine can occupy several slow wave cycles and in the cat can be associated with disappearance of slow waves.[7] Presumably the depolarization that occurs during these events is so great that the contraction escapes from the constraints of the myogenic slow wave and is controlled directly by enteric nervous programs. Small intestinal pacing in the dog can cause slow waves and associated contractions to appear to migrate in a reverse direction.[8]

Patterns of contractile activity are largely coordinated by the intrinsic nerves of the gut (the gut brain or the enteric nervous system) and generated by reflexes triggered by the interaction of food with chemoreceptors and tension receptors in the bowel wall. The observation that administration of tetrodotoxin to isolated segments of small intestine can induce contractions on every slow wave demonstrates the existence of a powerful inhibitory nervous influence within the enteric nervous system.[9]

Acetylcholine is thought to be the major excitatory post-ganglionic neurotransmitter. The identity of an inhibitory neurotransmitter is still not established, although vasoactive intestinal polypeptide (VIP) or ATP are strong candidates. Serotonin is an important neurotransmitter substance at interneuron sites; this probably explains why serotonin or serotonin blockers have such a profound effect on intestinal motor activity.

Extrinsic nerves: the small intestine is supplied by parasympathetic nerves from the vagus and by sympathetic nerves from the thoracolumbar outflow. Most of these nerves end at the level of the enteric plexus and are thought to modulate the activity of the intrinsic system in response to extraenteric influences. Thus exercise, anxiety and fear can suppress gut motor activity by interaction through the sympathetic nervous system and the ingestion of food can enhance intestinal motor activity via the vagus nerve. Most of the fibres in the vagus nerves supplying the gut are afferent rather than efferent and these provide a route whereby events in the gut can: (a) reach consciousness and influence behaviour; (b) influence the function of the other organs. The extrinsic nervous system is not essential for the organization of small bowel motility; extrinsic denervation of the small intestine does not inhibit propulsion of luminal contents or cause gross alterations in its contractile pattern.

Some intestinal reflexes, however, are mediated through the extrinsic nerves. The inhibition of intestinal motor activity caused by stimuli, such as gross intestinal distension, is mediated by the sympathetic nerves and relayed through the prevertebral ganglia.[10]

Substances injected into the spinal cord and cerebral ventricles can alter patterns of motor activity and influence transit via extrinsic nerve connections,[11,12] although in some instances humoral substances may be involved.[13]

Peptides: studies on the effects of peptides on the contractility of the small intestine indicate that gastrin, motilin and cholecystokinin (CCK) increase contractility whereas VIP, glucagon and secretin decrease contractility. Some of these agents may be present in enteric neurons and function as neurosecretions or neurotransmitters.[14]

Patterns of contractile activity

Migrating motor complex: under fasting conditions the motor activity of the small intestine in most mammalian species is organized into a recurrent pattern of different phases known as the migrating motor complex (MMC). This consists of a period of quiescence (Phase I), which is succeeded by a period of intermittent contractile activity resembling the activity that normally occurs after a meal (Phase II), and finally by a short period of intense contractile activity when contractions and spike bursts are superimposed upon every slow wave (Phase III). Phase III usually starts in the upper small intestine or the stomach but may start lower in the intestine; it migrates at a slow rate (less then 8 cm/minute) towards the ileum, but often dies away before reaching the ileocecal junction.

Phase II has been divided into two phases. Phase IIa consists of irregular contractions, many of which are not propagated. In Phase IIb, which occurs just before Phase III, the contractions are more likely to be organized into clusters which appear to be propagated down the small intestine. Phase II appears to be related to autonomic arousal as it may be absent during sleep and is very much reduced after vagotomy.[15]

The MMC is thought to clear the small intestine of bacteria and food residues between meals. For this reason, it has been called the intestinal housekeeper, sweeping away the debris of the last meal. Absence of MMCs are associated with evidence of bacterial overgrowth both in man and in the rat.[16,17] Simultaneous recordings of transmural potential differences and intraluminal pressure in humans suggests that

Phase III of the MMC is associated with a burst of intestinal secretion.[18] Thus, the housekeeper may wash as well as sweep the small intestine clean.

Evidence indicates that Phase III of the MMC, like other patterns of motor activity, is coordinated by the intrinsic nerve system. Isolated and extrinsically denervated loops of small intestine still show MMCs. Recent studies have shown that the MMC cycles in an isolated loop of intestine in a manner that appears independent of that in the rest of the small intestine.[19] It is possible to block propagation of Phase III down the intestine by a local intra-arterial injection of tetrodotoxin or ganglion blockers,[20] which block the continuity of the intrinsic nerves. The occurrence of Phase III can, however, be influenced by higher centres. Injection of peptides into cerebral ventricles, for example, can alter the frequency of Phase III activity.[21] Also, Finch and his colleagues have shown that the frequency of cycling of intestinal Phase III is very similar to that of EEG patterns during sleep.[22]

The peptide motilin is considered by some to be responsible for Phase III activity, although the evidence is not totally convincing. Infusions of motilin in physiologic concentrations can induce premature MMCs,[23] spontaneous peaks of blood levels of motilin are often associated with Phase III of the MMC in the upper gut,[25,26] and an antiserum to motilin can disrupt MMCs in the upper gut.[26] However, Phase III cannot be induced in fed animals by motilin infusions, but can be induced by morphine.[27] The infusion of acid and lipid into the small bowel will also induce premature Phase IIIs,[28] which are not associated with increases in motilin. Also, spontaneous episodes of Phase III can occur in the jejunum and ileum in the absence of a rise in motilin.[29] Thus, although motilin may be involved in the initiation of Phase III, its role may be permissive or modulatory.

The length of Phase II activity varies inversely with the length of Phase I and appears to be associated with the level of arousal. Vagotomy or freezing the vagus in the neck reduces the period of Phase II,[15] whereas splanchnectomy increases it.[30] Similar effects have been seen with atropine and adrenergic antagonists.

Fed pattern of motor activity: ingestion of a meal disrupts the MMC in man, dog and many other species, leading to a prolonged period of apparently irregular activity. The period over which the MMC pattern is disrupted is directly correlated with the size of the meal[31] and is influenced by its content. Meals containing fat, for example, will disrupt the MMC pattern for longer than meals that contain equivalent amounts of energy in the form of protein and carbohydrate.[31,32] The length of disruption may be related to the period of time it takes certain meals to empty from the stomach and hence the exposure of the upper small intestine to nutrient material.[33]

Recordings from multiple, closely spaced sites show that many of the irregular contractions that occur after ingesting a meal are propagated downstream, although the distance of propagation may be very small. It is as if the chyme is gently moved along by contractions that form and reform. The degree and type of activity can be influenced by the content of the food. For example, the number of spikes or contractions are greatest after meals containing glucose and least after meals containing fats.[34] Infusion of fats into the small intestine, particularly the distal part of the small intestine, reduces the post-prandial contraction rate, amplitude and degree of propagation.[35]

Intravenous infusion of secretin, insulin, CCK, gastrin and pancreatic polypeptide disrupt MMCs. Infusions of somatostatin may induce or suppress the occurrence of MMCs dependent upon the conditions of the experiments. The possible role of humoral agents in the suppression of MMCs induced by feeding is contradicted by studies showing that feeding dogs did not disrupt the MMCs in auto-transplanted loops of small intestine.[36] Also, dogs with isolated antral loops who secreted high levels of gastrin showed quite normal patterns of MMC activity.[37]

The conversion of the fasting to fed pattern and the length of the fed pattern can be inhibited by vagotomy[38] or vagal freezing, suggesting that vagal activity suppresses the interdigestive pattern. Local factors, however, are also important. Infusion of relatively small concentrations of glucose into an isolated denervated loop of small intestine can disrupt the fasting motor pattern.[39]

The return of the MMC after a meal occurs sooner if the meal is conveyed rapidly down the small intestine.[33]

Migrating clusters of contractions: ingestion of non-nutrient meals containing viscous polysaccharides such as guar gum or cellulose may induce clusters of contractions which are propagated downstream.[35,40] Mixing fat or protein into these meals or infusion of fat into the small intestine reduces the incidence of clusters and their degree of propagation.[35,60]

Propagated clusters of contractions can also be induced by other stimuli. Obstruction of the intestine can induce clusters proximal to the site of obstruction.[41] Many of the factors that cause diarrhea, such as laxative agents, enterotoxins, prostaglandins and VIPs, can induce propagated clusters of contractions.[42] Thus, contraction clusters can be seen as an adaptation of small bowel motor activity to clear the intestine of a bolus or to remove substances that can damage the intestine or the organism.

Prolonged propagated contraction: the prolonged propagated contraction (PPC) is a broad based high amplitude contraction that is usually seen only in the ileum (*Figure 2*). It may last up to 15 seconds and can occupy several slow wave cycles. It is highly propagative and can clear the ileum of its contents.[43] Such contractions can be caused by infusions of acetylcholine, bile acids, refluxed fecal material and laxative agents.[44]

Migrating action potential complexes: exposure of a loop of rabbit ileum to cholera toxin induces intense spiking activity that can occupy several slow wave cycles (*Figure 3*) and appears to propagate through the loop and can cause expulsion of fluid.[45] Migrating action potential complexes (MAPCs) may be the electrical counterpart of the PPC and can be induced by a number of enterotoxins, by bile acids and by laxative agents. Since these agents also cause intestinal secretion, it has been suggested that MAPCs are caused by luminal distension with secretions. Luminal distension can certainly induce a similar motor pattern, although substances that do not cause intestinal secretion are still able to induce MAPCs.[46] The observations that MAPCs only occur in loops exposed to toxins and not in the rest of the intestine, and that they can be blocked by tetrodotoxin and ganglion blockers, indicate that they are mediated by an enteric nervous reflex rather than the release of hormones. Abolition by indomethacin, however, suggests the involvement of prostaglandins.[47]

Repetitive bursts of action potentials: exposure of a loop of rabbit ileum to invasive bacteria or to certain enterotoxins can induce brief episodes of spike potentials which do not usually propagate, occupy only one slow wave cycle[48] and occur in a repetitive manner. Mathias has suggested that this pattern may induce stasis, leading to proliferation and invasion of bacteria.[48]

Aboral propagation during emesis: vomiting is often preceded by a broad contraction which frequently starts in the jejunum and sweeps up towards the pylorus, clearing

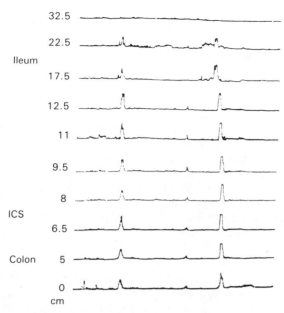

Figure 2 A recording of intraluminal pressure from the ileum, ileocecal sphincter (ICS) and colon of a healthy human showing large single phasic contractions that last 20–40 seconds and appear to migrate aborally. Reproduced with permission from Quigley EMM, Borody TJ, Phillips SF *et al*. Motility of the terminal ileum and ileocecal sphincter in healthy humans. *Gastroenterology* 1984; **87**: 857–66.

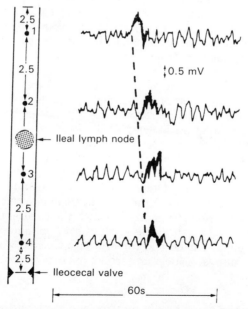

Figure 3 A migrating action potential complex recorded from a loop of ileum in an anesthetized rabbit. Electrode placement is indicated schematically as left. Note the prolonged burst of action potentials that appear to migrate distally. Reproduced with permission from Mathias JR, Carlson GM, DiMarino AJ *et al*. Intestinal myoelectric activity in response to live *Vibrio cholerae* and cholera enterotoxin. *J Clin Invest* 1976; **58**: 91–6.

intestinal contents into the stomach.[49,50] This retroperistaltic contraction can be abolished by section of the vagus or administration of atropine, indicating that it is modulated or mediated by the vagus nerve.

The ileocolonic junction
A high pressure zone exists at the end of the ileum as it projects into the cecum. The pressure in this zone can be relaxed by ileal distension and increased by colonic distension,[51] or by blocking intrinsic nerve activity with tetrodotoxin. These observations support the concept of a true ileocolonic sphincter.[52] It was initially considered that the ileocolonic reflux can be shown to occur in normal people and does not increase if the ileocolonic junction is removed.

The terminal ileum exhibits two types of propagated activity, discrete clusters of contractions and prolonged propagated contractions. The latter are highly propulsive and sweep ileal contents down into the colon. Phase III of the migrating motor complex often does not reach the terminal ileum.[43]

Small intestinal transit
It takes 2–12 hours for a solid meal to travel down the small intestine to the ileum. Small bowel transit time in humans is inversely correlated with the frequency of contractions in the upper small intestine,[33] though studies in dogs have suggested that the rate at which a meal travels down the small intestine is more closely related to the length of spread of propagation than the frequency of contractions.[40] The rate of transit of a meal is not directly related to gastric emptying[53] unless this is very rapid or very slow.

Although disruptible solids and liquids empty at different rates from the stomach, recent studies suggest that the small intestine does not discriminate between solid and liquids;[54] both travel down the small intestine at similar rates. Nondisruptible solids, such as drug capsules, have to wait for the next interdigestive migrating complex before they can empty from the stomach; consequently their arrival at the cecum depends more on the delay in emptying from the stomach than on their transit through the small intestine.[55]

Varying the composition of the meal can alter the transit rate through the small intestine. Increasing the amount of unabsorbable carbohydrate will accelerate small bowel transit probably by causing distension and inducing propagation.[56] Increasing the lipid content of a meal will delay small bowel transit (unpublished observations). This effect is probably related to an action of lipid on the ileum, since infusion of lipid into the ileum but not the jejunum delays small bowel transit.[57] The effect of lipid can be blocked by the specific opiate antagonist naloxone, suggesting mediation by opiate receptors.[58] Other studies have shown that the presence of an intestinal tube can accelerate transit through the small intestine, an important point to remember in any physiologic studies in which the small intestine is intubated.[59] Mental stress can also accelerate small bowel transit,[60] although physical stress such as repeatedly plunging the hand and forearm into ice cold water can delay transit (unpublished observations). Moderate exercise appears to have no effect on transit time.[61]

Relationship between small bowel motility and transport

Contact time:　the degree of absorption of nutrients from the meal depends on the time of exposure to the small intestinal epithelium. Under normal post-prandial conditions, exposure or contact time is equal to transit time.[42] The absorption of foods that are more slowly digested or transported across the epithelium will be limited more by transit time (*Figure 4*). Studies in ileostomy patients, who have had minimal ileal resection, have shown that administration of agents that accelerate small bowel transit decrease absorption of fat and other components of the meal.[62] Intubation experiments in normal volunteers have also shown that the degree of absorption from the small intestine can be increased when small bowel transit time is prolonged by infusing lipid into the ileum.[63]

Contact area: alterations in the area of the intestine exposed to luminal contents may have a large influence on the degree of absorption. Motor activity may increase the contact area in several ways. Propulsion of luminal contents may aid contact by spreading nutrients over a large area of epithelium; the spreading of the first part of the meal over a long length of small intestine may be responsible for an initial rapid rate of absorption. Rhythmic movements of the longitudinal muscle layer of small intestine are said to be responsible for maximum exposure of the enterocyte surface area to luminal contents,[64] because they stretch and open out the intestinal epithelium, exposing sites on the sides of the villi; in this respect, Lee has shown that stretching the intestine *in vitro* increases the rate of absorption.[65] Ring-like contractions of circular smooth muscle and rhythmic contractions of muscularis mucosae may have the same function. The piston-like movements of the intestinal villi may also expose sites on the sides of adjacent noncontracted villi to luminal contents.[66]

Mixing: mixing enhances absorption by increasing the interactions between food molecules and digestive enzymes and between products of digestion and the carrier sites on the absorptive epithelium. Intestinal motor activity is responsible for mixing luminal contents. Analysis of the effects of wall movements using a mechanical model has suggested that propagating circular contractions are most effective in increasing

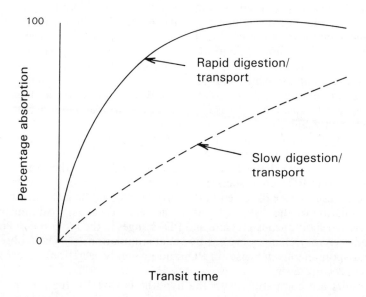

Figure 4   Relationship between transit time and absorption in the small intestine. The absorption of foods that are more slowly digested or transported are more likely to be limited by transit time.

the transport of material out of tubes constructed from dialysis membranes.[67] Although wall movements can bring nutrients close to the epithelial surface, they have to cross a relatively unstirred layer of fluid by diffusion before they can come into contact with the enterocytes.[68] This diffusion barrier limits the uptake of substances that are rapidly transported.[68] Movements of the intestinal villi[66] or microvilli or muscularis mucosae may stir this unstirred layer and increase uptake by reducing the functional dimensions of the diffusion barrier.[68] This hypothesis has yet to be tested. The reduction in the rate of nutrient absorption caused by feeding viscous polysaccharides is probably due to an inhibition of mixing.[69]

Intestinal tone: Naftalin provided evidence from *in vitro* studies which suggests that certain drugs such as theophylline may cause secretion and reduce absorption by reducing the permeability of a submucosal fluid barrier, whereas other drugs such as loperamide may reverse this effect.[1] The anatomical identity of this submucosal barrier is unknown but it is probably the muscularis mucosae. The relevance of these experiments to the small intestine *in situ* with an intact blood supply is not known, although Lee has recently demonstrated an inverse correlation between smooth muscle tone and fluid absorption in exteriorized loops of rat intestine *in vivo*.[70]

Reflex intestinal secretion: it is difficult to determine whether intestinal contractions may induce intestinal secretion because there is no simple direct means of recording fluctuations in intestinal fluid transfer in intact animals or humans over the same time period as contractions take place. However, under carefully controlled conditions, measurements of transintestinal potential difference (PD) may provide a useful on-line index of neurally induced secretion. Many but not all intestinal secretagogues elevate the PD, making the lumen more negative.[71] Distension of the intestinal lumen induces intestinal secretion[72] and increases the PD;[73,74] both effects can be blocked by hexamethonium and partially inhibited by atropine. Balloon distension of the intestine also releases transmitters such as acetylcholine,[75,76] serotonin[77] and prostaglandins,[76,78] all of which induce intestinal secretion and increase the PD. Finally, brief stimulation of the efferent fibres of the vagus nerve in the neck of the anesthetized ferret causes an increase in jejunal pressure activity, accompanied by a rise in PD and a burst of intestinal secretion.[79]

Recordings in the human small intestine showed that the repetitive spontaneous bursts of contractions that occurred at intervals of about 1 minute were associated with fluctuations in PD that peaked about 45 seconds after the pressure event.[73] Much larger rises in PD were associated with Phase III of the migrating motor complex.[18] Similar results were observed in the ferret and could be generated by low frequency stimulation of the distal cut end of the cervical vagus.[80] Administration of atropine blocked spontaneous pressure and PD changes in the ferret but did not block the PD and secretory changes evoked by vagal stimulation.[79,80] These observations suggest that spontaneous increases in PD (and probably secretion) occurred secondary to the pressure events.

These results are compatible with the hypothesis that fluctuations in PD (and presumably secretion) are triggered by stimulation of tension receptors by intestinal contractions, though they could also occur by stimulation of mucosal mechanoreceptors by food or the opposing mucosal surface. Rubbing the mucosal surface gently with the smooth end of a glass rod or a small balloon has been used for many years to induce secretion in the intestine of experimental animals.[78]

References

1 Naftalin RJ. The mechanism and control of fluid absorption and secretion. In: Den RJ, Stahl P, eds. *Developments of Cell Biology, Secretory Processes.* London: Butterworths 1985; 181-200.

2 Taylor AB, Kreulen D, Prosser CL. Electron microscopy of the connective tissue between longitudinal and circular muscle of the small intestine of the cat. *Am J Anat* 1977; **150**: 427-42.

3 Furness JB, Costa M. Types of nerves in the enteric nervous system. *Neuroscience* 1980; **5**: 1-20.

4 Hara Y, Kubota M, Szurszewski JH. Electrophysiology of smooth muscle of some mammals. *J Physiol* 1986; **372**: 501-20.

5 Thunberg L. Interstitial cells of Cajal: intestinal pacemaker cells? In: Beck F, Hild W, van Limbrorgh J, Ortmann R, Pauly JE, Schiebler F, eds. *Advances in Anatomy, Embryology and Cell Biology*, Vol 71. Berlin, Springer-Verlag 1982; 1-130.

6 Hara Y, Szurszewski JH. Effect of potassium and acetylcholine on canine intestinal smooth muscle. *J Physiol* 1986; **372**: 521-37.

7 Weisbrodt NW, Christensen J. Electrical activity of the cat duodenum in fasting and vomiting. *Gastroenterology* 1972; **63**: 1004-10.

8 Sarr MG, Kelly KA, Gladen HE. Electrical control of canine jejunal propulsion. *Am J Physiol* 1981; **240**: G355-60.

9 Biber B, Fara J. Intestinal motility increased by tetrodotoxin, lidocaine and procaine. *Experientia* 1973; **29**: 551-2.

10 Kreulen DL, Szurzewski JH. Reflex pathways in the abdominal prevertebral ganglia: evidence for a colo-colonic inhibitory reflex. *J Physiol (Lond)* 1979; **295**: 21-32.

11 Stewart JJ, Burks TF, Weisbrodt NW. Intestinal myoelectric activity after activation of central emetic mechanism. *Am J Physiol* 1977; **233**: E131-7.

12 Stewart JJ, Weisbrodt NW, Burks TF. Central and peripheral actions of morphine on intestinal transit. *J Pharmacol Exp Ther* 1978; **205**: 547-55.

13 Bardon T, Ruckebusch M. Changes in 5-HIAA and 5HT levels in lumbar CSF following morphine administration to conscious dogs. *Neurosci Lett* 1984; **49**: 147-51.

14 Furness JB, Costa M, Gibbons TL. Transmitters, contents and pathways of enteric neurons. *Proc Int Union Physiologic Sci* 1983; **61**: 103.

15 Ruckebush Y, Bueno L. Migrating myoelectrical complex of the small intestine. *Gastroenterology* 1977; **73**: 1309-14.

16 Vantrappen G, Janssens J, Ghoos Y. The interdigestive motor complex of normal subjects and patients with bacterial overgrowth of the small intestine. *J Clin Invest* 1977; **59**: 1158-66.

17 Scott LD, Cahall DL. Influence of the interdigestive myoelectric complex on enteric flora in the rat. *Gastroenterology* 1982; **82**: 737-45.

18 Read NW. The migrating motor complex and spontaneous fluctuations of transmural potential difference in the human small intestine. In: Christensen J, ed. *Gastrointestinal Motility.* New York: Raven Press 1980; 299-306.

19 Sarna S, Condon RE, Cowles V. Enteric mechanisms of initiation of migrating myoelectric complexes in dogs. *Gastroenterology* 1983; **84**: 814-22.

20 Sarna S, Stoddard C, Belbeck L, McWade D. Intrinsic nervous control of migrating myoelectric complexes. *Am J Physiol* 1981; **241**: G16-23.

21 Bueno L, Ferre J-P. Central regulation of intestinal motility by somatostatin and cholecystokinin octapeptide. *Science* 1982; **216**: 1427-9.

22 Finch PM, Ingram DM, Henstridge JD, Catchpole BN. Relationship of fasting gastroduodenal motility to the sleep cycle. *Gastroenterology* 1982; **83**: 605-12.

23 Itoh Z, Honda R, Hiwatashi K, Takeuchi S, Aizawa I, Takayanagi R, Couch EF. Motilin-induced mechanical activity in the canine alimentary tract. *Scand J Gastroenterol* 1976; **11** (Suppl 39): 93-110.

24 Lee KY, Chey WY, Yajim H. Radioimmunoassay of motilin: validation of studies on the relationship between plasma motilin and interdigestive myoelectric activity of the duodenum of dog. *Am J Dig Dis* 1978; **23**: 789-95.

25 Itoh Z, Takeuchi S, Aizawa I *et al.* Changes in plasma motilin concentration and gastrointestinal contractile activity in conscious dogs. *Dig Dis Sci* 1978; **23**: 929-35.

26 Lee KY, Chang T-M, Chey WY. Effect of rabbit antimotilin serum on myoelectric activity and plasma motilin concentration in fasting dog. *Am J Physiol* 1983; **245**: G547-53.

27 Sarna S, Condon RE, Cowles V. Morphine versus motilin in the initiation of migrating myoelectric complexes. *Am J Physiol* 1983; **245**: G217-20.
28 Lee KY, Chey WY, Tay HH, Wagner D, Yajima H. Cyclic changes in plasma motilin levels and interdigestive myoelectric activity of canine antrum and duodenum. *Gastroenterology* 1977; **72**: 1162.
29 Rees WD, Malagelada J-R, Miller LJ, Go VLW. Human interdigestive and postprandial gastrointestinal motor and gastrointestinal hormone patterns. *Dig Dis Sci* 1982; **27**: 321-9.
30 Marlett JA, Code CF. Effect of celiac and superior mesenteric ganglionectomy on interdigestive myoelectric complex in dogs. *Am J Physiol* 1979; **237**: E432-6.
31 DeWever I, Eeckhout C, Vantrappen G, Hellemans J. Disruptive effect of test meals on interdigestive motor complex in dogs. *Am J Physiol* 1978; **235**: E661-5.
32 Eeckhout C, DeWever I, Peeters T, Hellemans J, Vantrappen G. Role of gastrin and insulin in postprandial disruption of migration complex in dogs. *Am J Physiol* 1978; **235**: E666-9.
33 Read NW, Al-Janabi MN, Edwards CA, Barber DC. Relationship between postprandial motor activity in the human small intestine and the gastrointestinal transit of food. *Gastroenterology* 1984; **86**: 721-7.
34 Schang JC, Danchel J, Sara P *et al*. Specific effects of different food components on intestinal motility. *Eur Surg Res* 1978; **10**: 425-32.
35 Welch IMcL, Worlding J. The effect of ileal infusion of lipid on the motility pattern in humans after ingestion of a viscous non-nutrient meal. *J Physiol* 1986; **378**: 12P.
36 Sarr MG, Kelly KA. Myoelectric activity of the autotransplanted canine jejunoileum. *Gastroenterology* 1981; **81**: 303-10.
37 Russell J, Bass P, Shimizu M, Miyauchi A, Go VLW. Canine intestinal ulcer: myoelectric components and the effect of chronic hypergastrinaemia. *Gastroenterology* 1982; **82**: 746-52.
38 Weisbrodt NW, Copeland EM, Moore EP, Kearley RW, Johnson LR. Effect of vagotomy on electrical activity of the small intestine of the dog. *Am J Physiol* 1965; **228**: 650-4.
39 Eeckhout C, DeWever I, Vantrappen G, Hellemans J. Local disorganisation of the interdigestive migrating motor complex (MMC) by perfusion of a Thiry-Vella loop. *Gastroenterology* 1979; **76**: 1127.
40 Scheeman M, Erhlein MJ. Postprandial canine jejunal motility and transit of luminal content. *Gastroenterology* 1986; **90**: 991-1000.
41 Summers RW, Anuras S, Green J. Jejunal manometry patterns in health, partial intestinal obstruction and pseudo-obstruction. *Gastroenterology* 1983; **85**: 1290-300.
42 Read NW. Diarrhea motrice. *Clin Gastroenterol* 1986; **15**: 657-83.
43 Quigley EMM, Borody TJ, Phillips SF, Wienbeck M, Tucker RL, Haddad A. Motility of the terminal ileum and ileocecal sphincter in healthy humans. *Gastroenterology* 1984; **87**: 857-66.
44 Kruis W, Azpiroz F, Phillips SF. Contractile patterns and transit of fluid in canine terminal ileum. *Am J Physiol* 1985; **12**: G264-70.
45 Mathias JR, Carlson GM, DiMarino AJ, Bertiger G, Morton HE, Cohen S. Intestinal myoelectric activity in response to live *Vibrio cholerae* and cholera enterotoxin. *J Clin Invest* 1976; **58**: 91-6.
46 Sinar DR, Burns TW. Migrating action potential complexes occur independent of fluid secretion from cholera toxin. *Gastroenterology* 1979; **76**: 1249.
47 Mathias JR, Carlson GM, Bertiger G, Martin JL, Cohen S. Migrating action potential complex of cholera: a possible prostaglandin-induced response. *Am J Physiol* 1977; **232**: E529-34.
48 Mathias JR, Carlson GM, Martin JL, Sheilds RP, Formal S. *Shigella dysenteriae* I enterotoxin: proposed role in pathogenesis of shigellosis. *Am J Physiol* 1980; **239**: G382-6.
49 Gregory RA. The nervous pathways of intestinal reflexes associated with nausea and vomiting. *J Physiol (Lond)* 1947; **106**: 95-103.
50 Stewart JJ, Burks TF, Weisbrodt NW. Intestinal myoelectric activity after activation of central emetic mechanism. *Am J Physiol* 1977; **233**: E131-7.
51 Cohen S, Harris LD, Levitan R. Manometric characteristics of the human ileocecal junctional zone. *Gastroenterology* 1968; **54**: 72-5.
52 Conklin JL, Christensen J. Local specialization at ileocecal junction of the cat and opossum. *Am J Physiol* 1975; **228**: 1075-81.
53 Read NW, Cammack J, Edwards C, Holdgate AM, Cann PA, Brown C. Is the transit time of a meal through the small intestine related to the rate at which it leaves the stomach? *Gut* 1982; **23**: 824-8.

54 Malagelada J-R, Robertson JS, Brown ML *et al.* Intestinal transit of solid and liquid components of a meal in health. *Gastroenterology* 1984; **87**: 1255–63.

55 Davis SS, Hardy JG, Fara JW. Transit of pharmaceutic dosage forms through the small intestine. *Gut* 1986; **27**: 886–92.

56 Read NW, Miles CA, Fisher D *et al.* Transit of a meal through the small intestine and colon in normal subjects and its role in the pathogenesis of diarrhoea. *Gastroenterology* 1980; **79**: 1276–82.

57 Read NW, MacFarlane A, Kinsman R *et al.* Effect of infusion of nutrient solutions into the ileum on gastrointestinal transit and plasma levels of neurotensin and enteroglucagon in man. *Gastroenterology* 1984; **86**: 274–80.

58 Kinsman RI, Read NW. The ileal brake: a mechanism for controlling gastric emptying and small bowel transit, modulated by opiates. *Gastroenterology* 1984; **87**: 335–7.

59 Read NW, Al-Janabi MN, Bates TE, Barber DC. The effect of gastrointestinal intubation on the passage of a solid meal through the stomach and small intestine in humans. *Gastroenterology* 1983; **84**: 1568–72.

60 Cann PA, Read NW, Cammack J *et al.* Psychological stress and the passage of a standard meal through the stomach and small intestine in man. *Gut* 1983; **24**: 236–40.

61 Cammack J, Read NW, Cann PA, Greenwood B, Holgate AM. Effect of prolonged exercise on the passage of a solid meal through the stomach and small intestine. *Gut* 1982; **23**: 957–61.

62 Holgate AM, Read NW. The relationship between small bowel transit time and absorption of a solid meal: influence of metoclopramide, magnesium sulfate and lactulose. *Dig Dis Sci* 1983; **28**: 812–9.

63 Holgate AM, Read NW. The effect of ileal infusion of intralipid on gastrointestinal transit, ileal flow rate and carbohydrate absorption in humans after a liquid meal. *Gastroenterology* 1985; **88**: 1005–11.

64 Melville J, Macagno E, Christensen J. Longitudinal contractions in the duodenum, their fluid mechanical function. *Am J Physiol* 1975; **228**: 1887–92.

65 Lee JS. Effect of stretching and stirring on water and glucose absorption by canine mucosal membrane. *J Physiol (Lond)* 1983; **345**: 335–43.

66 Sessions JT, Viegas de Indrade SR, Kokas E. Intestinal villi. Forward motility in relation to function. In: Glass CBJ, ed. *Progress in Gastroenterology.* New York: Grune & Stratton 1968.

67 Macagno EO, Christensen J, Lee CL. Modelling the effect of wall movement on absorption in the intestine. *J Physiol (Lond)* 1982; **343**: G541–50.

68 Dietschy JM, Westergaard H. Effect of unstirred water layers on various transport processes in the intestine. In: Csaky TZ, ed. *International Absorption and Malabsorption.* New York: Raven Press 1975; 197–207.

69 Blackburn NA, Redfern JS, Jarjis M *et al.* The mechanism of action of guar gum in improving glucose tolerance in man. *Clin Sci* 1984; **66**: 329–36.

70 Lee JS. Relationship between intestinal motility and tone and water absorption and lymph flow in the rat. *J Physiol (Lond)* 1983; **345**: 489–99.

71 Read NW. Speculations on the role of motility in the pathogenesis and treatment of diarrhoea. *Scand J Gastroenterol* 1983; **81**: (Suppl 84): 45–63.

72 Caren JF, Meyer JH, Grossman MI. Canine intestinal secretion during and after rapid distension of the small bowel. *Am J Physiol* 1974; **227**: 183–8.

73 Read NW, Smallwood RH, Levin RJ *et al.* Relationship between changes in intraluminal pressure and transmural potential difference in the human and canine jejunum *in vivo. Gut* 1977; **18**: 141–51.

74 Fuller J, Hardcastle J, Hardcastle PT. Effect of intraluminal pressure on electrical activity on rat ileal mucosa. *J Physiol* 1980; **302**: 12.

75 Kazic T, Varagic VM. Effect of increased intraluminal pressure on the release of acetylcholine from the isolated guinea pig ileum. *Br J Pharmacol Chemother* 1968; **32**: 185–92.

76 Yagasaki O, Susuki H, Sohji J. Effects of loperamide on acetylcholine and prostaglandin release from isolated guinea pig ileum. *Jap J Pharmacol* 1978; **28**: 873–83.

77 Burke TF, Lang JP. 5-hydroxytryptamine release into dog intestinal vasculature. *Am J Physiol* 1966; **211**: 619–25.

78 Beubler E, Juan H. PGE-released blood flow and transmucosal water movement after mechanical stimulation of the rat jejunal mucosa. *Naunyn-Schmied Arch Pharmacol*

1978; **305**: 91–5.

79 Greenwood B, Read NW. The vagal control of fluid transport, transmural potential difference and motility in the ferret jejunum. *Am J Physiol* 1985; **249**: G651–2.

80 Greenwood B, Read NW. The neural control of jejunal and ileal motility and transmural potential difference in the ferret. *Can J Physiol Pharmacol* 1986; **64**: 180–7.

Physiology of colonic motility

S F Phillips

The complex nature of the motor physiology of the human hindgut is suggested by the comparative anatomy of mammalian colons.[1] Depending largely on the natural diet, carnivores have short, simple colons; monogastric herbivores show most specialization of the hindgut; man and other omnivorous beasts come in between. This marked species variability relates, presumably, to the need to establish residence times in the hindgut of sufficient length to allow bacterial degradation of complex dietary carbohydrates. These materials are resistant to digestion by mammalian enzymes, and species that rely on such nutrients have developed colons that deal with them.

A second perspective is obtained from a longitudinal examination of the gut. In man, esophageal transit occupies seconds, gastric emptying minutes to hours, and small intestinal transit requires several hours; but residence times in the colon are hours to days.[2] Further, like the stomach, which in effect functions as two organs (relaxatory storage proximally, with physical disintegration and emptying being finely controlled distally), the colon should perhaps be considered as more than one organ. Thus, the proximal colon may be an organ of capacitance,[3] whereas the rectosigmoid and anal canal have clear functions of expulsion.

Colonic motility

Motility is a blanket term covering:
- the cellular properties of smooth muscle in the tunica muscularis (myogenic functions)
- neurogenic coordination of smooth muscle by the intrinsic and extrinsic nervous systems (neurogenic functions)
- contractions of muscle which elevate intraluminal pressures
- propulsion of contents (the net effect of antegrade and retrograde movements).

The membrane potentials of intestinal smooth muscle cells display periodic fluctuations;[4] these are quantified most directly by recordings from intracellular microelectrodes. Signals can also be recorded by extracellular electrodes located in, or near to, the tunica muscularis. In many segments of the gut, these electrical fluctuations comprise a 'slow wave' or 'pacesetter potential'. Superimposed upon these fluctuations of baseline potential are the electrical equivalents of smooth muscle contraction. These also can be measured by intracellular techniques as 'action potentials', or their equivalent can be recorded extracellularly as 'spike bursts'.

Contraction of smooth muscle produces the mechanical manifestations of motility. These can be recorded as changes in the intraluminal pressure, as measured by perfused open-tip catheters or small balloons. Alternatively, movement of the wall can be monitored by strain gauges sewn on to the serosal surface of the bowel. When oriented in a circular direction, strain gauges record contractions of circular muscle as a shortening in this dimension. The next, and more visible, expression of motility is the transit of contents. Experimentally, transit can be measured by half-times of the movement of markers through a segment of bowel or, in the clinical setting, as the mean transit time for radio-opaque solids or radionuclides.[2,5]

The mechanisms whereby colonic motility is integrated such that chyme is moved through the large bowel and also converted to solid stool are complex. Thus, total residence time within the large bowel will influence contact time of chyme with the mucosa and will also regulate the time available for the action of bacterial enzymes on fecal contents. Both physiologic phenomena will be influenced by those components of colonic motility which facilitate storage. On the other hand, propulsion through the colon is normally slow and is programmed delicately, such that contents arrive distally only when they are ready for brief storage in the rectum before voluntary evacuation. Most segments of the large bowel probably have the capacity to store and also to propel contents; the key to integrated function is the colon's ability to prevent a too rapid progression in a distal direction. It has been estimated that healthy subjects with normal bowel habits move the contents of the colon, under resting conditions, at an average rate of only 1 cm/hour.[6]

Measurements of transit
The simplest index of colonic motility in man is the passage of radio-opaque markers, which can be assessed radiologically. Small radio-opaque particles are ingested and their excretion can be monitored in stools, providing an estimate of mean mouth-to-anus transit time.[7,8] The technique can be modified by obtaining abdominal x-rays and assigning markers to different segments of the colon; in this manner, total and/or segmental transit within the large intestine can be calculated.[2,9] Overall, approximately 12 hours is needed for markers to leave the stomach, pass through the small intestine and enter the colon; thereafter, transit through the large intestine occurs in 36–48 hours. One-third of this time is taken up in the right colon, one-third in the left and one-third in the rectosigmoid. Feces also move backwards and forwards,[6] and stools may be retained for long periods in the right half of the colon, even in patients with diseases associated with frequent defecation.[10] More recently, the application of gamma camera scintigraphy has allowed colonic transit to be defined more precisely.[3,11,12] Storage in the right colon also involves mechanisms that prevent reflux of contents into the ileum. The ileocecal sphincter provides such a barrier,[13] and its resistance to reflux is augmented by colonic distension.[14] However, sphincteric pressures in humans are of lesser magnitudes than in the dog.[15,16]

The mechanisms that control propulsion in the colon are poorly understood. During steady state perfusion of the colon with isotonic fluids, the right colon contracts at regular intervals, suggesting that a critical volume must be reached before the right colon propels fluids onward.[17] When infused with a fluid simulating colonic contents in steatorrhea, the right colon increases its 'tone', such that the cecum and ascending colon tolerate lesser volumes of fluid.[11] In addition, fat in the right colon provokes high pressure contractions which propel contents rapidly to the transverse and descending colons, sigmoid and rectum (*Figure 1*), prompting defecation. Both phenomena are blocked by morphine.[3] Such findings support the concept that the right colon is sensitive to critical volumes and also suggest that it responds to the chemical nature of the contents (*Figure 2*).

Measurements of pressure and myoelectrical activity
Assessments of colonic motility *in vivo* utilize one of two techniques of recording; intraluminal pressure or extracellular electrical sensors. Intraluminal pressure recordings have given insights into the mechanisms of storage in the right colon. Thus,

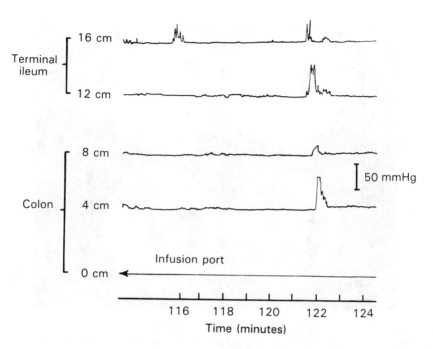

Figure 1 Pressure waves recorded from the cecum of a healthy volunteer, perfused with an emulsion of oleic acid, simulating chyme in steatorrhea. A high pressure wave began in the ileum and progressed to the proximal colon, associated with rapid transit of contents (see *Figure 2B*). Such waves were not seen when control saline was infused.

the transverse and descending colons generate pressure waves at greater frequencies[18] and more contractions can be observed radiologically[19] than in the right colon. Indeed, a 'pacemaker' in the mid-colon has been proposed.[20] The net effect of pacing from this location could be that the proximal colon would be paced along a retrograde vector, thus facilitating storage.

Recordings of intraluminal pressure *in vivo* also reveal at the rectosigmoid junction an area of high intraluminal pressure,[21] and a higher frequency of phasic contractions.[22] Specialized motility at this site could help prevent the uncontrolled aboral progression of stool from the sigmoid colon to the rectum. However, it is doubtful that a true physiologic sphincter exists at the rectosigmoid junction.

Intraluminal pressure recordings from the cecum suggest that cycles of interdigestive motility in the small intestine rarely propagate into the proximal colon.[15] On the other hand, there is an initial motor response of the colon to the ingestion of food, the 'gastrocolic reflex'. Though clearly demonstrable in the distal colon,[23] it is less prominent in the cecum and ascending colon.[24] Moreover, this response to food is neither a reflex nor does it require the presence of a stomach (for it occurs in gastrectomized subjects).[25] A more appropriate term is the 'colonic response to food'.[25]

The small intestine undergoes well-defined cycles of motor activity (interdigestive migrating electrical complexes, IDMEC) in the fasting state. It was logical, therefore, to seek parallel phenomena in the colon. In the dog[26,27] and man[15] cycles of small bowel motility occasionally pass into the cecum but not beyond. It is unlikely that progression of IDMECs into the colon is an important mechanism of coordination between the small and large bowels.[28] However, in the dog, Sarna has described a

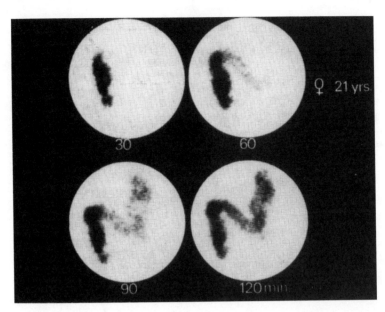

Figure 2A Scintiscan of healthy human colon perfused with saline. Transit of contents was slow; at 2 hours the ascending and transverse colons were filled. Reproduced with permission from Spiller RC, Brown ML, Phillips SF. Decreased fluid tolerance, accelerated transit and abnormal motility of the human colon induced by oleic acid. *Gastroenterology* 1986; **91**: 100–7.

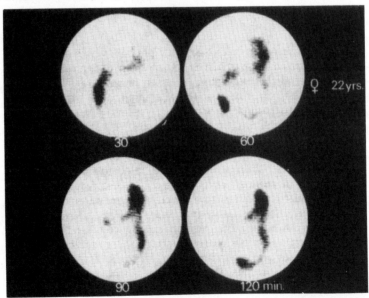

Figure 2B Scintiscan of healthy human colon perfused with oleic acid. Transit of contents was rapid; at 2 hours the rectum was filled. Note also that the proximal colon accommodates a lesser volume than with saline perfusions. Reproduced with permission from Spiller RC, Brown ML, Phillips SF. Decreased fluid tolerance, accelerated transit and abnormal motility of the human colon induced by oleic acid. *Gastroenterology* 1986; **91**: 100–7.

'colonic migrating complex' with a cycle length of 20–40 minutes; it features stationary and migrating bursts of electrical and mechanical activity.[28]

Huizinga and Daniel concluded that the "wiring of the intrinsic nervous system of human or animal colon is almost totally unknown based on structural studies".[29] Available data support the presence of excitatory cholinergic inputs, adrenergic inhibition and noncholinergic-nonadrenergic stimuli of both types. These transmitters are not identified, but immunochemically identifiable peptides, substance P, vasoactive intestinal polypeptide (VIP), somatostatin and enkephalins are present. Myogenic control is also defined incompletely, with apparent conflicts among species and different experimental preparations adding to the uncertainties. Slow waves can be recorded from longitudinal and circular muscle strips *in vitro*, but the frequencies differ and they appear to be much less stable than in comparable studies of stomach or small intestine. The site at which control signals (slow waves) are generated is also unclear.

Myoelectrical recordings in man have concentrated mainly on the frequency of slow waves in the distal colon and rectum. Rhythmic, electrical signals occur at two predominant frequencies; one averages 3 cycles/minute and the other 6–8 cycles/minute.[30-35] Some authors have proposed that patients with irritable bowel syndrome have a disproportion of electrical signals (and mechanical activity) at the slower frequencies,[30-34] though contrary evidence is also available.[35]

Colonic motility: studies *in vitro*

The electrophysiologic basis for contraction of intestinal smooth muscle is best established for the small intestine.[4] In most mammals, intestinal muscle shows an ever-present fluctuation of membrane potential ('slow waves', 'pacesetter potentials', 'electrical control activity'). These appear to be generated in longitudinal muscle and to pass rapidly and concentrically to circular muscle layers. When excitatory neurotransmitters act on the muscle, spiking and contractions are seen. Spikes are most likely to develop when the fluctuating membrane potential is most positive, i.e. when depolarization will be achieved by the least additional change in potential. In the small bowel, slow waves spread rapidly in a circumferential direction, presumably aided by the large number of 'gap junctions' which facilitate communication between cells. Circumstances are not so clear in the large intestine and more obvious differences between species complicate matters further.[5,36-42]

Thus, slow waves are present inconsistently in human colonic circular muscle, though they are recorded more regularly from the longitudinal muscle. Spiking occurs most often at the maximal depolarization of slow waves, suggesting that there may indeed be 'pacesetter' potentials. However, the rather constant frequency of slow waves seen in the small bowel varies much more widely in the colon; in some studies, this has fluctuated from as little as 4 to as many as 30/minute. Amplitude and frequency of slow waves are sensitive to stretch and to potential stimulatory or inhibitory transmitters.

Extrapolating from these *in vitro* observations to events *in vivo*, electrical signals may differ in frequency and amplitude, depending on the relative inputs from circular and longitudinal layers (which might be influenced by the exact positioning of electrodes in the muscle layers). Other modifying factors include the degree of stretch of the muscle, as well as local concentrations of neurotransmitters. Electrical and mechanical events may occur at different frequencies and, in practice, electrical signals are not easily recorded from the colon. For all of these reasons, an understanding of the control of colonic motility lags behind that of the small intestine.

When electrical oscillations of either muscle layer exceed a frequency of 12–14/minute, individual contractions may fuse, because relaxation between these frequent oscillations of membrane potential is incomplete. It is likely that 'long spike bursts' of electrical activity in the colon are due to such a phenomenon and the accompanying contractions are likely to be fused.[43-45] When electrical oscillations are slower, each may induce a monophasic (unfused) contraction, giving rise to individual contractile events which may be signalled by a sharp rise and fall of pressure in the lumen (*Figure 3*).

The relationships between electrical signals, contractions, pressures generated in the lumen and movement of contents are complex. Connell first drew attention to the decreased number of pressure waves in diarrheal states, suggesting that a colon which behaved more as an 'open pipe' would allow free flow of contents with minimal changes in pressure.[46] On the other hand, when mechanical activity is intense, the colon may be segmented actively and transit actually impaired.

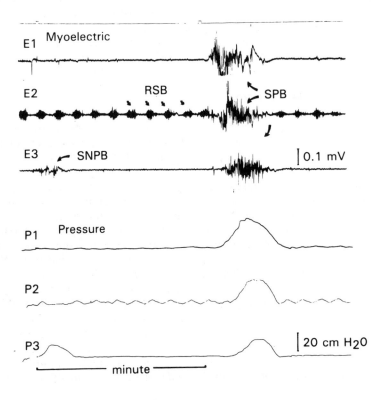

Figure 3 Simultaneous myoelectric and pressure recordings from human colon *in vivo*. Electrical activity consists of rhythmic spike bursts (RSB in E2) which are associated with small fluctuations in pressure (P2). Sporadic bursts may be either propagated (SPB) or nonpropagated (SNPB); these are also associated with changes in intraluminal pressure. Reproduced with permission from Schang JC, Devroede G. Fasting and postprandial myoelectric spiking activity in the human sigmoid. *Gastroenterology* 1983; **85**: 1048–53.

Neural control of colonic motility: in general, the vagus innervates the proximal colon and the pelvic nerves supply the distal colon and rectum. In addition to extrinsic, excitatory cholinergic and inhibitory adrenergic nerves, the noncholinergic, nonadrenergic system appears to have stimulatory and inhibitory inputs. Specific peptidergic nerves have been demonstrated,[47] including inhibitory VIP neurons to the muscularis mucosae.[48] The circuitry by which the enteric nervous system of the colon, those neural elements within the wall of the bowel, integrates and modulates contractile events is still unclear. However, what is certain is that many functions are controlled primarily at this level.[49] Thus, the enteric nervous system has been described by Wood as the 'mini-brain' of the gut.

Ways in which the extrinsic nervous system (perhaps by analogy, the 'big brain' of the CNS, and a 'mid-brain' in the abdominal plexuses) controls and modifies intrinsic control is even less well known. The prevertebral ganglia appear to act as sites of relay and coordination; afferent signals from mechanoreceptors in the colon proceed to ganglia and are processed there.[50-53] Sympathetic neurons, which are stimulated in ganglia, exert negative feedback control on other regions of the colon. The pelvic nerves in the dog reach the bowel at the level of the rectum but have been shown to progress in the orad direction for up to 50% of the length of the colon.[54] These 'ascending nerves' or 'shunt fascicles'[55] may be responsible for integrating colonic motility. In these ways, one segment of the colon may regulate the function of other segments; this is an important concept to grasp, even though more experimental data are needed before a cohesive picture is possible.

Colonic sphincters

The colon begins and ends at a sphincter. Entry of contents into the cecum and reflux of colonic contents into the ileum are modulated by the integrated actions of the ileocolonic junction and the ileocecal sphincter (ICS). Based on radiologic studies with barium, ileal emptying in man has been thought to be intermittent, presumably because of the specialized motility of the ileocolonic junction. Recent application of gamma scintigraphy has allowed ileal emptying to be examined by noninvasive techniques and under more physiologic conditions. In man and dog, one-third to one-half of ileal contents appear to empty intermittently, with the remainder moving in a more steady trickle.[56,57]

Other observations support the idea that the distal ileum, ICS and proximal colon act in concert to regulate ileocolonic transit in both directions.[26,27] In the dog, the ICS alone is insufficient to impede forward transit, except at very slow rates of flow.[58] The human and canine ICS exhibit resting tone, though the magnitude of this in man is small.[15,16] Nevertheless, muscle from the ICS exhibits specialized functions *in vitro*, corresponding physiologically with the properties of a 'true sphincter'.[59] The human ICS projects into the lumen of the cecum, providing an anatomical basis for the region to function as a 'flap valve'. This anatomy is maintained by external ligamentous attachments that ensure an acute angulation between the ileum and cecum, and so maintain the intraluminal position of the sphincter's labial flaps.[60] Thus, as with the lower esophageal sphincter, the mechanisms controlling ileocolonic transit and resisting coloileal reflux are probably multiple. These include intermittent but powerful peristaltic forces favouring ileal evacuation,[61] basal tone of the ICS and a potential 'flap valve'. Physiologic functions and dysfunctions of the ICS have not been well defined, though it can be argued that uncontrolled, rapid emptying of ileal contents could exceed the colon's capacity to absorb fluid and should lead to diarrhea.[62]

Anorectal function

Storage in the rectum results from several mechanisms. The rectal wall accommodates to distension by fecal residues; it has the viscoelastic properties which facilitate 'reservoir' continence.[63] The rate of distension and the degree to which the rectum accommodates are probably important in determining whether sensations are evoked such that an 'urge to stool' is appreciated. Often, however, the urge to defecate is ignored and stools are retained in the rectum. Rectal valves have been postulated to play a mechanical role in facilitating storage; in addition, the rectum and anal canal meet at an acute angle, a mechanical circumstance which favours the retention of solid stool above the anal canal. This mechanism, which doubtless contributes to fecal continence, relies upon the strong muscular pull of the puborectalis muscle, which helps form the pelvic floor and acts as a diaphragm.

The anal sphincters keep stool from the external environment. The smooth muscle of the internal sphincter is an extension of the circular muscular layer of the colon and rectum, whereas the external anal sphincter is composed of voluntary muscle. The internal sphincter contributes most to the zone of increased pressure. Based on studies using nerve blockade, about two-thirds of resting tone is contributed by the internal sphincter; one-third is thought to be due to the striated, external sphincter. Voluntary squeeze approximately doubles resting tone of the sphincter segment. Important also to the sphincteric mechanisms of continence is the anatomy featuring, as it does, the muscles of the pelvic diaphragm.[64] The puborectalis narrows the rectum side-to-side providing the basis for a 'flutter valve'.[65] The anterior pull of the puborectalis also contributes to the anorectal angle.

Rectal distension elicits the 'rectoanal inhibitory reflex', a decrement of tone in the upper anal canal attributed to relaxation of the internal anal sphincter.[66] The reflex often incorporates a contractile response distally, attributed to contraction of the external sphincter. The reflex, which is notably absent in aganglionosis coli (Hirschsprung's disease), has been claimed to permit the sensitive mucosa of the anal canal to be exposed to (and to discriminate between) gas, liquid or solid rectal contents. However, the importance of this putative function of the inhibitory reflex is uncertain, since discrimination is generally unimpaired after ileoanal anastomosis,[67] when the anorectal reflex is usually absent.

An interesting and important new concept of colonic pathophysiology relates to constipation. It seems likely that the 'constipation syndrome' includes several pathophysiologic processes. Thus, measurements of segmental colonic transit, in conjuction with neurophysiologic observations on the muscles of the pelvic floor,[68] can distinguish between constipation on the basis of slow colonic transit and that in which the final act of evacuation is faulty. In the latter, it is possible to demonstrate that the voluntary act of defecation may be accompanied by increased, rather than decreased, activity of the striated muscles involved in defecation. Should the pelvic floor not descend, the anorectal angle not be straightened and the sphincters not relax, defecation may be incomplete or even impossible.

Defecation

Bowel habits of a healthy population vary widely, but normal persons defecate from three times weekly to three times daily.[69] In general, fecal frequency in men is slightly greater than in women, but bowel habits differ considerably among cultures. The frequency of defecation, stool weight, the consistency of stools and intestinal transit times certainly are influenced by diet.[70-71] Daily stool weights are up to 250 g in Western societies, but in cultures in which the dietary intake of carbohydrate is greater, fecal weights may be considerably more.

The relevant unabsorbable carbohydrates in the diet are raw starches and complex fibres. Greater levels of these components in the diet leads to an increase in fecal bulk. Stephen and Cummings have proposed two mechanisms whereby fibre increases fecal bulk.[72,73] One of these involves a physicochemical trapping by fibre of stool water; the other proposes that carbohydrate in the colon provides substrates for maintenance of the fecal bacterial mass. Thus, increased levels of digestible fibre in the colon increase fecal bulk by stimulating the growth of the fecal flora, thereby increasing the mass of bacteria excreted.

References
1 Stevens CE. Comparative physiology of the digestive system. In: *Duke's Physiology of Domestic Animals.* Ithaca. Cornell University Press: 1977.
2 Metcalf AM, Phillips SF, Zinsmeister AR, MacCarty RL, Beart RW, Wolff BG. A simplified assessment of segmental colonic transit. *Gastroenterology* 1987; **92**: 40–7.
3 Kamath PS, Phillips SF, O'Connor MK, Brown ML. Capacitance of the proximal colon influences colonic function in man. *Gastroenterology* (In press).
4 Szurszewski JH. Electrophysiological basis of gastrointestinal motility. In: Johnson LR, ed. *Physiology of the Digestive Tract,* 2nd ed. New York: Raven Press 1987; 383–422.
5 Christensen J. Motility of the colon. In: Johnson LR, ed. *Physiology of the Digestive Tract,* 2nd ed. New York: Raven Press 1987; 665–94.
6 Ritchie JA. Colonic motor activity and bowel function. *Gut* 1968; **9**: 442–56.
7 Hinton J, Lennard-Jones J, Young A. A new method of studying gut transit times using radio-opaque markers. *Gut* 1969; **10**: 842–7.
8 Cummings JH, Jenkins DJA, Wiggins HS. Measurement of the mean transit time of dietary residue through the human gut. *Gut* 1976; **17**: 210–8.
9 Arhan P, Devroede G, Jehannin B *et al.* Segmental colonic transit time. *Dis Colon Rectum* 1981; **24**: 25–9.
10 Lennard-Jones JE, Langman MJS, Jones FA. Fecal stasis in protocolitis. *Gut* 1962; **3**: 301–4.
11 Spiller RC, Brown ML, Phillips SF. Decreased fluid tolerance, accelerated transit, and abnormal motility of the human colon induced by oleic acid. *Gastroenterology* 1986; **91**: 100–7.
12 Krevsky B, Malmud LS, D'Ercole F, Maurer AN, Siegel J, Fisher RS. Colonic transit scintigraphy. *Gastroenterology* 1986; **91**: 1102–12.
13 Kelley ML Jr, Gordon EA, Deweese JA. Pressure studies of the ileocolonic junctional zone in dogs. *Am J Physiol* 1965; **209**: 333–9.
14 Kelley ML Jr, Gordon EA, Deweese JA. Pressure responses of canine ileocolonic junctional zone. *Am J Physiol* 1966; **211**: 614–8.
15 Borody TJ, Quigley EMM, Phillips SF *et al.* Effects of morphine and atropine on motility and transit in the human ileum. *Gastroenterology* 1985; **89**: 562–70.
16 Nasmyth DG, William NS. Pressure characteristics of the human ileocecal region: A key to its function. *Gastroenterology* 1985; **89**: 345–51.
17 Chauve A, Devroed GJ, Bastin E. Intraluminal pressures during perfusion of the human colon *in situ. Gastroenterology* 1970; **70**: 336–40.
18 Torsoli A, Ramorino ML, Crucioli V. The relationships between anatomy and motor activity of the colon. *Am J Dig Dis* 1968; **13**: 462–7.
19 Gramiak R, Ross P, Olmsted WW. Normal motor activity of the human colon: combined radiotelemetric manometry and slow-frame cineroentgenography. *Am J Roentgen Rad Ther Nucl Med* 1971; **113**: 301–9.
20 Christensen J. Myoelectric control of the colon. *Gastroenterology* 1975; **68**: 601–9.
21 Hardcastle JD, Mann CV. Study of large bowel peristalsis. *Gut* 1968; **9**: 512–20.
22 Connell AM. The motility of the pelvic colon. *Gut* 1961; **2**: 175–86.
23 Snape WJ Jr, Matarazzo SA, Cohen S. Effect of eating and gastrointestinal hormones on human colonic myoelectrical and motor activity. *Gastroenterology* 1978; **75**: 373–8.
24 Kerlin P, Zinsmeister AR, Phillips SF. Motor responses to food of the ileum, proximal colon and distal colon of healthy humans. *Gastroenterology* 1983; **84**: 762–70.
25 Duthie HL. Colonic response to eating. *Gastroenterology* 1978; **75**: 527–9.

26 Quigley EMM, Phillips SF, Dent J, Taylor BM. Myoelectric activity and intraluminal pressure of the canine ileocolonic sphincter. *Gastroenterology* 1983; **85**: 1054–62.

27 Quigley EMM, Phillips SF, Dent J. Distinctive patterns of interdigestive motility at the canine ileocolonic junction. *Gastroenterology* 1984; **87**: 836–44.

28 Sarna SK. Cyclic motor activity; migrating motor complex. *Gastroenterology* 1985; **89**: 894–913.

29 Huizinga JD, Daniel EE. Control of human colonic motor function. *Dig Dis Sci* 1986; **31**: 865–77.

30 Snape WJ Jr, Carlson GM, Cohen S. Colonic myoelectric activity in the irritable bowel syndrome. *Gastroenterology* 1976; **70**: 326–30.

31 Snape WJ Jr, Carlson GM, Matarazzo SA, Cohen S. Evidence that abnormal myoelectrical activity produces colonic motor dysfunction in the irritable bowel syndrome. *Gastroenterology* 1977; **72**: 383–7.

32 Sullivan MA, Cohen S, Snape WJ Jr. Colonic myoelectrical activity in irritable bowel syndrome — effect of eating and anticholinergics. *N Engl J Med* 1978; **298**: 878–83.

33 Taylor I, Darby C, Hammond P, Basu P. Is there a myoelectrical abnormality in the irritable colon syndrome during relapses and remissions. *Gut* 1978; **19**: 391–5.

34 Taylor I, Darby C, Hammond P. Comparison of rectosigmoid myoelectrical activity in the irritable colon syndrome during relapses and remissions. *Gut* 1978; **19**: 923–9.

35 Latimer P, Sarna S, Campbell D, Latimer M, Waterfall W, Daniel EE. Colonic motor and myoelectrical activity: a comparative study of normal subjects, psychoneurotic patients and patients with irritable bowel syndrome. *Gastroenterology* 1981; **80**: 893–901.

36 Duthie HL, Kirk D. Electrical activity of human colonic smooth muscle *in vitro*. *J Physiol (Lond)* 1978; **283**: 319–30.

37 Chambers MM, Bowles KL, Kingma YL, Bannister C, Cote KR. *In vitro* electrical activity in human colon. *Gastroenterology* 1981; **81**: 502–8.

38 Huizinga JD, Stern H, Diamant NE, El-Sharkawy TY. The relationship between slow electrical oscillatory activity, spikes and contractions in human colonic circular muscle. *Gastroenterology* 1984; **86**: 1119 (abstr).

39 Huizinga JD, Chow E, Stern H, Diamant NE, El-Sharkawy TY. Alterations in electrical activity of human colon smooth muscle by adrenergic and cholinergic stimulation, *in vitro*. *Gastroenterology* 1984; **86**: 1119 (abstr).

40 Kubota M, Ito Y, Ikeda K. Membrane properties and innervation of smooth muscle cells in Hirschsprung's disease. *Am J Physiol* 1983; **244**: G406–15.

41 Sarna SK, Bardakjian BL, Waterfall WE, Lind JF. Human colonic electrical control activity (ECA). *Gastroenterology* 1980; **78**: 1526–36.

42 Sarna SK, Latimer P, Campbell D, Waterfall WE. Electrical and contractile activities of the human rectosigmoid. *Gut* 1982; **23**: 698–705.

43 Sarna SK, Waterfall WE, Bardakjian BL, Lind JF. Types of human colonic electrical activity recorded postoperatively. *Gastroenterology* 1981; **81**: 61–70.

44 Schang JC, Devroede G. Fasting and postprandial myoelectric spiking activity in the human sigmoid. *Gastroenterology* 1983; **85**: 1048–53.

45 Fioramonti J, Bueno L. Motor activity in the small intestine of the pig related to dietary fibre and retention time. *Br J Nutr* 1980; **43**: 155–62.

46 Connell AM. The motility of the pelvic colon: paradocecal motility in diarrhea and constipation. *Gut* 1963; **3**: 342–8.

47 Bloom SR, Polak JM. Clinical aspects of gut hormones and neuropeptides. *Br Med Bull* 1982; **38**: 233–8.

48 Angel F, Schmalz PF, Morgan KG, Go VLW, Szurszewski JH. Innervation of the muscularis mucosa in the canine stomach and colon. *Scand J Gastroenterol* 1982; **71**: 1–5.

49 Wood JD. Enteric neurophysiology. *Am J Physiol* 1984; **247**: G585–8.

50 Brown GL, Pascoe JE. Conduction through the inferior mesenteric ganglion of the rabbit. *J Physiol (Lond)* 1951; **118**: 113–23.

51 Job C, Lundberg A. Reflex excitation of cells in the inferior mesenteric ganglion by stimulation of the hypogastric nerve. *Acta Physiol Scand* 1952; **26**: 366–82.

52 Croweroft PJ, Holman ME, Szurszewski JH. Excitatory input from the distal colon to the inferior mesenteric ganglion in the guinea pig. *J Physiol (Lond)* 1971; **219**: 443–61.

53 Weems WA, Szurszewski JH. Modulation of colonic motility by peripheral neural inputs to neurons of the inferior mesenteric ganglia. *Gastroenterology* 1977; **73**: 273–8.
54 Fukai K, Fakuda H. The intramural pelvic nerves in the colon of dogs. *J Physiol (Lond)* 1984; **354**: 89–98.
55 Christensen J, Schultz-Debrieu K. Nerves in the colon: discovery and rediscovery. *Gastroenterology* 1985; **89**: 222–3.
56 Spiller RC, Brown ML, Phillips SF. Emptying of the terminal ileum in intact man: influence of meal residue and ileal motility. *Gastroenterology* 1987; **92**: 724–9.
57 Spiller RC, Brown ML, Phillips SF, Azpiroz F. Scintigraphic measurements of canine ileocolonic transit: Direct and indirect effects of eating. *Gastroenterology* 1986; **91**: 1213–20.
58 Kruis W, Phillips SF, Zinsmeister AR. Flow across the canine ileocolonic junction: Role of the ileocolonic sphincter. *Am J Physiol* 1987; **15**: G13–8.
59 Conklin JL, Christensen J. Local specialization at ileocecal junction of cat and opossum. *Am J Physiol* 1975; **228**: 1075–81.
60 Kumar D, Phillips SF. Reflux across the ileo-cecal junction: role of superior and inferior ileocecal ligaments. *Gastroenterology* 1986; **90**: 1059 (abstr).
61 Kruis W, Azpiroz F, Phillips SF. Contractile patterns and transit of fluid in canine terminal ileum. *Am J Physiol* 1985; **249**: G264–70.
62 Phillips SF. Diarrhea: role of the ileocecal sphincter. In: Barbara L, Miglioli M, Phillips SF, eds. *New Trends in Pathophysiology and Therapy of the Large Bowel.* Amsterdam: Elsevier Science Publishers 1983: 107–18.
63 Arhan P, Danis K, Dornic C, Faverdin C, Persoz B, Pellerin D. Viscoelastic properties of the rectal wall in Hirschsprung's disease. *J Clin Invest* 1978; **62**: 82–7.
64 Dickinson VA. Maintenance of anal continence: a review of pelvic floor physiology. *Gut* 1978; **19**: 1163–74.
65 Phillips SF, Edwards DAW. Some aspects of anal continence and defecation. *Gut* 1965; **6**: 396–406.
66 Schuster MM, Hendix TR, Mendeloff AI. The internal anal sphincter response: manometric studies on its normal physiology, neural pathway and alteration in bowel disorders. *J Clin Invest* 1963; **42**: 196–207.
67 Stryker SJ, Phillips SF, Dozois RR, Kelly KA, Beart RW. Anal and neorectal function after ileal pouch-anal anastomosis. *Ann Surg* 1986; **203**: 55–61.
68 Henry MM, Swash M. *Coloproctology and the Pelvic Floor.* Boston: Butterworths 1985.
69 Connell AM, Hilton C, Irvine C, Lennard-Jones JE, Misiewicz JJ. Variation of bowel habit in two population groups. *Br Med J* 1965; **ii**: 1095–9.
70 Wyman JB, Heaton KW, Manning AP, Wicks ACB. Variability of colonic function in healthy subjects. *Gut* 1978; **19**: 146–50.
71 Baird IM, Walters RL, Davies PS, Hill MJ, Drasar BS, Southgate DAT. The effect of two dietary fiber supplements on gastrointestinal transit, stool weight and frequency, and bacterial flora, and fecal bile acids in normal subjects. *Metabolism* 1977; **26**: 117–28.
72 Stephen AM, Cummings JH. Mechanism of action of dietary fiber in the human colon. *Nature* 1980; **284**: 283–4.
73 Stephen AM, Cummings JH. Effect of changing transit time on fecal bacterial mass in man. *Gut* 1980; **21**: A905–6.

II
Diagnosis

Diagnostic methodology of esophageal problems

G Vantrappen*

The accessibility of the esophagus and its relatively simple mechanical function have led to the development of a host of investigational techniques to diagnose problems in this region of the gut. There are three main symptoms of esophageal disease or disorder — heartburn, chest pain and dysphagia — and this article will discuss the diagnostic approach and techniques available to determine the cause of these symptoms.

Heartburn

Careful history taking of a patient who has typical heartburn should enable a physician to reach a diagnosis of gastroesophageal reflux without recourse to sophisticated investigations. Typical heartburn is characterized by the substernal upward movement of the burning sensation, its occurrence in relation to meals or posture and its relief by antacids. Clinical judgement should determine whether or not technical investigations are needed to prescribe rational treatment.

If heartburn is sufficiently severe for the patient to seek medical advice, esophagoscopy with biopsy should be the initial investigative step. It is important to determine what damage the gastroesophageal reflux has already caused. Epithelial changes that have not progressed beyond the stage of increased papillary length or basal zone hyperplasia may be treated symptomatically because complications in these cases are rare. However, once esophagitis has developed, with evidence of erosions on esophagoscopy and polymorphonuclear cell infiltration of the epithelium on biopsy, the aim of treatment no longer is merely to alleviate symptoms but to heal the lesions in order that complications do not develop. Therefore, do more sophisticated techniques such as manometry or pH measurements have a role in the evaluation of patients with gastroesophageal reflux?

pH measurements
pH measurements in the lower esophagus allow confirmation of the presence or absence of acid gastroesophageal reflux. A fall of pH below 4 at 5 cm above the lower esophageal sphincter (LES) is generally accepted as an indication of acid reflux. It is more difficult to determine alkaline reflux because saliva has a slightly alkaline pH and alkaline bile and pancreatic juice may be partially neutralized by gastric acid before entering the esophagus.

* Co-author: J Janssens

51

In addition, pH measurements allow gastroesophageal reflux to be assessed quantitatively. The parameters used for this numerical analysis include: the number of reflux episodes; the number of episodes lasting more than 5 minutes; the length of time the intraesophageal pH is below 4; and the mean pH during the time the pH is below 4.[1]

It is generally believed that the most accurate data are obtained if the pH measurements are taken over a period of 24 hours.[2,3] However, there is some evidence that equally reliable data can be obtained over shorter test periods, provided the recordings comprise both a post-prandial period and a period in the supine position.[4]

To the clinician an investigation is of value if it contributes appreciably to the diagnosis, if it helps to determine the prognosis and, particularly, if it affects the type of treatment to be given, either by facilitating the choice of the appropriate drug or by influencing the decision to use surgery.

Diagnostic value of pH measurements: esophageal pH measurements may contribute substantially to the diagnosis of gastroesophageal reflux if symptoms are atypical and if it can be shown that these ayptical symptoms coincide in time with reflux episodes. A simpler way, perhaps, to determine the esophageal origin of atypical symptoms is the acid perfusion test. At present, 24-hour combined pH and pressure recordings constitute the most reliable investigation to ascertain the esophageal origin of atypical symptoms, particularly chest pain.[5]

Quantitative analysis of reflux parameters is useful to determine the severity of gastroesophageal reflux. If one or more of the numerical reflux values are greater than the mean $\pm$ 2SD of the control population, the gastroesophageal reflux is said to be pathologic. pH measurements, therefore, may help to differentiate physiologic from pathologic reflux.

Problems arise when attempts are made to correlate these numerical pH data with either reflux symptoms or signs of reflux esophagitis. In a study[6] involving healthy subjects and patients with reflux symptoms exhibiting varying degrees of esophagitis, the following parameters were studied: the number of pH drops below 4; the number of pH drops below 4 lasting longer than 5 minutes; the length of time pH was below 4; the area on the plot and the mean pH when below 4. These parameters were calculated for the total 24-hour period, for the post-prandial period, the inter-prandial period and the night period when the patient was in the supine position. A total of 20 parameters were analyzed by a computer program of stepwise discriminant analysis.

The most discriminating factor in differentiating healthy individuals from patients with reflux symptoms or endoscopic signs of reflux esophagitis was the number of reflux episodes per 24 hours; 79% of cases were correctly classified by this parameter. The most important parameter to discriminate patients with reflux symptoms without esophagitis from patients with mild or severe esophagitis was the number of reflux episodes lasting more than 5 minutes during the night; 76% of cases could be correctly classified on the basis of pH values. The most important parameter the computer selected to discriminate between mild and severe esophagitis was the mean pH of reflux episodes in the post-prandial period, with 88% of cases being classified correctly. The most important factor to discriminate healthy individuals from patients with severe esophagitis was the number of reflux episodes lasting more than 5 minutes over the 24-hour period. The correctness of this discrimination was as high as 96%.

These results indicate that 24-hour pH measurements offer a highly accurate means of discriminating normal subjects from patients with severe esophagitis, but this diagnostic accuracy drops when all grades of severity are included in the discriminative analysis.

Prognostic and therapeutic value of pH measurements: the value of pH measurements in determining the future course of pathological reflux is unknown. Prospective, longitudinal studies are needed to ascertain their role here. There are no hard data to show that pH measurements are necessary in the preoperative evaluation of reflux patients. However, many physicians feel more confident in advising an antireflux procedure if their patient is a bad refluxer and if postoperative tests indicate that the procedure improved the reflux parameters. It is not clear whether this is more important for the comfort of the physician than for the success of treatment.

Esophageal manometry

The LES has an important role in the prevention of gastroesophageal reflux. A LES pressure of less than 6 mmHg is almost always accompanied by significant gastroesophageal reflux. However, reflux may occur in spite of a normal LES pressure, the mechanism being related to the so-called 'inappropriate' or 'transient' sphincter relaxations, i.e. relaxations not elicited by swallows.[7] Normal esophageal peristalsis has an important role in the clearance of reflux material from the esophagus.[8]

Manometry is not appropriate for diagnosing gastroesophageal reflux. Theoretically measurement of LES pressure could be important in guiding medical therapy if motor stimulating drugs were available which act selectively on one or the other mechanism of gastroesophageal reflux, i.e. LES tone and inappropriate LES relaxations. Manometry would also be clinically useful if the LES response to a drug regimen would predict the therapeutic outcome of that therapy. Unfortunately, studies to test these hypotheses have not been done. Manometry is carried out in patients with esophagitis who are not responding to H_2-blocker treatment. If the LES pressure is found to be low, motor stimulating drugs are added to the therapeutic regimen in the hope that an increased LES pressure will decrease reflux of alkaline secretions unaffected by H_2-blockers. Although such an approach may seem logical, its value remains to be proven.

Measurement of LES pressure could also be important in the pre-operative investigation of patients with gastroesophageal reflux. Patients with a low LES pressure are more likely to be submitted to an antireflux procedure than patients with normal LES pressure. This also seems quite logical to those who believe that the sphincter pressure is the single most important factor in the production of reflux and that an antireflux procedure results in an increased LES pressure. Here again, the effect of antireflux procedures on inappropriate sphincter relaxations is unknown. It could be that an antireflux procedure not only increases the LES pressure but also inhibits inappropriate relaxations. If this were so, manometry would lose some of its value as a tool of pre-operative investigation.

Manometric investigation of the peristaltic performance of the esophagus seems important in as much as absence of peristalsis is a relative contraindication for an antireflux procedure, because any reflux material will tend to stay in the gullet for long periods of time.

In conclusion, it seems that esophageal pH and pressure measurements are not needed for clinical purposes in the majority of patients with heartburn.

Dysphagia

Whereas heartburn and chest pain of esophageal origin are mostly caused by gastroesophageal reflux or by esophageal motor disorders, dysphagia is often due to organic, possibly malignant lesions. The investigation of dysphagia, therefore, must be conducted in a different fashion. The first step is to look for stenosing lesions.

Radiography and endoscopy

Many radiologists feel that the first examination should involve a barium x-ray, particularly full column examination in the prone and prone-oblique positions. Endoscopists often take the view that endoscopy is superior to radiology and that it will have to be performed anyway if a lesion is demonstrated by radiology. However, radiology probably is superior to endoscopy in the detection of upper esophageal webs and strictures that measure over 10 mm in calibre; it is safer for demonstrating large pharyngoesophageal diverticula and high stenoses; it can visualize the esophagus below a stricture that cannot be passed by the endoscope; and compression by extrinsic structures or mediastinal tumours and intramural submucosal tumours may also be more easily missed by endoscopy.

Radiologic examination should demonstrate almost all intraluminal malignant lesions that cause dysphagia because malignant lesions usually cause dysphagia only if more than half of the esophageal circumference is involved by the tumourous process. At that time visualization of the tumour should not be too difficult. It is important that the radiologist uses the appropriate technique. Here the gastroenterologist can play an important role, because the radiologic technique adopted will be determined by the patient's clinical signs and symptoms. In many cases the examination will have to be completed by endoscopy.

Manometry

If careful radiology, followed by endoscopy, fails to demonstrate stenosing lesions that can explain the dysphagia, the motor function of the esophagus should be investigated. Although radiology will often suggest the presence of functional abnormalities, manometry is the method of choice.

The manometric diagnosis of esophageal motility disorders is straight forward if typical patterns are obtained. Complete absence of peristalsis and of normal LES relaxations, with or without an increase in basal pressure of the LES and esophageal body, is typical for untreated achalasia. A deglutitive response characterized by frequent non-peristaltic contractions of high amplitude and long duration, which may be repetitive in nature, is compatible with diffuse esophageal spasm. Peristaltic contractions of high amplitude (with peak pressures greater than 200 mmHg and mean pressures greater than 120 mmHg) and long duration (more than 7.5 minutes) point to a diagnosis of symptomatic peristalsis or so-called nutcracker esophagus. The clinical significance of these giant peristaltic contractions remains controversial.[9]

Problems may arise when the manometric pattern is atypical. In a series of 156 consecutive patients with dysphagia of such a degree that treatment by pneumatic dilatation was deemed necessary,[10] the nature of the motility disorders was analyzed on the basis of very simple manometric criteria, i.e. the presence or absence of peristaltic contractions and the presence or absence of complete LES relaxations. Theoretically four different combinations were possible: absence of peristalsis and of LES relaxations, i.e. achalasia; presence of some peristalsis and of LES relaxations, i.e. diffuse spasm; and two intermediate types in which either peristalsis or LES relaxations are preserved. Typical achalasia was found in 70% of the 156 patients, typical diffuse spasm in 11% and intermediate types in 19%.

Problems also arise when manometric abnormalities are absent or trivial. Most patients with apparent functional dysphagia do not experience dysphagia during the manometric study, when they are lying down quietly and swallowing saliva or small boluses of liquid. The study conditions are quite different from the situation found in daily life where dysphagia occurs upon eating and drinking. Mellow showed that when esophageal manometry is performed during ingestion of a meal, motility disorders responsible for dysphagia are more likely to be determined than with routine manometry testing.[11] Not only is the nature of the swallowed material important; the esophageal response to swallows repeated at short intervals is quite different from that observed after isolated deglutitions. During a meal, when swallows are taken in relatively rapid succession, hidden disorders in the deglutitive inhibition of the esophageal body and LES may become apparent. Normally, the LES stays open during a sequence of rapid swallowing and contracts only intermittently in relation to an oncoming contraction. In patients with dysphagia, the meal manometry test may show LES relaxations to be absent or even replaced by sphincteric contractions during certain periods of the meal.

Similarly, strong contractions of the esophageal body occurring below the level of a descending bolus will hamper the passage of the bolus and cause dysphagia. Thus, both inappropriate contractions of the LES and precocious contractions of the esophageal body constitute a functional obstruction that is not always demonstrated by standard manometric tests. The interpretation of manometric tests during a meal is difficult. A standard eating test is required, with standard food and a standard sequence of swallows.

Another approach to the problem of functional dysphagia in patients with atypical or apparently insignificant esophageal motor abnormalities is the 24-hour recording of esophageal pressure in ambulatory patients. Episodes of more severe or more typical motor abnormalities are often observed in these patients when they are monitored over periods of 12–24 hours (G Vantrappen and J Janssens, unpublished data).

Chest pain

The two most frequent esophageal causes of angina-like chest pain are gastroesophageal reflux and esophageal motor disorders. The presence of reflux or esophageal motility disorders cannot be accepted as proof of the esophageal origin of the pain, unless it can be shown that either reflux or motor disorders or a combination of both coincide in time with the onset of pain. Unfortunately this will rarely occur during conventional pH or manometric recordings because of the limited duration of these tests.

Esophagoscopy
When looking for an esophageal cause of chest pain, upper gastrointestinal endoscopy should be performed initially to exclude ulcerated esophageal carcinoma, which is a rare but life-threatening cause of angina-like chest pain of esophageal origin. Endoscopy will also reveal an esophageal or a duodenal ulcer.

The main reason for beginning the investigation with endoscopy is the importance of erosive esophagitis as a cause of chest pain. If esophagitis is present, the esophagus may be regarded tentatively as the cause of the angina-like chest pain and, consequently, the effect of medical therapy may be awaited before proceeding to other investigations. In a study of 60 patients with non-cardiac chest pain, 15 patients were found to have erosive esophagitis.[5] Twenty-four-hour recording of esophageal pressure and pH showed the esophagus to be the definite cause of the pain in 60% of the patients and the probable cause in another 27%.

Manometry
The next step in determining the esophageal origin of chest pain is manometry. If conventional manometry reveals classical achalasia, severe diffuse esophageal spasm or nutcracker esophagus, the angina-like chest pain is probably of esophageal origin. However, these motor disorders are generally found in no more than 20% of chest pain patients.[5] Other motor abnormalities such as severe but non-specific motor disturbances, although more frequently present, can only be considered as the probable cause of the chest pain if a typical pain attack has been observed to coincide in time with the occurrence of the motor abnormalities.

To increase the chances of observing chest pain concomitantly with a reflux episode or severe motor disturbances, provocation tests should be conducted or the recording time prolonged.

Provocation tests
The Bernstein acid perfusion test is a simple provocation test that mimicks endogenous reflux.[12] Hydrochloric acid, 0.1 N, is perfused at a rate of 6-8 mL/minute in the middle third of the gullet via an intraesophageal catheter. If acid perfusion provokes the familiar angina-like chest pain, but perfusion of saline does not, the test result is termed positive-related and the pain is confirmed to be esophageal in origin. If the test provokes a sensation that is different from the familiar pain (e.g. heartburn), this result is termed positive-unrelated and the esophagus can only be suspected of being the cause of the pain. A negative test (acid not inducing pain, or pain induced by saline) has no diagnostic value and does not exclude an esophageal origin of the pain. In a series of 50 patients with angina-like chest pain of non-cardiac origin studied by Castell, the acid perfusion test produced a positive-related result in 10% of the patients.[13] In another study of 60 patients with non-cardiac chest pain, 27% had a positive-related acid perfusion test result.[5]

There is an important limitation in the interpretation of a positive-related acid perfusion test. While a positive-related test strongly suggests that the chest pain is esophageal in origin, it does not necessarily indicate that the pain is due to reflux. In a study of 21 patients with angina-like chest pain of esophageal origin 24-hour pH and pressure measurements showed the pain to be due to reflux (alone or in combination with motor disorders) in 13 patients and to esophageal motility disorders alone in 8 patients.[14] The acid perfusion test was positive-related not only in those patients who were found to have reflux at the time of their spontaneous pain attacks, but also in the patients who had motor disorders without reflux at the time of their spontaneous pain. These observations suggest that hypersensitivity of the esophagus to various stimuli has a role in the production of chest pain of esophageal origin. This condition can be termed 'irritable esophagus'.[15]

A positive-related acid perfusion test, therefore, seems to indicate an irritability of the esophagus rather than to prove the reflux-induced nature of the spontaneous chest pain.

Several investigators have tried to provoke esophageal motility disorders by the administration of pharmacologic agents such as pentagastrin, bethanechol, ergonovine and edrophonium. Although pentagastrin and bethanechol are known to increase the motor abnormalities in patients with diffuse esophageal spasm, their value is limited in patients with angina-like chest pain. Benjamin and co-workers reported that pentagastrin and bethanechol induced chest pain in only 3% and 6% of such patients, respectively.[16]

Ergonovine is probably the most effective agent at inducing esophageal abnormalities and chest pain.[17,18] Success rates ranging from 22–60% have been reported. However, the cardiac risks of this drug limit its use as a diagnostic test. Edrophonium may yield equivalent results and is much safer to use.[16] The intravenous injection of 80–200 µg/kg of edrophonium was reported to produce manometric changes and chest pain in 20–30% of the patients. The response occurs within 5 minutes and ceases quickly as the drug is rapidly metabolized. The edrophonium test can safely be performed in the office. A positive edrophonium response (motor abnormalities and symptoms) strongly suggests that the esophagus is the source of the chest pain. In contrast to the acid perfusion test, however, intravenous administration of a relatively high dose of a cholinergic agent cannot be considered to be a physiologic provocation. The edrophonium test may be positive in patients with angina-like chest pain due to esophageal motor disturbances, but may also identify patients in whom the pain is related to reflux problems.[15]

Recently Richter and co-workers used balloon distension in the lower esophagus as a provocation test.[19] Chest pain occurred in 60% of the patients and in only 20% of the controls. The chest pain patients experienced their pain at distension volumes lower than those of the controls, a finding analogous to that observed in the sigmoid colon of patients with irritable bowel syndrome. Obviously this simple and safe test warrants further study.

24-hour combined pH and pressure measurements

Prolonging the recording time increases the chances of recording chest pain concomitantly with an episode of gastroesophageal reflux or esophageal motor disturbances. A new sensing, recording and analyzing system has been developed that allows the continuous recording over a 24-hour period of intraesophageal pH and pressures in ambulatory patients.[5,20,21] The sensing probe comprises a pH glass electrode with an intraluminal reference electrode and three pressure transducers. The probe is positioned via the nose in order that pressures are measured at 3, 10 and 17 cm and the pH at 5 cm above the LES. All data are recorded on a portable cassette recorder. The system also comprises an event marker for the patient to indicate the pain episodes.

A group of 60 patients with angina-like chest pain of non-cardiac origin was studied using this technique. All appropriate investigations, including (if deemed necessary) coronarography and ergonovine stimulation during cardiac catheterization, were conducted initially to exclude a cardiac origin to the chest pain. The results of this study were compared with those obtained using conventional methods such as radiography, endoscopy with biopsy, conventional esophageal manometry and the acid perfusion test.

The following criteria were used. The esophagus was considered to be the source of the chest pain if the familiar pain sensation was reproduced by the acid perfusion test or if the pain occurred during an episode of gastroesophageal reflux, severe motor disturbances or both. The chest pain was considered to be of probable esophageal origin when severe motor abnormalities such as achalasia or diffuse spasm (or nutcracker esophagus) were observed on conventional manometry. The mere presence of pathologic reflux (on x-ray or on a 24-hour pH plot) or of its consequences (esophagitis on endoscopy and biopsy) was considered to be of less importance for the diagnostic scoring.

Figure 1 summarizes the results of this study. Based upon conventional investigations (radiology, endoscopy, conventional manometry and the Bernstein test), the esophagus was almost certainly the cause of the chest pain in 27% of the patients, a probable cause in 28% and a possible cause of the pain in 25% of the 60 patients. When the results of the 24-hour pH and pressure recordings with indication of pain periods were combined with those of the more conventional investigations, the final diagnostic score was as follows: the esophagus was suspected to be the cause of the

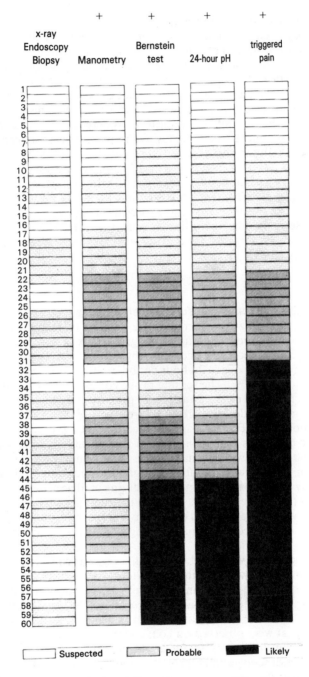

Figure 1 Diagnostic score calculated first after x-rays and endoscopy with biopsy, and then after adding successively the results of manometry, the Bernstein test, 24-hour pH analysis, and 24-hour combined pH and pressure recording triggered on pain. Each horizontal block represents one of the 60 patients included in the study. Thick stippled blocks = chest pain probably of esophageal origin. Thin stippled blocks = esophagus was suspected to be the cause of the chest pain. Black blocks = pain was almost certainly of esophageal origin.

pain in 14 patients (25%); it was a probable cause of the pain in 10 patients (17%); and the esophagus was almost certainly the cause of the pain in 29 patients (48%).

Ambulatory 24-hour recording of esophageal pH and pressure achieves better results in establishing the esophageal cause of non-cardiac chest pain than any other presently available technique. Moreover, it is the most physiologic test and the only one that allows motor disorders to be distinguished from reflux as the cause of the pain, an important factor when it comes to determining appropriate therapy.

Future developments

Esophageal tests are generally only performed in patients with angina-like chest pain after a cardiac cause of the pain has been excluded. This often requires invasive investigations such as coronary arteriography and ergonovine provocation tests of coronary spasms and can be conducted only at considerable cost.

As Rapaport stated: "It is reasonable to assume that in the absence of a conduction disturbance or other electrocardiographic causes that might obscure a detectable ischemic response, the failure of ST segment changes to occur in a patient complaining of chest discomfort at rest suggests an extracardiac source. When this is coupled with a normal resting ECG and no prior history of coronary heart disease nor any major risk factor, the likelihood approaches a high probability".[22] Therefore, if a 24-hour ambulatory recording system can be developed that allows the simultaneous recording of intraesophageal pH and pressures, and a continuous multichannel ECG recording with reliable ST segment registration, many unnecessary coronary arteriographies can be avoided and a positive diagnosis of angina-like chest pain of esophageal origin can be made.

References

1 Johnson LF. New concepts and methods in the study and treatment of gastroesophageal reflux disease. *Med Clin N Am* 1981; **65**: 1195–222.
2 Johnson LF, DeMeester TR. Twenty-four hour pH monitoring of the distal esophagus: a quantitative measure of gastroesophageal reflux. *Am J Gastroenterol* 1974; **62**: 325–32.
3 DeMeester TR, Johnson LF, Guy JJ, Toscano MS, Hall AW, Skinner DB. Patterns of gastroesophageal reflux in health and disease. *Ann Surg* 1976; **184**: 459–70.
4 Galmiche JP, Guillard JF, Denis P, Boussakr K, Lefrançoid R, Colin R. Etude du pH oesophagien en période post-prandiale chez le sujet normal et au cours du syndrome de reflux gastro-oesophagien. Intérêt diagnostique d'un score de reflux acide. *Gastroenterol Clin Biol* 1980; **4**: 531–9.
5 Janssens J, Vantrappen G, Ghillebert G. 24-hour recording of esophageal pressure and pH in patients with noncardiac chest pain. *Gastroenterology* 1986; **90**: 1978–84.
6 Janssens J, Vantrappen G, Peeters TL, Ghillebert G. How do 24-hour pH measurements distinguish the disease spectrum of reflux patients? *Gastroenterology* 1985; **88**: 1431.
7 Dent J, Dodds WJ, Friedman RH, Sekiguchi T, Hogan WJ, Arndorfer RC, Petrie DJ. Mechanism of gastroesophageal reflux in recumbent asymptomatic human subjects. *J Clin Invest* 1980; **65**: 256–67.
8 Stanciu C, Bennett JR. Oesophageal acid clearing: one factor in the production of reflux oesophagitis. *Gut* 1974; **15**: 852–7.
9 Cohen S. Esophageal motility disorders and their responses to calcium channel antagonists. Editorial. *Gastroentology* 1987; **93**: 201–3.
10 Vantrappen G, Janssens J, Hellemans J, Coremans G. Achalasia, diffuse esophageal spasm and related motility disorders. *Gastroenterology* 1979; **76**: 450–7.
11 Mellow MH. Esophageal motility during food ingestion: a physiologic test of esophageal motor function. *Gastroenterology* 1983; **85**: 570–7.
12 Bernstein LM, Baker LA. A clinical test for esophagitis. *Gastroenterology* 1958; **34**: 760–81.
13 Castell DO. Diagnosis of noncardiac chest pain in older patients. *Geriatrics* 1985; **40**: 61–86.
14 Vantrappen G, Janssens J, Ghillebert G. Angina-like chest pain of esophageal origin:

due to motor disorders, gastro-esophageal reflux or an irritable esophagus? *Gastroenterology* 1986; **90**: 1677.

15 Vantrappen G, Janssens J, Ghillebert G. The irritable esophagus — a frequent cause of angina-like pain. *Lancet* 1987; **i**: 1232-4.

16 Benjamin SB, Richter JE, Cordova CM, Knuff TE, Castell DO. Prospective manometric evaluation with pharmacological provocation of patients with suspected esophageal motility dysfunction. *Gastroenterology* 1983; **84**: 893-901.

17 Eastwood GL, Weiner BH, Dickerson WJ, White EM, Ockene IS, Haffajee CI, Alpert JS. Use of ergonovine to identify esophageal spasm in patients with chest pain. *Ann Intern Med* 1981; **94**: 768-71.

18 London RL, Ouyang A, Snape WJ Jr, Goldberg S, Hirschfield JW Jr, Cohen S. Provocation of esophageal pain by ergonovine or edrophonium. *Gastroenterology* 1981; **81**: 10-4.

19 Richter JE, Barish CF, Castell DO. Abnormal sensory perception in patients with esophageal chest pain. *Gastroenterology* 1986; **91**: 845-52.

20 Vantrappen G, Servaes J, Janssens J, Peeters T. Twenty-four hour esophageal pH- and pressure recording in outpatients. In: Wienbeck M, ed. *Motility of the Digestive Tract*. New York: Raven 1982; 294-7.

21 Vantrappen G, Janssens J. Angina and oesophageal pain — a gastroenterologist's point of view. *Eur Heart J* 1986; **7**: 828-34.

22 Rapaport E. Angina and oesophageal pain. *Eur Heart J* 1986; **7**: 824-7.

Diagnosis of gastric motility disorders

R W McCallum

Symptoms of disordered gastric motor function

Symptoms of gastric dysmotility can be divided into two broad categories — those which suggest slow emptying of the stomach and those indicating rapid emptying (*Table 1*).

The clinical manifestations of delayed gastric emptying form a constellation of symptoms. Occasionally, the patient may experience only one or two 'uncomfortable' symptoms. Nausea and vomiting are the most disquieting of all the symptoms. Some patients with gastric emptying disorders may complain only of post-prandial bloating or fullness, assumed to be caused by gastric distension. Anorexia and early satiety, although of possible constitutional origin, within the framework of appropriate signs and symptoms may suggest gastroparesis. Although some abdominal pain is present in gastric retention states (again probably owing to distension), a dominating presence of abdominal pain should arouse suspicion of other clinical entities, either anatomically independent of the stomach or mechanically related, that result in delayed gastric emptying. These entities include gastric ulcer, posterior penetrating duodenal ulcer, gastric cancer, smouldering pancreatitis, biliary tract disease, 'upset stomach' possibly related to gastritis or a viral insult, and pancreatic cancer.

When taking a history, one should look for important clues relating to the aggravation and provocation of symptoms with meals, deviation and timing of symptoms and other accompanying findings (*Table 2*). Vomiting and significant weight loss can vary and may not always be elicited. Patients may have learned that weight can be maintained with liquid caloric intake and that there is less chance of vomiting if small liquid-soft meals are the major form of nutrition. However, disordered motility of the duodenum and small bowel can also present with a symptom complex similar to that of gastric stasis or it can also accompany gastroparetic states. In this setting there may be more emphasis on abdominal pain and sometimes suspicion of biliary dyskinesia and sphincter of Oddi, particularly in patients with a past history of cholecystectomy. Alternatively, there may be a history of pain medication requirements reaching addictive proportions.

Patients with symptoms suggestive of rapid emptying complain of anxiety, weakness, dizziness, tachycardia, sweating, flushing and decreased consciousness, all of which will occur post-prandially, either immediately following the meal or within 2 hours.

	Symptoms suggesting:	
Slow emptying		Rapid emptying
Nausea		Anxiety
Vomiting		Weakness*
Bloatedness, fullness		Dizziness*
Early satiety		Tachycardia*
Epigastric pain		Sweating*
Heartburn		Flushing*
Anorexia		Decreased consciousness
Weight loss		Food avoidance

*Symptoms occur soon after ingestion of a meal

Table 1 Symptoms of gastric motor dysfunction.

Clinical aspects and findings

Patients with suspected gastric motor disorders must be questioned specifically about the timing and characteristics of their symptoms, as summarized in *Table 1* and *Table 2*.

Any prior surgical procedure involving either a vagotomy or gastric resection raises the possibilities of 'dumping syndrome' and chronic post-gastric surgery stasis for solids. 'Dumping', or rapid emptying of liquids, can occur simultaneously with vomiting and slow emptying of solids. A fundoplication for gastroesophageal reflux disease and reduction of a hiatal hernia in which there was inadvertent vagotomy or vagal nerve damage can result in dumping for liquids and delayed gastric emptying of solids.

Some patients present with a history of acute onset of gastroenteritis. The diarrhea resolves but the upper gastrointestinal (GI) symptoms persist. Viral infections have often been suspected of causing alterations in gut myenteric plexus and/or smooth muscle function. Whether patients presenting with diarrhea may have underlying bacterial overgrowth of the upper GI tract with or without jejunal diverticula has been considered. There is evidence that antibiotic treatment of bacterial overgrowth has resulted in improved small bowel motility.[1]

When profound weight loss occurs the question of malignancy may arise. Infiltrative disorders such as lymphoma may have to be considered as well as the possibility of paraneoplastic syndromes.[2] Computerized tomographic (CT) scanning of the brain to exclude cerebellar tumours, meningiomas and other space-occupying lesions should be given due consideration.

A careful assessment of the patient's psychological profile and personality, as well as current lifestyle and psychosocial background, may have to be considered if no other obvious etiologies appear to be diagnostic. Acute stress can give rise to nausea and vomiting, but it is not known whether chronic stress can in fact lead to recurrent nausea and vomiting. Certainly, anorexia nervosa and bulimia are associated with disturbances in gastric emptying. Medications such as anticholinergics, antidepressants, levodopa and narcotic-containing agents also exert a retarding effect on GI motility (*Table 3*).

The physical examination should include evaluation for orthostatic hypotension, which, if found, might raise the question of autonomic neuropathy. Urinary dysfunc-

Finding	Implication
Timing of symptoms	
Minutes after meals	Psychoneurotic vomiting, bulimic vomiting, vomiting due to gastric outlet obstruction (channel ulcer), early dumping syndrome
Hours after meals	Mechanical obstruction, gastroparesis
Before breakfast	Pregnancy, uremia, alcoholism, increased intracranial pressure, after gastric surgery
Duration of symptoms	
Hours — days	Acute infections, drugs, toxins/poisons, acute inflammatory conditions, pregnancy
Weeks — months	Mechanical obstruction, gastroparesis, brain tumour, psychogenic vomiting
Quality of vomitus	
Partially digested old food	Gastroparesis, esophageal obstruction
Undigested food	Obstruction or diverticulum
Bile present	Gastric outlet patent
Feculent odour	Gastroparesis with stasis, intestinal obstruction, gastrocolonic fistula
Blood present	Cancer or inflammation
Amenorrhea	Pregnancy, anorexia nervosa
Headache	Brain tumour
Previous surgery	Post-vagotomy gastroparesis, dumping syndrome, other post-gastrectomy syndromes, mechanical obstruction

Table 2   Historical findings and their implications in patients with suspected gastric motor dysfunction. Reproduced with permission from Schiller. *Pract Gastroenterol* 1982; 7: 309.

tion and gustatory sweating should prompt a search for further symptoms and signs relevant to diabetes, dysproteinemias and collagen vascular disorders, as well as porphyria.

The patient's abdomen should be examined carefully and the presence of a succussion splash, which would indicate excess fluid in the stomach, noted. The presence of a succussion splash more than 4–5 hours after a meal would support the diagnosis of delayed gastric emptying (gastroparesis), although it would provide no evidence as to the condition's etiology.

Acute conditions

Abdominal pain/trauma/inflammation
Postoperatively
Acute infections/gastroenteritis
Acute metabolic disorders:
  acidosis, hypokalemia, hyper- or hypocalcemia, hepatic coma, myxedema
Immobilization
Hyperglycemia (glucose >200 mg/dL)

Pharmaceutical agents and hormones

Opiates, including endorphins and narcotics (eg, morphine)
Anticholinergics
Tricyclic antidepressants
Beta-adrenergic agonists
Levodopa
Aluminum hydroxide antacids
Gastrin
Cholecystokinin
Somatostatin

Chronic conditions

Acid-peptic disease
  Gastroesophageal reflux
  Gastric ulcer disease, nonulcer dyspepsia
Gastritis
  Atrophic gastritis ± pernicious anemia
  Viral gastroenteritis (acute — ? chronic)
Metabolic and endocrine
  Diabetic ketoacidosis (acute)
  Diabetic gastroparesis (chronic)
  Addison's disease
  Hypothyroidism
  Pregnancy?
  Uremia
Collagen vascular disease — scleroderma
Pseudo-obstruction
  Idiopathic
  Secondary, eg, amyloidosis, Chagas' disease, muscular dystrophies,
  cancer-associated syndrome
Post-gastric surgery
  Post-vagotomy and/or post-gastric resections
Medications
  Anticholinergics, narcotic analgesics, levodopa
Hormones (pharmacologic studies)
  Gastrin, cholecystokinin, somatostatin
Anorexia nervosa — bulimia
Idiopathic
  a) Isolated or part of diffuse GI motor
  b) Gastric dysrhythmias — tachygastria
  c) Gastroduodenal dyssynchrony
  d) Central nervous system — disturbance depression

Table 3 Conditions producing symptomatic gastric motor dysfunction.

Investigational procedures

Laboratory tests

Hematologic and biochemical profiles may provide supportive evidence of impaired nutrition, electrolyte imbalance or acidosis. Blood glucose levels should be evaluated for evidence of glucose intolerance and diabetes mellitus in patients with slow gastric emptying and for evidence of hyperglycemia and reactive hypoglycemia in patients with suspected dumping syndrome (delayed gastric emptying). Standard blood counts and chemistries provide supportive evidence, but a glucose tolerance study is necessary to define the severity of the problem. The presence of hypokalemia or hypocalcemia may provide important clues to the condition's etiology. Addison's disease can present as abdominal crisis involving pain and, in some cases, unexplained nausea and vomiting.[3]

Radiology and endoscopy

At this stage of the evaluation, some patients may require no further tests. Such patients would include those who have undergone gastric surgery and have clear-cut evidence of rapid gastric emptying, and pregnant women suffering from morning sickness.

Most other patients, however, especially those whose symptoms are compatible with delayed gastric emptying, require further diagnostic studies to be performed, initially to exclude the possibility of mechanical obstruction and then to focus on the motor abnormalities present. The first step is a barium contrast study.

Barium contrast studies: the diagnosis of gastric retention is supported by poor emptying of barium from the stomach, gastric dilatation and the presence in the stomach of retained food or bezoars. If barium passes out of the stomach freely, mechanical obstruction is not present. It should be noted, however, that such a result does not indicate that disease is absent, only that there is no mechanical obstruction. A substantial defect in the emptying of solids or nutritive liquids may still be present. Even the development of the barium 'burger' meal has not helped in addressing solid food gastric emptying. The barium 'burger' is difficult to quantitate objectively because the 'burger' quickly dissociates from the barium. Furthermore, significant radiation exposure limits its role for following the therapeutic results in patients.[4]

Endoscopy: endoscopy is always necessary in all patients to establish fully the anatomical status of the upper GI tract. In addition, biopsies of any observed lesions can be obtained. This is especially indicated when atrophic gastritis may be suspected, suggesting achlorhydria, or when significant antral gastritis appears to be present, raising the possibility of bacterial gastritis related to *Campylobacter pylori*.[5]

In the postoperative stomach, endoscopy is the procedure of choice to evaluate the role of bile reflux and also the ease of passage of the instrument into the efferent limb or the Roux-en-Y. In systemic disorders such as scleroderma and amyloidosis, there will be evidence of impaired esophageal motility or strictures, or both. Culture of the duodenum should be considered routinely. Duodenal dilatation may be seen, particularly in patients with diabetic neuropathy, scleroderma and a myopathic form of chronic idiopathic intestinal pseudo-obstruction. Unfortunately, mucosal biopsies by endoscopic or suction techniques in patients with chronic intestinal pseudo-obstruction will not be adequate because only a full-thickness biopsy with specimens several centimetres long are adequate to show neural disease. These are usually ob-

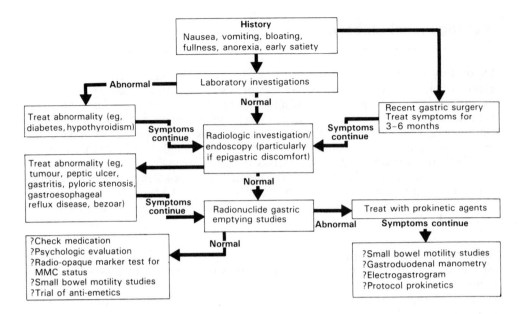

Figure 1   An approach to the evaluation of gastroparesis indicating the sequential evaluation of a patient with symptomatic gastroparesis, with emphasis on the laboratory investigations that are appropriate in reaching a diagnosis and providing a base for therapy.

tained at laparotomy. Therefore, if surgery is being contemplated in such patients, it is crucial that tissue be obtained for full histologic study and special stains.

Categorization of patients and additional diagnostic tests

At this point in the investigation, patients can be classified into two categories — those presenting with a clear clinical picture and those in whom the clinical picture is still confusing (*Figure 1*). An example of the first category is a patient with long-standing insulin-dependent diabetes mellitus (> 10 years) presenting with nausea and vomiting, residual food present on upper GI x-rays and poor emptying of barium from the stomach. Such a patient should undergo endoscopy to exclude gastric outlet obstruction, but further investigation should not be necessary. A diagnosis of diabetic gastroparesis could be made and therapy initiated.

Alternatively, another patient might be equally symptomatic but have normal barium study findings, no abnormalities upon endoscopy, no systemic disease, no medications which might affect motility and no history to suggest a cause. Additional studies are therefore indicated (*Table 4, Figure 1*).

Assessment of gastric emptying
Intubative techniques have helped to reveal a great deal about the role of liquids in gastric emptying.[6,7] The saline load test of Boyle and Goldstein[8] can still contribute to decisions on nasogastric tube aspiration in gastric outlet obstruction and provide some early predictions on the potential for surgical intervention. More recently, extensive work with the fractional test meal and intubative techniques have disclosed

1 Radioscintigraphy — gastric emptying and intestinal transit of radiolabelled solid and liquid components of a meal

2 Radiologic techniques

3 Fluoroscopy method

4 Intubation approaches

5 Impedance techniques

6 Abdominal ultrasound

7 Intraluminal pressure recordings — fasting and fed patterns of phasic pressure activity in the antrum and upper small bowel, as well as responses to pharmacologic provocation

8 Electrogastrograms — fasting and fed patterns

9 Endoscopy with antral biopsies for routine and special histological studies; specimens for bacterial overgrowth, including culture for *Campylobacter pylori*

10 Esophageal function testing including motility pH monitoring and Bernstein test

11 Gastric analysis (looking for hypersecretory or achlorhydric settings)

12 Psychological evaluation

Table 4   Diagnostic studies in patients with a suspected gastric motility disorder.

much about the contributions of gastric acid and other gastric constituents to the final emptied effluent.[9] Phenol red and other nonabsorbable markers can identify constituents of the pyloric effluent. In general, the invasive aspect of this test makes demands on patient tolerance and so repetition is limited. Such tests, at one time quite popular, are not used now in clinical practice. This is primarily because they are insufficiently standardized, may show normal results even when an emptying problem (eg, poor solid emptying) is present and are not 'patient friendly'. Modification of these tests to include a solid food aspect (homogenized meal) is very complex and clinically impractical.[10] However, intubation tests continue to play a role in research settings.

Radionuclide measurements of gastric emptying
The effort to quantitate gastric emptying with greater reliability and accuracy has been spurred on in part by the advent of drugs effective in treating gastric stasis syndromes. Radioisotopes, or radionuclides, have gone far in recent years toward achieving this goal. Being noninvasive, radionuclide testing is more physiologic than intubative methods, and the ability of radionuclides to 'tag' a solid test meal yields quantitative results not possible with barium radiography.

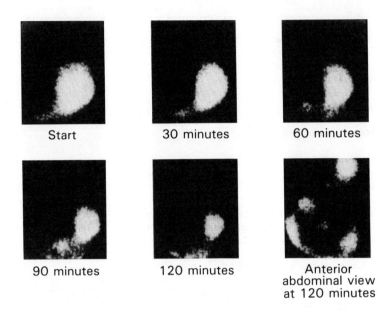

Figure 2 A series of abdominal scintiscans depicting the normal gastric emptying occurring after ingestion of an isotope-labelled solid test meal (chicken liver). Note the movement of isotope from the proximal stomach to the antrum, and in the final scan the decreasing intensity of gastric gamma counts as the small intestine is filled.

The current status of radionuclide applications to the study of gastroparesis may be appreciated more in the light of experience gained over the past 10 years with isotope 'tagging' of test meals. Radioactive technetium or chromium in some form was in general use and was presumed to remain steadfastly bonded to the test meal, even well into the final phase of digestion, regardless of the type of meal (meat, porridge, cornflakes). However, it was discovered that the isotopes readily strayed from the meals to which they were bound and became associated at random with other liquids such as mucus and bile. The isotopes even became attached to the gastric mucosa. Serious doubts were thus cast over what was being measured.[11]

These early studies led to the use of isotope-labelled chicken liver, a technique pioneered by Meyer and colleagues.[11] Technetium-99m (^{99m}Tc) bound to sulphur colloid is injected into the wing of a chicken; most of the ^{99m}Tc becomes bound to cytoplasmic protein in the chicken's Kupffer cells, which retain the isotope. Thirty minutes later the chicken is killed, its liver resected and sectioned into 1 cm cubes which are then mixed with stew, heated and fed to the patient together with crackers and liquids. The patient lies under a gamma camera linked to a computer to help interpret the data. A series of scintigrams reveal the movement of the isotope into the antrum and the subsequent arrival of the test meal in the small bowel (*Figure 2*). The computer is used to outline the stomach as the defined area of interest, and gamma counts are monitored from the region for a period of at least 2 hours or until 50% of the stomach contents have emptied.

The next phase of the development of this technique led to the use of two isotopes to monitor simultaneously the gastric emptying of solids and liquids (*Figure 3*). Indium (^{111}In)-DTPA was selected for the liquid or water phase of the meal because of its distinctive gamma spectrum.[12,13]

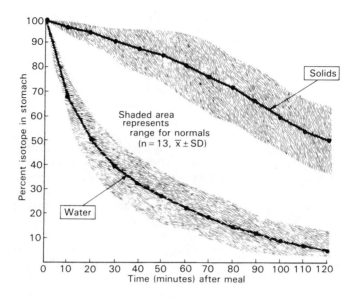

Figure 3   Gastric emptying rates of solids and liquids using dual isotope methodology. The ^{111}In-labelled water empties in exponential fashion representing fundic motility, while the chicken liver-labelled ^{99m}Tc sulphur colloid empties in a linear fashion, representing antral motility. Note the initial lag phase in the solid emptying process before definite emptying is obvious.

Use of commercial chicken livers, cut into cubes and injected with ^{99m}Tc sulphur colloid, eliminates the need to use live chickens. When ^{111}In is added to the water, gastric emptying results are comparable to those obtained using the *in vivo*-labelled technique.[14] Moreover, the affinity of ^{99m}Tc sulphur colloid for commercial chicken liver is reasonably good, with approximately 10% leaching of the isotope per hour following its injection into the liver. [99m]Tc sulphur colloid labelling of an omelette is also used to study gastric emptying of solids. There is very little isotope loss and the gastric emptying rate is only slightly faster than that following a chicken liver meal.[15] For vegetarians, an isotope-labelled egg salad sandwich provides an adequate clinical evaluation of solid emptying.[16]

Gastric emptying is influenced by a number of factors, including the size, consistency and caloric content of the meal[17], body position and concurrent drug administration. Therefore, whatever radionuclide technique is used, uniformity of method is of critical importance. Furthermore, the numerical results obtained will vary according to the method of analysis. Before establishing measurement of gastric emptying as a clinical test, a method must be decided upon and a normal range established for a particular laboratory; the technique must thereafter remain consistent. Any substantial changes in method must be taken into account in the analysis of the data.

Interpretation of radionuclide gastric emptying data
How should gastric emptying tests be analyzed? Percent of gastric emptying as a function of time is one way of expressing the data, either in terms of isotope retained in the stomach (*Figure 3*) or of isotope leaving the stomach. Another method

acknowledges the lag phase or lag period of gastric emptying. A lag period of 15–30 minutes occurs upon ingestion of a meal and is caused by receptive relaxation and the time it takes the antrum to begin actively functioning as a grinding and mixing organ. At the conclusion of the lag period, gastric emptying of the solid component occurs in a linear fashion (*Figure 3*). At this point, the solid meal is now triturated and homogenized, and the emptying rates of the solid and liquid markers follow a similar pattern. Thus, the gastric emptying curve comprises two distinct phases, the lag period and the linear gastric emptying period.

The time it takes for 50% of the contents of the stomach to empty provides a useful measure of liquid emptying, as this is a rapid process. However, for measuring solid food emptying in patients with severe gastric stasis, this approach is not meaningful. Interest is developing in the generation of mathematical curves and exponential functions to describe the emptying process.[18,19]

It is important that the patient is in a stable metabolic state when undergoing a gastric emptying test. Metabolic imbalance associated with sepsis, hyperglycemia, electrolyte disarray, acidosis, parenteral and hyperosmolar states and immediately post-surgery must be corrected. Total parenteral nutrition has been demonstrated to cause significant gastric stasis by an unknown mechanism.[20] Elemental diets take longer to empty from the stomach than blended 'whole' food of comparable caloric composition, probably due to the high amino acid content and hyperosmolality of the former.[21]

Medications that influence motility must be withdrawn 12–24 hours before a gastric emptying test, particularly opiates, anticholinergics, levodopa, beta-adrenergic agonists and, to a lesser degree, aluminum hydroxide antacids.[22] Cigarette smoking should also be stopped as it has been shown to delay emptying of solids.[23] Alcohol, in social doses, does not affect gastric emptying.[24] GI transit varies during the course of a woman's menstrual cycle, with prolongation during the luteal phase.[25] It is recommended that, in premenopausal women, gastric emptying studies be performed during the first 14 days of the menstrual cycle to minimize progesterone input. Studies in pregnant women show normal gastric emptying rates from 16 weeks of pregnancy to term.[26] However, there are no reports of gastric emptying studies in women during the early stages of pregnancy, when vomiting most often occurs. Finally, beta-blockers may stimulate gastric emptying.[27]

Another important application of the radiolabelled test meal technique is in the assessment of therapeutic agents for gastric stasis. If the dual isotope test shows that a prokinetic agent accelerated both liquid and solid emptying to a normal rate, then a therapeutic trial with the agent would be indicated. Alternatively, a patient could be studied while receiving chronic oral medication to determine whether a gastric emptying effect is present or sustained.

Nonradionuclide assessment of gastric emptying

Fluoroscopic screening: a radiographic technique using a radio-opaque marker and fluoroscopic equipment has been reported recently.[28] Emptying of indigestible solids relies upon the antral contractions occurring during late Phase II and Phase III of the migrating motor complex (MMC) which occurs only during the fasted state. Ten pieces of nasogastric tubing are ingested and emptying from the stomach is followed during the subsequent 6 hours with abdominal films. Feldman and colleagues showed that delayed emptying of radio-opaque markers (indigestible solids) may be a more sensitive test for diabetic gastroparesis than the radionuclide methods.[28] This should be investigated further. The problem of excess radiation exposure prevents more frequent observations and will limit the ability to repeat observations in individual patients. McCallum and co-workers have overcome this liability while retaining the uniqueness of the technique. Pieces of nasogastric tubing containing ^{111}In can be scanned at various times to ascertain more accurately the exact emptying rate with a radiation risk equivalent to only two abdominal flat plates.

Computerized tomography: in the animal model, CT studies of gastric emptying are being obtained using the dynamic spatial reconstructor. Multiple gastric images at the rate of 10/second are used to formulate cross-sectional and longitudinal reconstructions of the stomach and duodenum. Information obtained includes gastric and duodenal volumetric determinations which have been found to be within 5% of post mortem measurements. The method can also measure the frequency, velocity and amplitude of peristalsis. Computerized tomography has already demonstrated promise in physiologic studies and may, in the future, have a clinical application.

Impedance techniques: the measurement of changes in the electrical impedance in the epigastric region following the ingestion of liquids of low conductivity allows for an accurate determination of liquid emptying.[29] This technique represents an inexpensive and reproducible method which may gain wider acceptance as experience with it increases.

Abdominal ultrasound: the use of real-time ultrasound has been shown to provide an accurate method of measuring gastric emptying.[30] However, it is technically difficult to perform, time consuming and cannot be used in obese patients, following a gastrectomy or when excessive air is in the stomach. These limitations, plus the fact that it is suitable only for the measurement of liquid emptying, have so far prevented ultrasound from becoming widely accepted in gastric emptying studies.

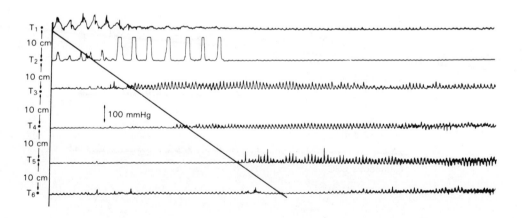

Figure 4 Normal propagation of a migrating motor complex (MMC) from the antrum, where the rate of contraction is 3 cycles/minute, to the proximal and distal duodenum and eventually the jejunum, where contraction rates have increased to 11 cycles/minute. This smooth orderly progression of the MMC allows for gastric emptying of nondigestible solids through an open pylorus.

Techniques for measuring gastric motility

Techniques to measure gastric motility include use of perfusion catheters and probes containing transducers. Perfusion catheters are cheaper than transducers and easy to assemble or buy; however, they are thicker than the usual transducer tube and hence more difficult to pass through the patient's nose. A further disadvantage is that infusing a constant rate of water over time may perturb motility and hence change the physiologic environment. On the other hand, although transducers are more expensive, the probes are thinner and do not disturb the luminal content; thus they provide a more accurate record of the physiologic status of the stomach.

Both methods have their limitations. They both require the patients under investigation to be attached to machinery, although more recently telemetry techniques allow recordings outside the hospital setting. The most recent advance in the area of transducer recording is the ultraminiature silicone pressure sensor device.[31] The transducers are arranged along a very narrow 2.7 mm probe contained within a flexible polyurethane sheath which passes easily through the nose and can be tolerated for long periods of time. The transducers are positioned at appropriate sites in order to detect pressure changes in the antrum, duodenum and small bowel. Measurements can be made for up to 24 hours, enabling a number of MMCs to be sampled (*Figure 4*) and providing greater opportunity to observe disturbed or disrupted complexes. (A tracing taken over a 2-6 hour period may only contain one or two such complexes.) Disrupted MMCs showing impaired propagation into the duodenum with some higher amplitude contractions may be observed in patients with gastroduodenal dyssynchrony synonymous with gastroduodenal motor dysfunction, nonulcer dyspepsia or a gastric and/or duodenal dysrhythmia (all entities predominantly observed in symptomatic female patients).

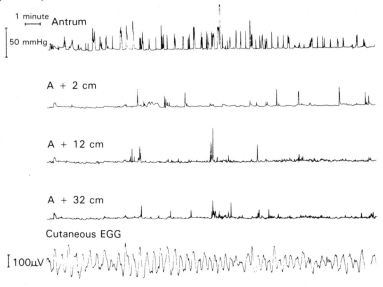

Figure 5 Recording of upper gastrointestinal motility using a probe with transducer sensors. Soon after ingestion of the meal, note the increased antral activity with a predictable contraction rate of 3/minute and increased contraction amplitudes averaging around 55 mmHg. In addition, there is evidence of increased motor activity in the duodenum and jejunum (sites antrum + 2 cm, antrum + 12 and 32 cm). There is a simultaneous recording of the cutaneous electrogastrogram (EGG) and the amplitude of the 3 cycle/minute activity is increased in the postprandial period compared to the fasting study.

Correlations of emptying and motility studies

In healthy individuals there is a positive correlation between post-cibal antral contractile activity and the rate of emptying of a radiolabelled meal measured radioscintigraphically.[32] Whether there is also a quantitative relationship between impairment of post-cibal gastrointestinal motility and gastric stasis is not completely known. A motility index or area under the curve estimates total activity based on contraction amplitudes and duration, and the calculation can be applied to the antral and duodenal response to a meal, usually over a 2-hour period (*Figure 5*).[32] Such measurements should be derived from a sample of two or three meals rather than one. While the observation of a hypomotility response does not allow for a specific diagnosis, or the distinction of a myopathy from a neuropathy, it does indicate that normal propagation of solid food from the antrum into the duodenum is unlikely.

Post-prandial hypomotility in patients with delayed gastric emptying by a radionuclide method could help distinguish a problem with antral motility from increased duodenal impedance and motor resistance (eg, duodenal dyscoordination). In a series of studies in which simultaneous measurements of gastroduodenal motility and gastric emptying were made during cold stress of labyrinthine stimulation, Malagelada and colleagues identified delayed gastric emptying in association with an altered post-prandial pattern of duodenal motility which resembled the fed pattern in some individuals. In addition, these studies and others[34] have consistently shown a relationship between delayed gastric emptying of digestible solids and decreased antral motility in both the fed and fasted states.

Settings in which reduced antral motility and delayed emptying are found most consistently include diabetic and post-vagotomy gastroparesis, and in patients with idiopathic gastroparesis.[19] Similarly, abnormal small intestinal motility manifested by prolonged bursts of nonpropagated contractions have been associated with impaired gastric emptying in some clinical settings, including diabetes, sympathetic autonomic neuropathy and idiopathic gastroparesis.[40] The association of abnormal gastroduodenal transit and altered gastric or duodenal electrical patterns has been less well established. Gastric dysrhythmias, most notably tachygastria, have been identified in patients with delayed gastric emptying from various causes including idiopathic gastroparesis.[35]

The discordance between gastric emptying and upper GI tract symptoms raises a question: how well does impaired gastric emptying correlate with symptoms of nausea, vomiting, bloating or abdominal pain in other clinical settings?

Pellegrini and co-workers evaluated 48 patients with clinically suspected gastroparesis, mostly secondary to surgery or diabetes, using radionuclide emptying studies.[36] They found that 50% of the patients had normal or rapid gastric emptying. Similarly, Malagelada and Stanghellini studied 104 patients with functional upper GI symptoms using a manometric probe as described previously.[32] They found that specific symptoms did not predict the presence or site of GI manometric abnormalities, although patients with known neurologic, urologic or metabolic diseases (eg, Parkinson's disease, hollow visceral myopathy, diabetes and post-vagotomy) did usually have manometric abnormalities when upper gut symptoms were present.

Some treatment trials in patients with significant diabetic gastroparesis have shown a poor correlation between improvement in gastric emptying and symptoms, while other studies have shown a fairly good correlation, particularly with symptoms of nausea and post-prandial fullness.[19] In cases of severe gastric stasis and bezoar formation in, for example, post-vagotomy states, it is most likely that upper tract symptoms parallel alterations in gastric emptying, particularly symptoms of post-prandial fullness, nausea and vomiting. Similarly, in cases of the dumping syndrome, which occurs most commonly after vagotomy and partial gastrectomy, symptoms of epigastric discomfort, nausea, diarrhea, palpitations, sweating and weakness may correlate fairly well with rapid gastric emptying.[19] However, the overall difficulty in identifying a consistent relationship between alterations in gastric emptying and symptoms results from the fact that small bowel and/or colonic motility abnormalities can be involved.

The value of recording motility of the antrum and duodenum is in predicting responses to a potential therapeutic agent. Such response assists the physician in prescribing therapy. Contractile responses to agents such as metoclopramide, bethanechol, domperidone or cisapride indicate that the problem is a neuropathy of the enteric nervous system rather than a myopathy.

Electrogastrography

The electrogastrogram measures the gastric electrical rhythm (the basal electrical rhythm or the gastric slow wave). Silver-silver chloride electrodes are placed on the epigastrium with a limb reference lead (*Figure 6*).[37] Correlations with surgically placed electrodes have been excellent (*Figure 7*).[38] Gastric dysrhythmias have been found in patients with symptoms of abnormal gastric motility[39,40] but they have also been observed in asymptomatic individuals. Antral motor activity has been shown to increase markedly the amplitude of the gastric slow wave; this technique may, therefore, eventually become a clinically useful tool in diagnosing impaired antral motor functions after meals.

Although gastric dysrhythmias have been described in a variety of clinical conditions, most studies have involved only isolated case reports. Therefore, the role of gastric dysrhythmias has yet to be examined with careful scientific scrutiny.

The first well-documented report of tachygastria in humans was published in 1978.[41] The case concerned a 5-month-old infant who was debilitated as a result of severe gastric retention and had symptoms of intractable nausea, vomiting and weight loss. Subsequently, the patient underwent resection of the distal three-quarters of the stomach and gastrojejunostomy, after which the symptoms dramatically subsided. When the surgical tissue was carefully studied *in vitro* by means of intracellular

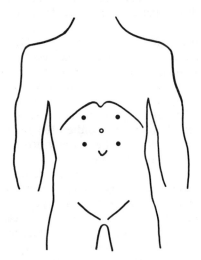

Figure 6 Positioning of the silver-silver chloride surface electrodes on the abdomen when measuring cutaneous electrogastrograms. A reference lead is usually attached to the leg. Abdominal positioning of the electrodes may vary a little in order to maximize the best signal-to-noise ratio.

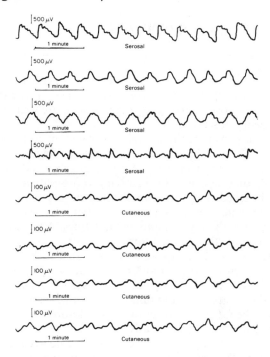

Figure 7 Simultaneous recording of the gastric slow wave activity by surgically implanted electrodes on the gastric serosa (at intervals from the body to the antrum) of the stomach and the cutaneous recordings of the same electrical slow wave with positioning of the electrodes on the skin of the abdomen as depicted in *Figure 6*. Note that the cutaneous EGG can provide an accurate and reproducible gastric slow wave providing verification of the fidelity of the cutaneous recording site. Note also the difference in voltage between the two recordings contributed to by the fat pad between the surface electrode and the serosa of the stomach.

microelectrode techniques, an abnormally fast electrical rhythm (occurring at a rate of 5–20 cycles/minute) was detected.

The association between tachygastria and abnormal gastric motor function was described in a 26-year-old woman with persistent nausea, vomiting and abdominal pain who was found to have antral tachygastria and severe impairment of antral motor function.[42] Her symptoms were relieved following a subtotal gastrectomy. Subsequent studies have revealed gastric dysrhythmias in 9 of 14 patients with unexplained nausea, vomiting and epigastric bloating for periods that ranged from 5 months to 10 years.[39] The significance of gastric dysrhythmias in certain human disease states is further suggested by their presence in some patients suffering from gastroparesis in association with diabetes mellitus or anorexia nervosa.

Gastric dysrhythmias are not restricted exclusively to stomachs with impaired motor function. They are present in asymptomatic individuals[43], during the immediate postoperative period and in a variety of unrelated clinical conditions. Under such circumstances, however, these dysrhythmias tend to be transient. Whether they are directly responsible for abnormal motor function of the stomach and/or dyspeptic symptoms is unclear. However, their persistent presence in a patient with dyspeptic symptoms may indicate an underlying motor dysfunction of the stomach which may warrant further investigation using techniques such as manometry and radioscintigraphy.

Etiology of delayed gastric emptying states

One of the most common causes of delayed gastric emptying is diabetes. Although many diabetics have neuropathy, an increasing number of younger patients with juvenile-onset diabetes whose gastric emptying problems are well in advance of other complications are being observed.

Post-surgical patients constitute the second most common group with gastric emptying disorders. Although most individuals who undergo vagotomy and antrectomy for peptic ulcer disease have rapid gastric emptying of solids and liquids, gastric stasis occurs in about 5% of cases, usually involving those patients with a Billroth II anastomosis. It is believed that this complication occurs because the patient had obstructive peptic ulcer disease for some months before surgery and distension of the stomach has impaired the smooth muscle mechanics. A vagotomy further denervates the muscle, and function never returns.

Pseudo-obstruction (so-called because it is associated with dilated, nonfunctioning bowel) involves the entire GI tract and may occur as a primary idiopathic entity or in the setting of diffuse and usually recognizable systemic disorders. Scleroderma, amyloidosis, muscular dystrophies and tumour syndromes associated with metastatic cancer not involving the GI tract can result in pseudo-obstruction and GI problems of varying degrees, including gastric stasis.

Up to 80% of patients with anorexia nervosa have delayed gastric emptying of solids.[12] In some cases this problem responds to prokinetic agents. Whether this represents a primary, secondary or epiphenomenon is unclear. Many patients with a diagnosis of nonulcer dyspepsia also have delayed gastric emptying with impaired antral motility. Overall, the syndrome is associated with less vomiting and more post-prandial discomfort, nausea, heartburn, belching and indigestion than classic gastric stasis. Because vomiting may be minimal and complaints of acidity or burning sensations are more marked, the diagnostic workup often focuses initially on ulcer disease rather than gastric motility; however, symptoms of acidity are not unusual in patients with delayed gastric emptying because food and acid remain in the stomach longer. At least 50% of nonulcer dyspepsia patients referred to the author's unit have delayed gastric emptying with impaired antral motility.

Gastroesophageal reflux is another common disorder frequently associated with delayed gastric emptying.[16] Much of the current research into the pathophysiology of reflux indicates that delayed gastric emptying plays a significant role by causing a gastrosphincteric reflex resulting in a transient relaxation of the lower esophageal sphincter. Although patients may complain primarily of heartburn, when questioned specifically about gastric symptoms a surprising number will report post-prandial bloating, fullness, belching and discomfort. A smaller percentage may have nausea and vomiting.

Gastritis is also worth considering in those patients with no apparent cause of delayed gastric emptying. Impairment of gastric motility in gastritis is believed to reflect interference with smooth muscle function correlated with the depth of inflammation on the mucosal surface. Atrophic gastritis can cause disordered motility limited to the stomach and commonly associated with achlorhydria. Approximately 5% of the population is achlorhydric at some time or other; therefore, measurement of stomach pH at endoscopy in patients with no other readily identifiable cause of delayed emptying is worthwhile.

Another possible cause of delayed gastric emptying is viral gastritis, particularly in those patients whose histories include a suggestion of chronic, active, infectious gastritis. Typically, these patients report that they had a sudden onset of gastritis while on vacation that still persists weeks or months later. The Norwalk agent has been shown to infiltrate gastric smooth muscle. Recently, a role for *Campylobacter pylori* has been proposed, but although this organism can cause antral gastritis, most studies to date have not found it to be a cause of delayed gastric emptying.

The 1980s have seen the emergence and acceptance of a new disease concept — idiopathic gastric stasis. This condition sometimes seems to be approaching epidemic proportions. Indeed the patient with idiopathic gastric stasis may already be a familiar visitor to practices across the country. Such patients have all the symptoms of gastric stasis, normal endoscopic findings and show delayed emptying (usually solid food) upon gastric scintigraphy. However, they have no history of surgery, are not taking medications which affect gut motility and have no evidence of an underlying condition. For reasons which are not yet clear, the condition occurs more commonly in women; 80–90% of patients are women under the age of 50. No correlation has been found between occurrence of symptoms and the menstrual cycle. There is a possibility that these patients are supersensitive to normal levels of estrogen. The preponderance of women with this disorder may also be a reflection of an increased willingness on their part to discuss their symptoms and to consult with their physicians. In the past, this subset of patients was dismissed as either neurotic or suffering from disorders ranging from peptic ulcer to irritable bowel syndrome.

In up to 50% of patients with idiopathic gastric stasis, the entire GI tract is involved to some degree. This finding is consistent with what is known about neuropathies in general; diabetes, scleroderma and amyloidosis are all associated with colonic and small bowel dysfunction. The difference is that here it is presenting in an idiopathic form.

Some patients may present with a gastric motility disturbance but in fact have a more diffuse impairment of GI smooth muscle, including duodenal gastric dyscoordination, intestinal pseudo-obstruction and colonic involvement. When lower abdominal pain and a relationship to base stools is elicited, the syndrome has often been called the 'irritable gut syndrome' and there has been a tendency to regard it primarily as a psychological problem. However, the preponderance of evidence suggests that these patients have underlying motor disorders that may be exacerbated by psychological factors but nonetheless are worthy of being detected and recognized.

Constipation is often an important clue to a diffuse impairment, and many patients present with it idiopathically. Careful questioning, however, will elicit symptoms of a diffuse myopathy or neuropathy—heartburn, dysphagia and other symptoms of motor disorder in the esophagus as well as profound post-prandial bloating and fullness. Patients have diffuse general symptoms of stasis and stagnation and may even have intermittent diarrhea from bacterial overgrowth in the small intestine.

In some patients with diffuse idiopathic disease, abdominal pain is very prominent and difficult to manage. The pain tends to occur after meals and to be concentrated in the periumbilical area or right upper quadrant. The cause is assumed to be bowel distension. There is some suggestion that this particular subgroup of patients may have a problem with pain threshold. Not uncommonly, they have undergone surgical procedures such as cholecystectomy and hysterectomy. Many are receiving narcotics or other pain-relieving medications which confuse the clinical picture further.

One area currently under investigation which may play a role in patients with idiopathic motility disorders is gastric dysrhythmia. In view of the fact that the GI tract is the largest generator of electrical activity in the body, the possibility that the electrical rhythm of the gut may become disturbed is not beyond reason. Whether dysrhythmia precedes or follows delayed gastric emptying and whether or how much dysrhythmia is a normal physiologic event are questions which remain unanswered. Nevertheless, a potential role for 'gastric pacing' in the treatment of motility disorders is being investigated.

Psychological factors may contribute to gastric dysmotility in some patients, and psychiatric evaluation is almost always worth pursuing. Even when psychological factors do not cause the disorder, many patients change considerably from their normal baseline by the time their condition is diagnosed; they have consulted with numerous physicians and have subsequently become anxious or depressed. Therefore, the physician must show patience and understanding in order to give these patients the faith to remain hopeful of more diagnostic findings and effective therapy.

Conclusion

The differential diagnosis section of this chapter included an effort to develop the concept that a gastric motor disturbance can be part of a diffuse neuropathy or myopathy involving smooth muscle throughout the GI tract. In the case of the diabetic this diffuse neuropathy is generally appreciated. In the case of idiopathic gastroparesis, the following approach might be considered.

The full symptom complex of irritable bowel syndrome could be hypothesized to represent the total accumulation of symptoms arising from a number of regions in the GI tract, each termed 'irritable' (*Figure 8*). In patients being evaluated for chest pain who have essentially a normal manometric pattern, but have painful responses to the acid infusion test (Bernstein test) and/or intravenous edrophonium, an 'irritable esophagus' is sometimes hypothesized, suggesting an esophagus with a low pain threshold or increased sensitivity of mucosal receptors (in the case of the Bernstein test) or muscarinic receptors (in the case of an edrophonium injection). External stress can also be superimposed upon this setting. It is also reasonable to accept the notion of the 'irritable stomach'. This is typically a setting of 'idiopathic' gastric stasis,

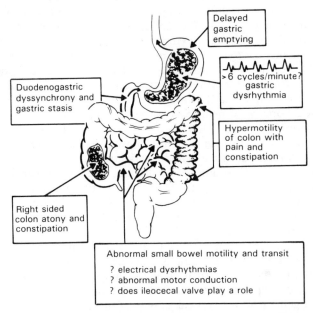

Figure 8 A theoretical approach to the concept of a neuropathy or myopathy involving different parts of the gastrointestinal tract with variable symptomatic manifestations in a given individual patient. It provides an hypothesis for the concept of the potential for more proximal manifestations of what was previously referred to as the 'irritable bowel syndrome'.

sometimes gastric stasis in a patient termed as 'nonulcer dyspepsia', gastric stasis representing the motor sequelae of tachygastria or bradygastria, or gastric stasis also occurring with disordered small bowel motility. Finally, the symptoms of nausea, bloating, fullness and vomiting may represent an overlap with a small bowel motor disturbance (irritable small bowel) or a colonic motility abnormality (irritable colon) and here the gastric emptying may or may not be abnormal. This finding of a normal gastric emptying may be confusing, but it is a reminder also to consider other origins for these symptoms.

References

1 Vantrappen G, Janssens J, Ghoos Y. The interdigestive motor complex of normal subjects and patients with bacterial overgrowth of the small intestine. *J Clin Invest* 1977; **59**: 1158-66.
2 Shivshanker K, Bennett RW, Haynie TP. Tumor-associated gastroparesis: correction with metoclopramide. *Am J Surg* 1983; **145**: 221-5.
3 Smalley WE, Valenzuela G, McCallum RW. Nausea and vomiting with adrenocortical insufficiency: is it central in origin or a gastrointestinal motility disturbance? *Am J Gastroenterol* 1987; **82**: 1066-8.
4 Perkel MS, Fajman WA, Hersh T *et al.* Comparison of the barium test meal and the gamma camera scanning technique in measuring gastric emptying. *So Med J* 1981; **74**: 1065-8.
5 Marshall BJ. *Campylobacter pyloridis* and gastritis. *J Infect Dis* 1986; **153**: 650-7.
6 Hunt JN, Spurrell WR. The pattern of emptying of the human stomach. *J Physiol (Lond)* 1951; **113**: 157-68.
7 George JD. A new clinical method for measuring the role of gastric emptying: the double sampling test meal. *Gut* 1968; **9**: 237-42.
8 Goldstein H, Boyle J. The saline load test — a bedside evaluation of gastric retention. *Gastroenterology* 1965; **49**: 375-80.
9 Dubois A, VanEerdewegh P, Gardner JD. Gastric emptying and secretin in Zollinger-Ellison syndrome. *J Clin Invest* 1977; **59**: 255-63.
10 Malagelada JR, Longstretch GE, Summerskill WHJ *et al.* Measurement of gastric function during digestion of ordinary solid meals in man. *Gastroenterology* 1976; **70**: 203-10.
11 Meyer JH, McGregor MB, Gueller R *et al.* Tc-tagged chicken liver as a marker of solid food in the human stomach. *Am J Dig Dis* 1976; **21**: 296-304.
12 McCallum RW, Grill BB, Lange RC, Plankey M, Glass E, Greenfeld DG. Definition of a gastric emptying abnormality in patients with anorexia nervosa. *Dig Dis Sci* 1985; **30**: 713-22.
13 Collins PJ, Horowitz M, Cook DJ *et al.* Gastric emptying in normal subjects — a reproducible technique using a single scintillation camera and a computer system. *Gut* 1983; **24**: 1117-25.
14 Christian PE, Moore PE, Dante FL. Comparison of Tc-labeled liver and liver pate as markers for solid phase gastric emptying. *J Nucl Med* 1984; **25**: 364-6.
15 Knight LC, DeVegvar ML, Fisher RS *et al.* Tc-sulfur-colloid scrambled eggs versus *in vivo* chicken liver normal subjects. *J Nucl Med* 1983; **23**: 21.
16 McCallum RW, Berkowitz DM, Lerner E. Gastric emptying in patients with gastroesophageal reflux. *Gastroenterology* 1981; **80**: 285-91.
17 Moore JG, Christian PE, Coleman RE. Gastric emptying of varying meal weights and composition in man. Evaluation by dual liquid and solid phase isotopic method. *Dig Dis Sci* 1981; **26**: 16-22.
18 Elashoff JE, Reedy TJ, Meyer JH. Analysis of gastric emptying data. *Gastroenterology* 1982; **83**: 1306-12.
19 Minami H, McCallum RW. The physiology and pathophysiology of gastric emptying in humans. *Gastroenterology* 1984; **86**: 1592-610.
20 MacGregor IL, Wiley ZD, Lavigne ME *et al.* Total parenteral nutrition slows gastric emptying of solid foods. *Gastroenterology* 1978; **74**: 1059 (abstr).
21 Bury KD, Jambunathan G. Effects of elemental diets on gastric emptying and gastric secretion in man. *Am J Surg* 1974; **127**: 59-64.
22 McCallum RW, Caride V, Prokopf E. Effect of sucralfate and an aluminum hydroxide gel on gastric emptying in solids and liquids. *Clin Pharmacol Ther* 1985; **37**: 629-32.
23 Harrison A, Ippoliti A. Effect of smoking on gastric emptying. *Gastroenterology* 1979; **76**: 1152(abstr).

24 Barboriak JJ, Meade RC. Effect of alcohol on gastric emptying in man. *Am J Clin Nutr* 1970; **23**: 1151–3.

25 Wald A, Van Thiel DH, Hoechstetter L *et al*. Gastrointestinal transit: the effect of the menstrual cycle. *Gastroenterology* 1981; **80**: 1497–500.

26 Hunt JN, Murray FA. Gastric function in pregnancy. *J Obstet Gynaecol Br Commonwealth* 1978; **65**: 78–83.

27 Rees MR, Clark RA, Holdsworth CD. The effect of beta-adrenoreceptor agonists and antagonists on gastric emptying in man. *Br J Clin Pharmacol* 1980; **10**: 551–4.

28 Feldman M, Smith HJ, Simon JR. Gastric emptying of solid radio-opaque markers: studies in healthy subjects and diabetic patients. *Gastroenterology* 1984; **87**: 895–904.

29 Sutton JA, Thompson S. Measurement of gastric emptying rates by radioisotope scanning and epigastric impedance. *Lancet* 1985; **i**: 888–90.

30 Holt S, Cervantes J, Wilkinson A *et al*. Measurement of gastric emptying rate in humans by real-time ultrasound. *Gastroenterology* 1986; **90**: 918–23.

31 Mathias JR, Sninsky CA, Millar HD *et al*. Development of an improved multi-pressure sensor probe for recording muscle contraction in human intestine. *Dig Dis Sci* 1985; **30**: 119–23.

32 Malagelada JR, Stanghellini V. Manometric evaluation of functional upper gut symptoms. *Gastroenterology* 1985; **88**: 1223–31.

33 Stanghellini V, Malagelada JR, Zinsmeister AR *et al*. Stress-induced gastroduodenal motor disturbances in humans: possible humoral mechanisms. *Gastroenterology* 1983; **85**: 83–91.

34 Camilleri M, Brown MC, Malagelada JR. Relationship between impaired gastric emptying and abnormal gastrointestinal motility. *Gastroenterology* 1986; **9**: 94–9.

35 Kim CH, Malagelada JR. Electrical activity of the stomach: clinical implications. *Mayo Clin Proc* 1986; **61**: 205–19.

36 Pellegrini CA, Broderick WC, Dyke DV *et al*. Diagnosis and treatment of gastric emptying disorders: clinical usefulness of radionuclide measurements. *Am J Surg* 1983; **145**: 143–50.

37 Bellahsene BE, Hamilton JN, Reichelderfer M. An improved method for recording and analyzing the electrical activity of the human stomach. *IEEE Trans Biomed Eng* 1985; **BME-32**: 911–5.

38 Bellahsene BE, Schirmer B, McCallum RW. Validation of cutaneous EGG recordings from intragastric surgically implanted electrodes. *Gastroenterology* 1987; **92** (abstr).

39 You CH, Lee KY, Chey WY *et al*. Electrogastrographic study of patients with unexplained nausea, bloating and vomiting. *Gastroenterology* 1980; **79**: 311–4.

40 Abell TL, Lucas AR, Brown ML *et al*. Gastric electrical dysrhythmias in anorexia nervosa. *Gastroenterology* 1985; **88**: 1300.

41 Telander RL, Morgan KG, Kreulen DL, Schmalz PF, Kelly KA, Szurszewski JH. Human gastric atony tachygastria and gastric retention. *Gastroenterology* 1978; **75**: 497–501.

42 You CH, Chey WY, Lee KY, Menguy R, Bortoff A. Gastric and small intestinal myoelectrical dysrhythmia associated with chronic intractable nausea and vomiting. *Ann Intern Med* 1981; **95**: 449–51.

43 Stoddard CJ, Smallwood RH, Duthie HL. Electrical arrhythmias in the human stomach. *Gut* 1981; **22**: 705–12.

Diagnostic methodology of small bowel motility problems

J-R Malagelada

Motility disorders affecting the small bowel are currently subject to intense research and clinical scrutiny. This interest in motility disorders can be explained on several counts. First, there is evidence that gastrointestinal motility is abnormal in a number of patients with functional-type symptoms. Another reason is the ever increasing sophistication of those methods used for quantifying motility. These physiologic methods include manometry, electromyography and radioscintigraphy, as well as special histopathologic approaches. Manometry evaluates the fasting and fed patterns of phasic pressure activity in the antrum and upper small bowel. Electromyography (serosal and mucosal) records electrical signals, determining their rhythm and the occurrence of action potentials. Radioscintigraphy makes it possible to quantify the intestinal transit of radiolabelled solid and liquid components of a meal. Esophageal, gastric and anorectal manometry can provide complementary information on contractile patterns at both ends of the gut.

Morphologic and *in vitro* electrophysiologic studies of myoneural elements on the gut wall can sometimes establish the nature of the intestinal motility disorder (e.g. visceral myopathy, myenteric plexus disease). However, these tissue techniques must be regarded as invasive, since at the present time they are only applicable to full thickness biopsies of the gut obtained at surgery. Furthermore, only a handful of histopathologic laboratories possess the necessary expertise to utilize them reliably.

Clinical evaluation of gastrointestinal motility disorders
A topographic diagnosis of a gut motility disorder rarely can be made on clinical grounds alone.

Symptoms such as chronic nausea, vomiting, abdominal distension and pain are the most common manifestations and the usual reason for requesting physician consultation. However, such symptoms are quite non-specific and may reflect a gastric, intestinal and often colonic disturbance. A more objective diagnosis of gut motility disorders requires appropriate tests to be performed. Barium contrast studies may show dilatation, stasis or, rarely, evidence of abnormal peristaltic activity. However, they can be normal in up to 50% of patients.[1] Endoscopy may suggest gastric stasis in the form of retained food and secretions but direct endoscopic assessment of motility is usually unreliable because of air distension and short observation periods.

Both radiology and endoscopy are obviously important in excluding a structural lesion which, by definition, precludes the diagnosis of gut motility disorder. Even non-obstructive lesions, for instance, severe mucosal inflammation, can potentially affect motility and if such lesions are present abnormal motility studies must be interpreted with caution. Computer-assisted tomography (CAT) scans of the abdomen, ultrasonography and other imaging procedures can assist in the detection of retroperitoneal lesions or other forms of intra-abdominal disease which also need to be excluded before a diagnosis of a primary gastrointestinal motility disorder can be made.

Having established the absence of structural abnormalities the laboratory diagnosis of intestinal motility disorders relies on the assessment of intestinal contractile and propulsive function.

Intestinal manometry

Intestinal manometry assesses contractile activity in the small bowel by measuring the frequency in amplitude of the phasic pressure waves caused by contractions of the gut wall. Manometry can be performed with different systems: miniature strain gauges, perfused catheters, balloons, and others. The author's institution employs a perfused pneumohydraulic manometric system which consists of a multilumen polyvinyl probe incorporating 8–12 thin catheters arranged around a central core which slides over a guiding wire. The lumens of each catheter (internal diameter 0.8 mm) have a side opening for perfusion. The external diameter of the probe should not exceed 5–6 mm, and the catheter should be smooth and flexible to avoid stretching or compression of the gut wall (*Figure 1*).

The manometric ports are grouped into two sections: the antroduodenal section, consisting of 3–6 ports, 1 cm apart; and the intestinal section, consisting of 3–6 ports, 10 cm apart. It is important to evaluate manometrically the antrum at the time an intestinal manometric study is performed because gastric and small bowel motility disorders often occur simultaneously.[2] The perfusion lumens are connected via strain gauge transducers and steel capillary tubes to a pneumohydraulic pump containing distilled water. The perfusion pressure is 11 pounds per square inch and the perfusion rate can vary (depending on the length of the capillary tube and its diameter)

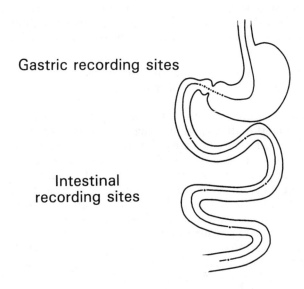

Gastric recording sites

Intestinal recording sites

Figure 1 Schematic representation of gastrointestinal manometry showing position of recording sites.

from 0.1–0.5 mL/minute. Electrical impulses from the strain gauges are registered on a paper chart recorder which is operated usually at a speed of 0.25 mm/second. Before each study, the manometric system needs to be calibrated using either a pneumatic or a water-driven calibration device.

Preparation begins at least 2 days before the study when any medication with known effects on gut motility, such as opiates or anticholinergics, are stopped. If the patient is narcotic addicted, he should be withdrawn under an appropriate protocol before undertaking motility studies. Depending on the degree of associated gastric stasis, the patient may need to be either on prior continuous gastric suction, no oral feedings or simply have a liquid supper the evening preceding the study.

In the morning of the test the manometric assembly is introduced into the proximal small bowel over a guiding wire that has already been advanced through the pylorus using either a steerable catheter or a pediatric-sized endoscope. The position of the manometric assembly needs to be verified fluoroscopically to ensure that the more proximal recording sites are straddled across the antroduodenal junction and that no slack of the tube is present in the stomach. Further adjustments in the position of the probe can be performed after the manometric recording has been started. Patients are moved to a quiet room where they remain supine in bed, head-end elevated at a 45° angle for the remainder of the study.

Gastrointestinal motor activity is monitored for 3 hours and then the patients are fed a solid-liquid meal which consists of chicken, potato and water. The total caloric value of the meal is 511 kcal. At the time the meal is ingested the tube is repositioned so that the most distal of the antroduodenum 1 cm sequential sites registers duodenal-type activity (up to 11 waves/minute). This manoeuvre is designed to ensure that the more proximal recordings are indeed located in the distal antrum. Pressure activity is then monitored post-prandially for an additional 2 hours.

Currently, analysis of manometric tracings is performed manually. Nevertheless, computer systems to facilitate pattern recognition and quantification are under development.

In the intestine, fasting intestinal pressure activity is first analyzed quantitatively by determining the number of interdigestive migrating motor complexes (MMCs) and whether they originate in the stomach or in the proximal small bowel. The manometric criteria used by the author for defining interdigestive MMCs are as follows: Phase I equals less than 3 waves over 12 mmHg during a 10-minute period; Phase II equals 3 or more waves over 12 mmHg in 10 minutes at less than the maximal rate (3 minutes in the antrum and 11/minute in the duodenum and jejunum); Phase III equals at least 32 consecutive waves within 1 minute in the antrum and 11 consecutive waves within 1 minute in the intestine. Migration of Phase III is defined as the sequential onset of Phase III with an interval exceeding 2 minutes in at least two nonadjacent sites (for instance, antrum and ligament of Treitz, or duodenum and jejunum). After a meal, the duration of the fed pattern is determined by the interval from ingestion of the meal to the first post-prandial Phase III. The fed pattern is defined by the same criteria as for Phase II except it occurs after the meal.

Abnormal intestinal motility can be identified manometrically.[2-4] However, manual calculation of an intestinal motility index would be impractical because of the large number of pressure waves occurring at multiple sites. Although computer methods are being developed, at the present time visual analysis by pattern recognition is the standard method of analysis. Some investigators rely on measurement of the frequency of interdigestive MMCs.

This approach has the potential disadvantage of requiring long observation periods, since the variability in cycle frequency between individuals and even within the same individual is considerable. Overnight studies are ideal for determining the frequency of MMCs since that is when they occur physiologically. However, overnight studies require hospitalization and they are expensive.

On the other hand, with the 3-hour fasting observation period, the frequency of interdigestive MMCs cannot be estimated accurately. Therefore, the criteria used for diagnosing intestinal dysmotility at the author's laboratory are based on alterations of the configuration and pattern of pressure wave activity and not on the basis of MMC frequency. The criteria for abnormality were developed by reference to a large population of patients with idiopathic and secondary intestinal pseudo-obstruction syndromes.[5] The main four criteria are:

• abnormal propagation or configuration of the interdigestive MMCs, if present;
• incoordinated intestinal bursts of phasic pressure activity;
• sustained (over 30 minutes) incoordinated intestinal pressure activity;
• failure of the meal to induce a fed pattern.

None of these patterns is seen in healthy individuals.

Other abnormal patterns have been described.[6,7] Furthermore, in patients with 'pure' muscular disorders, manometry may show a normal pattern of activity (suggesting intact neural control) with striking reduction in the amplitude of phasic pressure waves (*Figure 2*).

Measurement of small intestinal transit time

Radioscintigraphic methods are the most practical, at present, for measuring quantitatively the small bowel transit of chyme. These measurements must be performed in conjunction with measurements of gastric emptying because of the close relationship between motor disorders of the stomach and of the small bowel.[2]

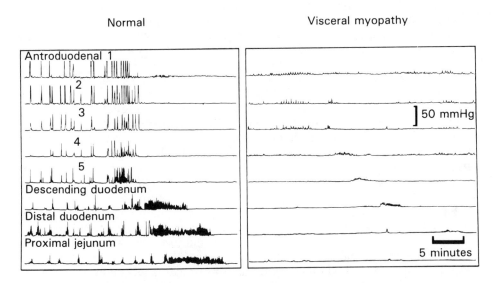

Figure 2 Examples of intestinal manometric pattern in a normal individual (left) and in a patient with myogenic pseudo-obstruction syndrome (right). Note the low amplitude of phasic pressure waves with preservation of the normal pattern of migration of the interdigestive motor complex.

The test meal used in intestinal transit studies consists of cheese, crackers and water (200 kcal) whose solid-liquid phases are radiolabelled with ^{131}I-fibre and ^{99m}Tc-DTPA respectively.[8] The liquid phase binding of ^{99m}Tc-DTPA needs to be stabilized by addition of 1% (w/v) bovine serum albumin.[9] The imaging is performed on a tilt table at an angle of 45°. A large field-of-view camera with high-energy collimation is placed over the subject's abdomen. Time 0 is defined as the start of ingestion of the meal. Imaging is started 10 minutes after subjects begin eating their meal and is repeated at 10-minute intervals during the first hour, at 20-minute intervals during the second hour, and at 30-minute intervals during the third and fourth hours. After 4 hours, a standard hospital meal (chicken, potato, water; 300 kcal) is given to maintain a physiologic meal schedule. The frequency of imaging again starts at 10-minute intervals during the first hour, 20-minute intervals during the second hour, 30-minute intervals during the third hour and hourly thereafter until at least 90% of the markers has entered the colon. Three minutes of acquisition are used for each radionuclide. The ^{131}I activity is recorded using a 20% window around the 364 keV peak and the ^{99m}Tc activity is recorded using a 20% window around the 140 keV peak.

Data are stored on a small on-line computer for later analysis. Subjects are ambulatory after 1 hour of imaging after the two meals.

Quantification of radioactivity and corrections are performed as follows. Two well-defined areas of interest (stomach and colon) are identified in the scans. In each sequential scan, the gastric and colonic outlines are drawn as regions of interest, using a variable region of interest program.[8] The stomach and colon are easily identified in virtually all scans, since the operator can display sequential scans forwards and backwards in time, showing the radiolabel movement through both viscera and thereby identifying the outline. Furthermore, the gastric outline can be accurately drawn in scans of solid marker and can thus be used to separate stomach from contiguous small bowel loops in the liquid marker scans. The activity of each isotope is determined in each scan, and corrections made for crossover (assuming 41% of iodine counts in the technetium window, as shown in previous publications) and physical decay.

The analysis of transit data must be carried out by quantifying gastric emptying and small bowel transit as two separate functions. The gastric emptying data for solids are analyzed by a dual-phase model consisting of a lag phase and an emptying phase.[10,11] The duration of the lag phase is determined by the first appearance of detectable amounts of ^{131}I in the proximal small intestine. The emptying part of the solid emptying curve is linearized by logistic transformation and the slope of the linearized plot determined. Liquid emptying data are submitted to power exponential analysis.[12]

To calculate small bowel transit two methods with degrees of complexity may be used. For the simpler method, the half-life for gastric emptying (t½) is subtracted from the t½ for colonic filling.[13] t½ for gastric emptying is obtained from the proportionate gastric emptying data whereas the t½ for colonic filling is obtained from the plotted colonic filling curves. The more complex method involves deconvolution analysis (*Figure 3*). First the gastric emptying and colonic filling curves are computer-fitted by a polynomial regression to obtain the equation for each curve. These two curves, which represent small bowel input and output of labelled chyme, are then deconvoluted using an iterative numerical process to obtain the small bowel transit spectrum.[8] This spectrum, unlike the simpler mean transit time obtained from t½ values, represents the movement of the entire meal along the small bowel. It therefore reflects not only how fast chyme moves but also how it spreads in the intestine during digestion.

Experience with measurements of transit time in disease states is limited. In a re-

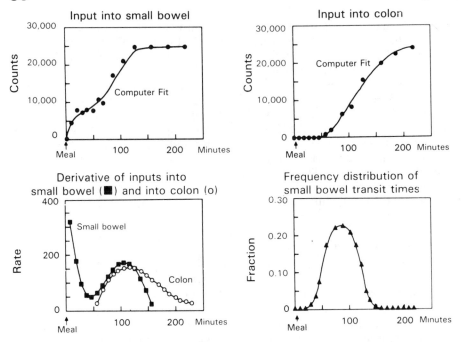

Figure 3 Method for measuring small bowel transit based on deconvolution analysis. The process includes obtaining input curves for small bowel and colon, calculating the corresponding rates and finally deconvoluting them to obtain the transit spectrum. Reproduced with permission from Malagelada J-R, Robertson JS, Brown ML *et al*. Intestinal transit of solid and liquid components of a meal in health. *Gastroenterology* 1984; **87**: 1255–63.

cent study performed in patients with the intestinal pseudo-obstruction syndrome a significant prolongation of transit of chyme along the small bowel was demonstrated.[14] The delay in transit was more pronounced for the solid than for the liquid component of chyme (*Figure 4*). In this group of patients gastric emptying was delayed but not to the extent observed in a separate group of patients with the gastroparesis syndrome whose motility disturbance was limited to the stomach. Delayed gastric emptying in patients with intestinal dysmotility could be attributed to either the abnormal small bowel impeding flow out of the stomach or to simultaneous involvement of the stomach and the intestine.

In this group of patients with intestinal pseudo-obstruction transit measurements obtained with the radioscintigraphic method were compared with transit estimates obtained from conventional barium fluoroscopy. It was found that barium small bowel transit time was not appreciably delayed. The disparity may be due to the fact that barium fluoroscopy measures fasting transit time whereas the radioscintigraphic method measures fed transit time. Alternatively it could be that barium suspension, being a liquid, is affected to a lesser extent than the solid component of chyme by intestinal dysmotility.

Measurement of small bowel transit in patients with intestinal dysmotility is a useful method for evaluating the efficacy of therapeutic drugs that stimulate propulsive activity. The prokinetic agent cisapride helps normalize impaired intestinal transit of chyme in patients with chronic idiopathic pseudo-obstruction syndrome. This drug was shown to stimulate transit of both the liquid and the solid phases of chyme: Gastric emptying was also stimulated although the effect was most noticeable during the post-lag emptying phase.

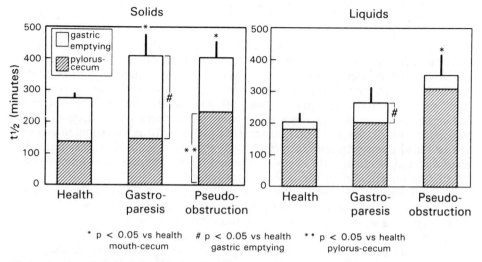

Figure 4 Gut transit in regional motor dysfunction defined manometrically. Note that prolongation of orocecal transit of the solid phase of a meal is comparable in gastroparesis and pseudo-obstruction. In the former this is due to delayed gastric emptying whereas in the latter this is due to prolonged small bowel transit. Reproduced with permission from Camilleri M, Brown ML, Malagelada J-R. Impaired transit of chyme in chronic intestinal pseudo-obstruction. *Gastroenterology* 1986; **91**: 619–26.

Interpretation of manometric and radioscintigraphic measurements — potential pitfalls

The methods described here for evaluation of small intestinal motor function are relatively new procedures and as such are subject to potential technical and interpretative pitfalls.

Technical problems associated with gastrointestinal manometry occur primarily in relation to the configuration and positioning of the manometric assembly. The pneumohydraulic and strain-gauge systems generally cause no problems. For successful intestinal manometry, particularly of the distal small bowel, perfusion tubes must be both thin and flexible enough to adapt to the shape of the bowel without stretching it, but firm enough to prevent bending at sharp angles. Positioning of the manometric assembly must be accomplished within a reasonable period of time to prevent fatigue and nausea.

As it is usually important to obtain antral manometric recordings at the same time as intestinal recordings, care must be taken to place several recording ports across the antroduodenal junction. The variation in the lengths of small bowel from patient to patient makes it usually impossible to simultaneously place recording sites at the pylorus and at the ileocecal valve. The most practical approach is to position the tube by reference to the antroduodenal junction and to eliminate any tube slack in the stomach that could result in later displacement of the recording sites.

Interpretation of intestinal manometric tracings can be hampered by artefacts caused by some of these technical problems. It is risky to attempt to draw conclusions from poor quality recordings, particularly those which show a 'wandering baseline' or fail to demonstrate the fine respiratory movement characteristic of good tracings. More substantial difficulty is posed by the correct interpretation of abnormal patterns of motility recorded by manometry. Whereas reasonable experience has been gained with motility patterns in healthy individuals, an adequate number of 'disease controls' is still lacking, i.e. individuals with illnesses apparently unrelated to the gut who may nevertheless exhibit motility patterns at variance with those observed in healthy volunteers. Pathologic patterns in some conditions, for instance in intestinal pseudo-obstruction, have been analyzed in relatively large numbers of affected subjects.[5] Unfortunately, such conditions are defined on the basis of clinical criteria and it is unknown whether they involve one or several different pathologic entities. Important and common conditions, such as diarrhea syndromes, barely have been studied. Also, alterations of intestinal motility due to lesions at different levels of control (for instance brain tumours, autonomic neuropathy or myenteric plexus disease) may be associated with similar abnormal manometric patterns. Thus, intestinal manometry can be relied upon primarily to establish whether contractile activity is normal or abnormal and to identify the segment affected by the disorder. It is less helpful in elucidating the etiology of the motor disturbance.

Radioscintigraphic transit studies may also be hampered with technical and interpretative difficulties. Input of radiolabelled markers into the small bowel can usually be determined accurately by measuring disappearance of activity from the stomach area. On the other hand, input into the colon is subjected to potential error (particularly in the early phases) since ileal loops may overlap with the cecal area. Computer fitting of the curves can help minimize the problems by taking into account the entire profile of the transfer of marker from one compartment into the other. Estimation of depth presents another important problem since stomach and colon are not on the same plane. A possible solution is to use a dual camera system (anterior and posterior). Another possibility is the mathematical adjustment of the input and output curves.[8]

Realistic interpretation of transit studies needs to take into account the special conditions under which the studies were performed. Test meals for transit studies tend to be small. Markers, unlike ordinary food, are not absorbed. Thus, liquid-phase markers travel along the gut dissolved in intraluminal fluid which is continuously renovated by absorption and secretion. When solid-phase markers are incorporated into a digestible food such as liver or egg they are gradually released into the aqueous intestinal phase thus becoming liquid-phase markers. This latter problem can be circumvented by employing a radiolabelled solid marker such as ^{131}I-fibre that passes through the gut intact.[8,14]

It is theoretically possible to perform simultaneous manometric and radioscintigraphic transit studies. In practice most human volunteers find it uncomfortable, particularly if solid meals are to be ingested and the studies last over 6 hours. Performing manometric and transit studies on two different days is an acceptable compromise. Technology, in any event, is not at the point where minute-to-minute correlations between motility and movement of content over short segments of gut can be performed in humans, as is already possible in experimental animals. Progress, however, is rapid and such fine measurements perhaps with the assistance of sophisticated computers may become feasable in the near future.

References
1 Malagelada J-R, Stanghellini V. Manometric evaluation of functional upper gut symptoms. *Gastroenterology* 1985; **88**: 1223–31.
2 Malagelada J-R, Camilleri M, Stanghellini V. *Manometric Diagnosis of Gastrointestinal Motility Disorders*. New York: Thieme-Stratton Inc. 1986.
3 Summers RW, Anuras S, Green J. Jejunal manometry patterns in health, partial intestinal obstruction and pseudo-obstruction. *Gastroenterology* 1983; **85**: 1290–300.
4 Kummar D, Wingate DL. The irritable bowel syndrome: a paroxysmal motor disorder. *Lancet* 1985; **ii**: 973–7.

5 Stanghellini V, Camilleri M, Malagelada J-R. Chronic idiopathic intestinal pseudo-obstruction: clinical and intestinal manometric findings. *Gut* 1987; **28:** 5–12.

6 Reese WD, Leigh RJ, Christofides ND, Bloom SR, Turnberg LA. Interdigestive motor activity in patients with systemic sclerosis. *Gastroenterology* 1982; **83:** 575–80.

7 Mathias JR, Fernandez A, Sninsky CA, Clench MH, Davis RH. Nausea, vomiting and abdominal pain after Roux-en-Y anastomosis: motility of the jejunal limb. *Gastroenterology* 1985; **88:** 101–7.

8 Malagelada J-R, Robertson JS, Brown ML *et al.* Intestinal transit of solid and liquid components of a meal in health. *Gastroenterology* 1984; **87:** 1255–63.

9 Thomforde GM, Brown ML, Malagelada J-R. Practical solid and liquid phase markers for studying gastric emptying in man. *J Nucl Med Tech* 1985; **13:** 11–4.

10 Jacobs F, Akkermans LMA, Yoe OH, Hoekstra A, Wittebol P. A radioisotope method to quantify the function of fundus, antrum and their contractile activity in gastric emptying of a semi-solid meal. In: Weinbeck EM, ed. *Motility of the Digestive Tract.* New York: Raven Press 1982; 233–40.

11 Camilleri M, Malagelada J-R, Brown ML, Becker G, Zinsmeister AR. Relation between antral motility and gastric emptying of solids and liquids in humans. *Am J Physiol* 1985; **249:** G580–5.

12 Elashoff JD, Reedy TJ, Meyer JH. Analysis of gastric emptying data. *Gastroenterology* 1982; **83:** 1306–12.

13 Read NW, Al-Janabi MN, Edwards CA, Barber DC. Relationship between postprandial motor activity in the human small intestine and the gastrointestinal transit of food. *Gastroenterology* 1984; **86:** 721–7.

14 Camilleri M, Brown ML, Malagelada J-R. Impaired transit of chyme in chronic intestinal pseudo-obstruction. *Gastroenterology* 1986; **91:** 619–26.

Investigation and diagnosis of colonic motility disorders

W J Snape Jr

Recent studies have shown that slow waves, spike potentials and accompanying contractions control the flow of luminal contents from the cecum to the rectum.[1] As a result of these studies, further work has been conducted whereby myoelectric activity recorded from human subjects using different types of electrodes has been evaluated using computer technology. *Figure 1* shows a graphical printout of digitized slow wave activity recorded from a patient. Using the digitized data, various slow wave frequencies can be calculated. The slow wave is the pacemaker which sets the frequency at which contractions occur. Spike potentials occur on specific portions of the slow wave cycle. The spike potential initiates contractions by increasing calcium influx into the cell.

From the digitized record, the slow wave activity in various specific frequency bins can be calculated, using Fourier analysis or peak analysis.[2] In this way, it is possible to calculate either an average slow wave frequency over a long period of time or a minute-to-minute slow wave frequency over a short period of time. The information obtained from recording slow wave activity may be extended by the use of various analytic techniques.

Recently, studies have been performed to correlate movement of luminal contents using scintigraphy with changes in manometry and myoelectric activity. During the fasting post-prandial period, the radioisotope that is injected into the splenic flexure remains in the splenic flexure. However, post-prandially, the material moves both proximally and distally.[3] These observations confirm and extend the observations that pellets ingested on different days become mixed in the right side of the colon and are excreted together at various different time periods.[4] The movement of the colonic contents is dependent upon the pressure activity within the colon. The higher pressure within the descending colon pushes material into the transverse colon. Thus, the pressure differential between different areas within the colon determines the movement of material through the colon.

Diagnosing disease

Measurement of myoelectric activity, intraluminal pressure and transit can be used to diagnose certain diseases. Healthy individuals and patients with irritable bowel syndrome or diverticular disease have different patterns of motility. The alteration in motility may be responsible for the abdominal discomfort and alteration in bowel habit associated with the irritable bowel syndrome or diverticular disease. The mean slow wave frequency differs between the groups. However, there is a large scatter of the data. The data suggest that the patients within the irritable bowel syndrome and diverticular groups are not homogeneous. This heterogeneity within each patient population creates a difficulty in characterizing and cataloguing patients with various motility patterns.

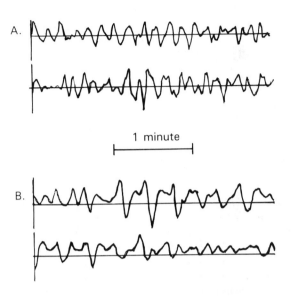

A.

1 minute

B.

Figure 1   Graphical representation of digitized wave activity from (A) a
healthy subject and (B) a patient with the irritable bowel syndrome.

The question arises whether changes in slow wave frequency influence the changes
in the physiologic function of the organ. It is expected that a change in the overall
rhythm of the slow wave activity in an organ will change the pattern and frequency
of the contractile activity. The change in the contractile pattern which occurs in the
irritable bowel syndrome may initiate an abnormal contractile pattern. The increase
in the 3 cycle/minute slow wave activity can be translated into an increase in 3 cy-
cle/minute contractile activity.[5] This may have some significance in the overall
pathologic or pathophysiologic component of a given patient's disease. As more is
understood about the transit of luminal contents within the colon, these changes in
motility and their role in diseases of the colon may become more significant.

Another important component of colonic physiology is the colonic motor response
to a meal. *Figure 2* shows slow wave activity with the spike potential superimposed
upon slow wave activity and the concomitant increase in intraluminal pressure which
occurred 20 minutes after a 10 kcal meal. Fat is the dietary component which is most
responsible for stimulating post-prandial colonic motility.[6]

Neural control of the GI tract
Myoelectric recordings allow general observations to be made about the control of
colonic motility by the brain, the spinal cord and other parts of the gastrointestinal
tract. There are neural connections between the brain and the colon.[7] An increase
in stress increases motility in the distal and most probably in the proximal regions
of the colon.[8] After eating a meal, an increase in motility occurs in the transverse
and distal colon, and probably in the more proximal regions of the colon also. The
increase in motility can be mediated by two effects. First, circulating neuropeptides
can be released into the plasma. Second, a local neurotransmitter can be released
through a spinal reflex. Glick and co-workers showed that transection of the spinal

Myoelectrical

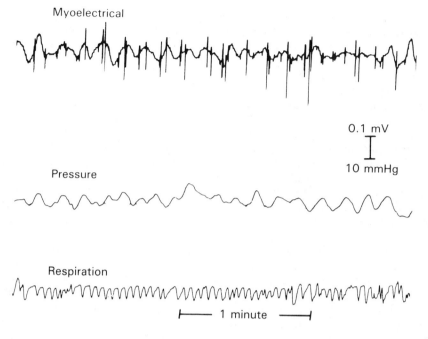

0.1 mV

10 mmHg

Pressure

Respiration

├─── 1 minute ───┤

Figure 2 Myoelectrical and intraluminal pressure tracing from a healthy subject who had eaten a 10 kcal meal 20 minutes before.

column abolished the gastrocolonic response.[9] This reflex may be mediated by various neurotransmitters, acetylcholine, substance P, enkephalin or bombesin, released locally. The complexity of this system is expanded since each of the stimulatory compounds, such as substance P, neurotensin, bombesin, the enkephalins and acetylcholine, affect smooth muscle cells in a different manner. They alter different membrane functions and alter different ionic functions through the ionic channels.[10,11] The agents can change both the rhythm and also potentially the contractility of these smooth muscle cells.[12]

Colonic motility diseases

Since the control mechanisms are very complex, it is not surprising that various disease states occur as one or more limbs of the controls of colonic motility are altered. When a healthy subject eats a 1000 kcal meal, there is an immediate increase in spike activity during the first 30 post-prandial minutes. In patients with the irritable bowel syndrome, there is a different pattern of increase of colonic spike and contractile activity.[13] The motor activity is delayed, occurring from 60–90 minutes after the meal. The abnormal response is not caused by slow gastric emptying, because in these particular patients no abnormality in gastric emptying is found. It appears that an abnormality may exist within either the spinal cord or the myenteric plexus which control the function of the smooth muscle organ.

In another group of patients constipation occurs secondary to colonic inertia. This group of patients shows no increase in the post-prandial response of colonic spike activity or contractile activity. Two disease states associated with colonic inertia are progressive systemic sclerosis and diabetes mellitus.[14,15]

Patients with progressive systemic sclerosis can be divided into two groups. There are those patients who, when stimulated directly through neostigmine by blocking acetylcholine-esterase function, or metoclopramide, can respond; these patients have normal smooth muscle. The second group of patients have the myopathic form of scleroderma in which the collagen tissue has replaced the smooth muscle. Colonic motility studies must be performed to differentiate these two groups of patients with progressive systemic sclerosis.

The same type of gastrocolonic response can be seen in patients with diabetes mellitus. In patients with severe constipation, who move their bowels less than two times a week, the gastrocolonic response is absent, whereas a normal gastrocolonic response is found in those patients who have no constipation. This difference in the response to colonic motility gives an indication as to whether the patient can be treated or not. Patients who have severe constipation and an abnormal gastrocolonic response show an improvement in their bowel habit when given a prokinetic agent.

Colonic motility may be disturbed in patients with inflammatory bowel disease, specifically ulcerative colitis.[16,17] In patients with ulcerative colitis the gastrocolonic spike response is slightly decreased. However, there is a marked lack of contraction of the smooth muscle in these patients. It is uncertain whether this response is an abnormality in the smooth muscle itself, or there is an inability of the smooth muscle to contract because of inflammatory cells or an alteration in the passive elastic components within the muscle wall. In colonic smooth muscle removed from patients with ulcerative colitis there is a decrease in the contraction. Under certain characteristics of electrical field stimulation the muscle of these patients will contract. However, the pharmacologic stimulation of this tissue, with either bethanechol or potassium, is decreased. In this group of patients, there may well be a very specific abnormality in the membrane or post-membrane event which is necessary to initiate a contraction. Binding of acetylcholine or another neurotransmitter to a receptor or the initiation of the actin-myosin cross bridge system may be disturbed in muscle from these patients.

Abnormalities in anal sphincter control may predispose patients to an alteration in their bowel habit which stimulates changes in colonic motility. Following an appearance of the fecal bolus within the rectum, the internal anal sphincter relaxes and the external anal sphincter contracts. Disturbance of this spinal reflex will produce symptoms of constipation.

Studies evaluating the presence of the myenteric plexus and the intact neural reflex controlling the anal sphincter can be performed using motility recordings. A motility probe is placed at both the internal and the external anal sphincter. Distension of a rectal balloon initiates the normal anorectal reflexes of internal anal sphincter relaxation and external sphincter contraction.

This reflex can be disturbed in patients with Hirschsprung's disease and occasionally in some patients with a form of irritable bowel syndrome.

Using the techniques of scintigraphy, manometry and myoelectric activity recording, it is possible to predict the response of various broad patient groups with various broad disease states and to classify these patients. Such techniques may, in time, allow further drugs to be developed which will specifically treat these conditions.

References

1 Christensen J. Myoelectric control of the colon. *Gastroenterology* 1975; **68**: 601–9.
2 Suchowiecky M, Clarke DD, Bhsker M, Perry RJ, Snape WJ Jr. Effect of secoverine on colonic myoelectric activity in diverticular disease of the colon. *Dig Dis Sci* (In press).
3 Moreno-Osset E, Lo S, Lambert P, Ristow E, Mena I, Snape WJ Jr. Correlation between colonic transit and colonic motility in normal human volunteers. *Gastroenterology* 1987; **92**: 1540.
4 Wiggins HS, Cummings JH. Evidence for the mixing of residue in the human gut. *Gut* 1976; **17**: 1007–11.

5 Snape WJ Jr, Carlson GM, Matarazzo SA, Cohen S. Evidence that normal myoelectric activity produces colonic motor dysfunction in the irritable bowel syndrome. *Gastroenterology* 1977; **72**: 383-7.
6 Wright SH, Snape WJ Jr, Battle W, Cohen S, London RL. Effect of dietary components on gastrocolonic response. *Am J Physiol* 1980; **238**: G228-32.
7 Rostad H. Colonic motility in the cat/IV. Peripheral pathways mediating the effects induced by hypothalamic and mesencephalic stimulation. *Acta Physiol Scand* 1973; **89**: 154-68.
8 Narducci F, Snape WJ Jr, Battle WM, London RL, Cohen S. Increased colonic motility during exposure to a stressful situation. *Dig Dis Sci* 1985; **30**: 40-4.
9 Glick ME, Meshkinpour H, Haldeman S, Hoehler F, Downey N, Bradley WE. Colonic dysfunction in patients with thoracic spinal cord injury. *Gastroenterology* 1984; **86**: 287-94.
10 Sims SM, Walsh JV Jr, Singer JJ. Substance P and acetylcholine both suppress the same K+ current in dissociated smooth muscle cells. *Am J Physiol* 1986; **251**: C580-7.
11 Snape WJ Jr, Tan ST, Kao HW. Mechanism of neurotensin depolarization of rabbit colonic smooth muscle. *Regul Peptides* (In press).
12 Snape WJ Jr, Tan ST, Kao HW. Effects of bethanechol and the octapeptide of cholecystokinin on colonic smooth muscle in the cat. *Am J Physiol* 1987; **252**: G654-61.
13 Sullivan MA, Cohen S, Snape WJ Jr. Colonic myoelectrical activity in irritable bowel syndrome: effect of eating and anticholinergics. *N Engl J Med* 1978; **298**: 878-83.
14 Battle WM, Snape WJ Jr, Wright S, Sullivan MA, Cohen S, Myers A, Tuthill R. Abnormal colonic motility in progressive systemic sclerosis. *Ann Int Med* 1981; **97**: 749-52.
15 Battle WM, Snape WJ Jr, Alavi A, Cohen S, Braunstein S. Colonic dysfunction in diabetes mellitus. *Gastroenterology* 1980; **79**: 1217-21.
16 Snape WJ Jr, Matarazzo SA, Cohen S. Abnormal gastrocolic response in patients with ulcerative colitis. *Gut* 1980; **21**: 392-6.
17 Cohen JD, Kao HW, Tan ST, Lechago J, Snape WJ Jr. Effect of acute experimental colitis on rabbit colonic smooth muscle. *Am J Physiol* 1986; **251**: G538-45.

Histopathology of gastrointestinal motility disorders

M D Schuffler

Throughout its length, the gastrointestinal tract is invested with smooth muscle coats. The contractions of the smooth muscle are necessary to produce a variety of functions:
- transport in the esophagus
- prevention of gastroesophageal reflux through competence of the lower esophageal sphincter
- mixing and emptying in the stomach
- mixing and transport in the small intestine
- mixing, storage and transport in the colon
- anal continence
- defecation.

Each of these functions requires that the smooth muscle be programmed when to contract, how strongly to contract and in which direction to contract. The duration of contraction, the length of intestine over which the contraction is propagated and the timing of relaxation must also be programmed. The computer system which regulates this contractility is the nervous system innervating the smooth muscle. Most of this nervous system is located in the myenteric plexus (located between the circular and longitudinal muscles) and the submucosal plexus within the intestinal wall. These plexuses contain millions of neurons and nerve fibres.

The extrinsic nervous system which innervates the gastrointestinal tract is also important in the regulation of contractility. The vagus nerves play a role in esophageal peristalsis, the opening of the lower esophageal sphincter and gastric emptying. Recent animal experiments have revealed that the prevertebral ganglia (celiac, superior and inferior mesenteric ganglia) play an important role in processing and integrating information from the central nervous system and intestine, particularly from the colon. These ganglia help to modulate colonic transport.

On a morphologic basis, extrinsic innervation in man is prominent in the esophagus, stomach and rectum, but is not at all prominent in the small intestine or in the colon proximal to the rectosigmoid. Thus, intrinsic control mechanisms would seem to be of great importance in the regulation of motility throughout the small intestine and most of the colon, whereas intrinsic plus extrinsic control mechanisms would be of more importance in the esophagus, stomach and rectosigmoid.

Abnormalities of the smooth muscle or myenteric plexus result in a number of neuromuscular disorders of the gastrointestinal tract depending on the location and distribution of the abnormalities. When the myenteric plexus of the esophagus is damaged, the clinical syndrome of achalasia is produced and when the myenteric plexus of the rectum or rectosigmoid is congenitally absent, Hirschsprung's disease results. Damage of the myenteric plexus of the stomach produces gastroparesis and damage of the myenteric plexus of the small intestine produces intestinal pseudo-obstruction. Abnormalities of the myenteric plexus throughout the colon produce severe constipation with or without colonic pseudo-obstruction. These abnormalities of the myenteric plexus may be localized, as in achalasia or Hirschsprung's disease, or may be diffuse throughout the gastrointestinal tract, as in a number of pseudo-obstruction syndromes. In addition, disorders of the myenteric plexus may be limited to the gastrointestinal tract, or they may be but one component of generalized neurological illnesses affecting the central, peripheral and/or autonomic nervous systems.

Disorders of gastrointestinal smooth muscle may be easily recognized by light microscopy. They may be part of systemic illnesses, such as progressive systemic sclerosis, polymyositis or amyloidosis; or they may be limited to the gastrointestinal tract, as in some cases of familial or sporadic visceral myopathies.

Structure of the normal myenteric plexus and smooth muscle

The myenteric plexus (Auerbach's plexus) is a mesh-like structure located between the circular and longitudinal muscles. It contains millions of neurons which congregate in ganglia, which are the areas at which the arms of the mesh come together. The arms of the mesh contain hundreds of nerve fibres relaying information from one ganglion to another and to the smooth muscle. The submucosal plexus (Meissner's plexus) is considered to relay afferent information to the myenteric plexus and smooth muscle as well as playing a role in the mucosal regulation of salt and water absorption and secretion.

In conventional hematoxylin and eosin (H & E) sections of the gastrointestinal tract, the myenteric plexus is visualized in cross-section between the two muscle layers. The myenteric plexus is oriented in a longitudinal direction and its neurons are congregated within ganglia which are separated from one another. Therefore, conventional light microscopy is ill-suited to study this structure because the perpendicularly cut sections allow only a tiny amount of plexus to be visualized. Neuronal morphology is also difficult to evaluate with this technique and neuronal processes and nerve fibres remain unstained.

If, on the other hand, thicker, larger sections are cut in the plane of the plexus, and then stained with silver, a large sample size of well-stained neurons and nerve processes is obtained. The layout of the mesh can be seen and nerve tracts full of fibres can be followed from one ganglion to another. Neuron morphology is sharply defined and abnormalities can be readily appreciated. This technique was developed by Smith, who applied it to a large number of motility disorders.[1] Neurons, axons, dendrites and nerve fibres vary in staining from light tan to deep black in colour; background muscle stains brown. Esophageal nerve fibres are a mixture of fine intrinsic fibres and thick, darker staining extrinsic fibres. Neurons vary in stain uptake from intense (argyrophilic) to weak (argyrophobic). Argyrophilic neurons in the esophagus are full bodied, round to elliptical in shape and have many short dendrites and occasional long axons. Argyrophobic cells are generally round, vary in size and have no visible processes. Small intestinal neurons are more pleomorphic and contain fewer dendrites; colonic neurons are even more pleomorphic. Small intestinal and colonic nerve tracts are composed mainly of fine intrinsic fibres; the lower sigmoid and rectum have more extrinsic fibres as well.

The muscularis propria of the esophagus, small intestine and colon is organized into two layers, an inner circular muscle and an outer longitudinal muscle. The stomach is more complex, with three layers in the fundus gradually merging into two layers in the antrum. The longitudinal muscle of the colon is thicker within the three taenia and may be quite thin between the taenia.

When cut in cross section, smooth muscle fibres have distinct borders which vary from round to irregular, depending on the state of contractility at the time of fixation. If completely relaxed, they will be round, and if contracted, irregular. Post mortem autolysis creates changes varying from swollen, densely stained fibres to ill-defined, poorly stained fibres. When visualized in longitudinal section, the fibres are of variable length and smooth to irregular in contour.

Normally, there may be some strands of collagen breaking the circular muscle up into bundles. However, this should be minimal in amount and have the appearance of septae. Collagen should not be present diffusely throughout the muscle.

The morphologic study of smooth muscle cells requires that the sections be thin (4 μm) and well-stained. Fixing the tissue in Hollande's solution and use of a modified H & E stain intense in eosin brings out the colour of the muscle cells. Because collagen may be difficult to distinguish from smooth muscle cells, some sections are stained with Masson's trichrome. This distinguishes between the scarlet staining muscle and blue staining collagen. Proper interpretation of smooth muscle is impossible unless these techniques are adhered to.

The classification of neuromuscular disorders with recogniable abnormalities of the myenteric plexus or smooth muscle are listed in *Tables 1* and *2*, and described in detail below.

Sporadic visceral neuropathies
  Idiopathic achalasia
  Chagas' disease
  Intestinal pseudo-obstruction
    — Noninflammatory degenerative neuropathies
    — Inflammatory degenerative neuropathies
      (i) Paraneoplastic, associated with small cell carcinoma or carcinoid of the lung
      (ii) Inflammatory axonopathy
  Myotonic dystrophy

Familial visceral neuropathies
  With neuronal intranuclear inclusions, autosomal recessive
  With mental retardation and basal ganglia calcifications, autosomal recessive
  With neither of above, autosomal dominant

Developmental abnormalities
  Hirschsprung's disease
  Total aganglionosis of colon ± the small intestine
  Neuronal intestinal dysplasia
  Maturational arrest at varying stages of development, ± mental retardation or other neurologic abnormalities.

Severe, idiopathic constipation

Diffuse small intestinal diverticulosis
  With neuronal intranuclear inclusions
  Fabry's disease

Amyloidosis

Toxic damage
  Laxatives
  Phenothiazines?
  Vinca alkaloids? } Little is known about these disorders
  Anticholinergics?

Table 1 Disorders of the myenteric plexus.

Primary
   Familial visceral myopathies
      — Autosomal dominant
      — Autosomal recessive (with ptosis and external ophthalmoplegia)
      — Autosomal recessive (with total GI tract dilatation)

   Sporadic visceral myopathies

Secondary
   Progressive systemic sclerosis/polymyositis
   Progressive muscular dystrophy
   Amyloidosis
   Ceroidosis?

Diffuse lymphoid infiltration

Diffuse small intestinal diverticulosis
   With muscle resembling visceral myopathy
   With muscle resembling progressive systemic sclerosis

Table 2 Disorders of smooth muscle.

Disorders of the myenteric plexus

Achalasia

A variety of pathologic abnormalities have been described in achalasia, including degenerative changes in the dorsal vagal nucleus, the vagus nerve and the esophageal myenteric plexus. The changes in the myenteric plexus are the most convincing and consist of a variable loss of neurons, sometimes accompanied by round cell infiltration. Using the silver technique, there is a loss of both argyrophilic and argyrophobic neurons.[1] Residual neurons appear degenerated, ie, they may have waxy or vacuolated cytoplasm and swollen, irregular, clubbed processes. Intrinsic nerve fibres are reduced in number, with the nerve tracts containing argyrophilic debris and a proliferation of Schwann cells.

It is probable that achalasia has a number of etiologies and a continuum of pathologic changes. It is possible that during the early course of the illness, round cells attack the plexus. As the plexus is destroyed, it may be replaced by Schwann cell scar, with no evidence of the abnormal cells which were present earlier. This hypothesis is difficult to prove and would require study of a large number of post mortem esophagi from patients with achalasia.

Chagas' disease

Chagas' disease is caused by the parasite *Trypanosoma cruzi*, which elicits an immune cell response which cross reacts with the myenteric plexus and thereby injures it. All areas of the intestine may be involved, with the esophagus and colon being most frequently affected. An achalasia-like illness is produced from the esophageal involvement, intractable constipation and megacolon results from the colonic involvement, and intestinal pseudo-obstruction is produced from small intestinal involvement. Pathologic processes include smooth muscle hypertrophy, infiltration of the myenteric plexus by lymphocytes and plasma cells, loss of both argyrophilic and argyrophobic neurons, degenerated argyrophilic neurons with swollen and irregular processes, and axonal destruction and dropout.[1] Thus, Chagas' disease produces an inflammatory neuropathy of the myenteric plexus, which is similar in appearance to the paraneoplastic visceral neuropathy described below.

Intestinal pseudo-obstruction syndromes

Noninflammatory degenerative sporadic visceral neuropathy: this is an imperfect term used to designate a form of chronic idiopathic intestinal pseudo-obstruction caused by at least two degenerative disorders of the myenteric plexus of the entire gastrointestinal tract.[2-4] It is not familial and does not involve the nervous system extrinsic to the gastrointestinal tract. The following case example illustrates the histologic findings. The patient was a 63-year-old man who had a subtotal colectomy and ileorectal anastomosis in an attempt to relieve severe obstipation and gaseous distension that was elevating his diaphragm to the point of respiratory compromise.

H & E serial sections appeared to show a decrease in the number of neurons, but this decrease could not be determined positively. Neuronal morphology was also difficult to interpret by this technique. Silver stains of longitudinal sections of the myenteric plexus, on the other hand, demonstrated a number of abnormalities which were patchy in occurrence, with some sections containing a normal or near normal plexus. Abnormalities consisted of neuronal swelling and fragmentation, neuron dropout, fragmentation and dropout of axons, and replacement of areas of the plexus by a proliferation of Schwann cells. Such areas were devoid of neurons and only a few axons remained.

Normally by this technique, neurons are irregular, often pyramidal in shape and have cell boundaries that are sharply defined and slightly concave. A number of distinct tapering processes emanate from the nerve bodies. In contrast, in this patient some neurons were swollen 2–3 times the size of control neurons, their cell boundaries were rounded and indistinct, and fewer processes were present. Many processes which were present were thickened and disorganized.

A second distinct type of sporadic visceral neuropathy was recently encountered in which degeneration of both the argyrophilic and argyrophobic neurons imparted a clearing to the neuronal cytoplasm, producing an appearance somewhat like signet ring cells.[4] Axonal degeneration was also present, but there were no intranuclear inclusions, no dendritic swellings, no inflammatory cells and no proliferation of Schwann cells.

Paraneoplastic visceral neuropathy associated with lung cancer: there have been several reports of this type of visceral neuropathy, usually in association with other neurologic manifestations of small cell carcinoma of the lung.[5,6] In 6 cases associated with small cell carcinoma of the lung and 1 case associated with a pulmonary carcinoid, all had intestinal pseudo-obstruction and obstipation/constipation; 6 had gastroparesis; 4 had esophageal peristaltic abnormalities; 2 had neurogenic bladders, autonomic insufficiency and peripheral neuropathy; 5 had dilated small bowel, 6 exhibited slow barium transit; 2 had dilated colons and 2 had slow colonic transit. Five of the patients died 4 to 9 months after onset of GI symptoms, while 2 survived. In 6 patients the myenteric plexus showed neuron and axon degeneration and dropout, lymphoplasmacytic infiltration and Schwann cell proliferation. An antrectomy from the seventh patient showed inflammatory cells without neuron dropout. Many nerve fibre abnormalities were present, consisting of axonal swellings, axonal fragmentation and frank dropout of axons. In some nerve tracts, axons were completely replaced by a Schwann cell 'scar'.

It is hypothesized that the plasma cells and lymphocytes mediated the injury to the plexus. This intestinal neuropathy may be the explanation for Ogilvie's syndrome, a colonic pseudo-obstruction originally described by Ogilvie in 1948 in association with metastatic cancer.

Inflammatory axonopathy: this recently encountered disorder proved fatal to a 39-year-old man just 3 months after his initial symptoms of pseudo-obstruction.[7] The myenteric plexus contained lymphocytes and plasma cells throughout the gastrointestinal tract. Although neurons were normal in appearance and numbers, axons demonstrated beading, fragmentation and dropout. There was no distant carcinoma. Thus, pseudo-obstruction was produced by axonal destruction within the plexus, in the absence of significant damage to neuron bodies.

Familial visceral neuropathy with neuronal intranuclear inclusions: this condition occurred in the only two children of a non-consanguineous marriage.[8] Both patients had diffuse neurologic abnormalities, mild autonomic insufficiency, symptoms of pseudo-obstruction of 40 years' duration and denervation hypersensitivity of pupillary and esophageal smooth muscles. Radiography showed chaotic, repetitive and spontaneous contractions of the entire esophagus; hyperactive contractions of dilated small intestine; and extensive diverticular disease of the colon.

Both patients eventually died and autopsies were performed. Smooth muscle throughout the intestinal tract was normal and no fibrosis was evident. The myenteric plexus, on the other hand, was characterized by diffuse abnormalities. Conventional light microscopy of serial sections of samples from the esophagus, stomach, small intestine and colon showed a significant reduction of neurons, approximately one-third of which contained a prominent intranuclear inclusion which was mildly eosinophilic. These inclusions were shown by histochemistry to contain protein, but no DNA or RNA. By electron microscopy, they were found to be composed of a random array of straight to slightly curving filaments, which were somewhat indistinct, but seemed to have beading at a periodicity of 15–30 nm and a diameter of 17–27 nm. They did not resemble any known viral inclusions. The inclusions were also present in the neurons of the submucosal plexus and could be found on mucosal rectal biopsy. Neuropathologic examination of the brain, spinal cord, peripheral nerves and autonomic nervous system revealed the same type of neuronal inclusions.

Silver stains of longitudinal sections of the myenteric plexus showed markedly decreased numbers of neurons and nerve fibres. Some nerve tracts contained only one or two axons whereas normal nerve tracts contain 50–100 axons. Most neurons were abnormally shaped and virtually none had a normal number of axons and dendrites. Particularly striking was the presence in the esophagus of some neurons with swollen, clubbed dendrites. No inflammatory cells were seen within the plexus and no proliferation of Schwann cells was apparent.

Thus, these two patients presented with intestinal symptoms caused by an abnormal process within the myenteric plexus. This process was but one component of a more generalized neurologic illness. The intestinal symptoms were the first to appear and remained the patients' most prominent source of disability throughout their lives. Eight additional cases of neuronal intranuclear inclusion disease have been reported subsequently in the neurology literature. In contrast to the above two patients, these additional cases have presented with extraintestinal neurologic symptoms. Two additional cases with intestinal involvement have been evaluated personally, one of whom had diffuse small intestinal diverticulosis.

Familial visceral neuropathy with mental retardation and calcifications of the basal ganglia: this condition was described in four siblings of a sibship of 16.[9] They had malabsorption, mental retardation, calcifications of the basal ganglia and episodes of pseudo-obstruction. The smooth muscle was of normal to reduced thickness. On silver staining, argyrophilic neurons were reduced in number and argyrophobic neurons were degenerated. Axons appeared normal.

Autosomal dominant visceral neuropathy: two families have been reported with this syndrome.[10] In both reports patients had intestinal pseudo-obstruction affecting predominantly the small intestine, without evidence of central, autonomic or peripheral nervous system involvement.

Upon H & E staining, the intestinal smooth muscle layers were found to be slightly thickened and the neurons did not contain any inclusions. Silver stains showed degeneration and a decrease in the number of neurons and axons. Many ganglia contained only one or two neurons, some of which were swollen, distorted, vacuolated and had decreased argyrophilia. Some nerve fibres were hypertrophied and had swellings, or were beaded and distributed haphazardly through the muscle. No inflammatory cells or glial cell proliferation was noted.[10]

Maturational arrest: arrested development of the myenteric plexus *in utero* can produce severe hypomotility in infants, requiring prolonged hospitalization and a long-term commitment to home parenteral nutrition. The pathologic findings vary, depending on the degree of immaturity. There may only be clusters of rudimentary neurons in areas corresponding to ganglia without development of nerve processes or nerve tracts; or there may be further development with nerve tracts in place but with few axons in them and few neurons with well developed processes; or there may be greater development of both neurons and nerve tracts but without a normal number of fully developed neurons. These abnormalities can be associated with neurologic abnormalities, including mental retardation in older children.

Hirschsprung's disease

Hirschsprung's disease is probably the most commonly encountered disorder of the myenteric plexus. It is caused by a failure *in utero* of the myenteric plexus to develop within the rectosigmoid. The plexus can be absent from a short segment of the rectum to virtually the entire colon. Most commonly, the plexus is abnormal within the rectum and distal sigmoid and normal above that. The involved segment of colon is contracted and has thickened muscle and the colon proximal to this is dilated and also has thickened muscle. Neurons are absent from the contracted segment and the rudimentary plexus which is present contains only an unmyelinated nerve fibre network that is extrinsic in origin.

Because the submucosal plexus of the rectum is also abnormal, mucosal rectal biopsy can be used as a diagnostic test. Two suction rectal biopsies are taken and serially sectioned. The absence of submucosal neurons in 120 H & E serial sections is a strong indicator of Hirschsprung's disease. If the diagnosis is still uncertain, a full thickness rectal biopsy can be taken in order to sample the myenteric plexus.

Severe idiopathic constipation and cathartic colon

A small proportion of those patients with constipation suffer severely with the condition, i.e. they may pass only one stool every 2–4 weeks despite cathartics and enemas.

Barium enemas will show some of these patients to have elongated, redundant colons; others have colons which are normal in appearance but which fail to evacuate the barium. In colectomy specimens taken from 20 such patients studied by B Smith, (unpublished data) 8 had abnormalities of the myenteric plexus which were ascribed to cathartic-induced damage in 5 cases.

These findings are consistent with a study of over 30 cases of severe constipation ± megacolon ± laxatives.[11] However, it was difficult to determine whether myenteric plexus damage existed in these 30 cases before laxative use or whether plexus damage was induced by laxatives. All the patients had a history of severe constipation before laxative use and the pathology did not resemble that described in the animal model of laxative injury.[12]

The myenteric plexus abnormalities found in these patients with severe idiopathic constipation included a loss of argyrophilic neurons, those remaining tending to be small and irregular and to have fewer processes.[11] They stained less intensely and more unevenly than normal and the edges of the cells tended to be indistinct. The ganglia contained numerous prominent, variably sized nuclei, many of which had very active chromatin. The cell bodies of these nuclei proved difficult to identify. They could be Schwann cells or immature neurons. Axons were also decreased in number and in some nerve tracts, slight axonal fragmentation and debris were apparent.

These features are common in these patients and may serve to distinguish this problem from other disorders of the myenteric plexus, including the visceral neuropathies producing intestinal pseudo-obstruction.

Amyloidosis

Amyloidosis can involve the myenteric plexus and thereby produce motility disturbances, particularly intestinal pseudo-obstruction.

Toxic damage

Evidence has been presented that mice given atropine, chlorpromazine or vinca alkaloids develop variable types of damage to the myenteric plexus (B Smith, unpublished data). It is well recognized that phenothiazines, vinca alkaloids, anticholinergics and tricyclic antidepressants can produce severe constipation in man. However, to what extent this constipation is caused by drug induced damage to the plexus is not yet known, and clinical studies are needed to determine whether such damage occurs in patients given these drugs.

Disorders of the smooth muscle

Primary disorders

Familial visceral myopathy (hereditary hollow visceral myopathy): the pathology of familial visceral myopathy is characterized by degeneration and thinning of smooth muscle, which can be readily appreciated on conventional H & E and trichrome stains.[13-19] Affected smooth muscle cells have a continuum of abnormalities including loss of stain intensity and indistinct cell boundaries which produce a smudged appearance in some areas. Frank cell fragmentation and dropout create spaces containing cell debris. Closely associated with this process is a variable amount of collagen deposition, ranging from mild to severe. When severe, an area of muscle is completely replaced by collagen, with no muscle cells or cell debris seen. Collagen is sometimes deposited around degenerating cells in such a way that the muscle takes on a distinctive honeycombed appearance readily appreciated at low magnification. This process is called 'vacuolar degeneration'. The severity and distribution of abnormalities vary from one sample site to another. In general, the longitudinal muscle is more affected than the circular and, in some areas, only the longitudinal muscle is affected. In addition, the same process may affect the smooth muscle of the bladder and ureters.

Electron microscopy shows a number of abnormalities which better define the process seen by light microscopy.[13] The earliest changes consist of dropout and disarray of myofilaments within the smooth muscle cells, such that the myofilaments do not align themselves in an orderly way with the dense bodies. This makes the cells appear electron lucent. As cells degenerate, their mitochondria swell, cell membranes disintegrate and cells lyse such that the muscle layer becomes filled with cellular debris. These areas fill in with collagen fibres and eventually areas are left which are extensively replaced with collagen.

Neurons, nerve processes and nerve terminals are normal in familial visceral myopathy. No acute inflammatory cells, lymphocytes or plasma cells are seen in the muscle coats and no vasculitis is present. Thus, visceral myopathy seems to be a pure disorder of smooth muscle, not mediated by inflammatory cells, vasculitis or neural disease.

Twelve families with familial visceral myopathies have been reported. Although the morphological abnormalities are identical in all families, the pattern of gastrointestinal and bladder involvement and the mode of genetic transmission has made several different expressions recognizable.

Type I familial visceral myopathy is transmitted as an autosomal dominant trait. It is characterized by esophageal dilatation, megaduodenum, redundant colon and megacystis. The stomach and small intestine distal to the duodenum are usually normal, although occasionally the jejunum may also be distended.

Type II familial visceral myopathy is transmitted as an autosomal recessive trait. It is characterized by dilatation of the stomach and small intestine along with numerous diverticula of the entire small intestine. Patients also have ptosis and external ophthalmoplegia, but they do not have a megacystis.

A third type of visceral myopathy occurred in a family with two involved siblings who had gastroparesis, a tubular, narrow small intestine and a normal esophagus and colon.

A fourth type of visceral myopathy occurred in a family with marked dilatation of the entire gastrointestinal tract from the esophagus to the rectum. The family history was suggestive of an autosomal recessive inheritance and no extraintestinal manifestations were observed.

Another family has members of three generations with the dysplastic nevus syndrome, visceral myopathy and multiple basal cell carcinomas. Affected family members have megaduodenums and bladder involvement.

Sporadic visceral myopathy: sporadic visceral myopathy can occur in individuals with no evidence of familial involvement.[20] The pathologic findings by light microscopy are identical to that of familial visceral myopathy. Sporadic visceral myopathy has also been identified in infants who died as a result of severe gastrointestinal hypomotility.

Undefined myopathies: there have been cases of myopathy that have not had familial involvement or the vacuolar degeneration described above. In these patients, smooth muscle coats are thin and fibrotic but they have no evidence for disorders such as progressive systemic sclerosis, polymyositis or myotonic dystrophy. Whether these cases represent progressive systemic sclerosis limited to the gastrointestinal tract or other yet undefined smooth muscle disorders remains to be determined.

Secondary disorders

Progressive systemic sclerosis/polymyositis: progressive systemic sclerosis (PSS) commonly involves intestinal smooth muscle and is the most common cause of intestinal pseudo-obstruction.[18,21] Although reports of gut involvement in polymyositis are rare, the pathology appears to be identical to that of PSS.

As in visceral myopathy, smooth muscle cells in PSS are fewer in number and the muscle layers are thinner than normal.[18] PSS can be differentiated usually from visceral myopathy, however. PSS is characterized by fibrosis of intestinal smooth muscle, but vacuolar degeneration is absent. Those muscle cells remaining are normal in appearance or are atrophied. In addition, the circular muscle is more involved in PSS whereas the longitudinal muscle is more involved in visceral myopathy. PSS also seems to be characterized by more patchy involvement; totally normal muscle may exist immediately adjacent to severely fibrotic muscle.

Progressive muscular dystrophy: gastrointestinal symptoms sometimes occur in patients with progressive muscular dystrophy.[22] In one case, a 15-year-old boy had dysphagia and attacks of intestinal pseudo-obstruction.[23] Radiography revealed a non-contractile esophagus, a lower esophageal diverticulum and a dilated small intestine. Upon autopsy, it was found that the intestinal smooth muscle had been replaced by collagen. This process was most prominent in the esophagus and stomach, but also involved the small intestine and colon. The condition appeared to be similar in appearance to PSS.

Amyloidosis: in addition to involving the myenteric plexus, amyloid can also infiltrate smooth muscle and thereby interfere with smooth muscle contractility. The muscularis mucosa, submucosal blood vessels and muscularis propia can all be involved.

Diffuse lymphoid infiltration
This syndrome was seen in four young women who presented with diarrhea, malabsorption and intestinal pseudo-obstruction.[24] Full thickness intestinal biopsies showed flat small intestinal mucosa, sparsity of crypts and widespread infiltration of lymphoid cells in the lamina propria, submucosa, serosa and muscularis propria. Although there were also scattered lymphoid cells in the myenteric plexus, there was no neuron or axon damage or loss. Absence of muscle cells in the vicinity of lymphoid cell infiltration in the muscularis propria probably accounts for the pathogenesis of pseudo-obstruction. Immunochemical stains showed that the infiltrate was polyclonal, and none of the patients has since developed lymphoma on clinical follow-up of 4 to 16 years.

Small intestinal diverticulosis
Small intestinal diverticulosis is a heterogenous disorder characterized by multiple diverticula which are most often located in the jejunum but which can also be present in the duodenum and ileum. There is evidence that the diverticula result from structural abnormalities of either the intestinal smooth muscle or myenteric plexus. These structural abnormalities often produce intestinal pseudo-obstruction.

Small intestinal diverticulosis is caused by at least four disorders of the smooth muscle and myenteric plexus.[25,26] One of the muscle disorders resembles progressive systemic sclerosis and the other visceral myopathy.[25] One familial form of visceral myopathy is also associated with small intestinal diverticulosis. Whether these represent separate and distinct disorders or whether they are just different manifestations of either PSS or visceral myopathy is unknown.

Two types of myenteric plexus disorders are associated with jejunal diverticulosis. In one type, the smooth muscle layers appear hypertrophied and the myenteric plexus is degenerated with some of the neurons containing eosinophilic intranuclear inclusions similiar to those described in one type of familial visceral neuropathy.[25] The other is associated with Fabry's disease in which there is accumulation of the glycolipid, ceramide trihexoside, within the neurons of the myenteric plexus.[26] Conventional stains show foamy vacuolation of the neurons of the submucosal and myenteric plexuses. A PAS-Luxol blue stain is diagnostic, with demonstration of blue staining granules within the affected cells. Silver stains of the myenteric plexus show a decrease of argyrophilic neurons which are enlarged and foamy and have cytoplasmic distortion. Argyrophobic neurons are also enlarged and granular, presumably from the glycolipid deposition. Mild axonal degeneration may be present with glial cell proliferation in some areas. No inflammatory cells are present within the plexus.

In those smooth muscle disorders which produce small intestinal diverticulosis, fibrosis of the muscle layers causes localized areas of atrophy and weakness of the intestinal wall which then protrude out. This creates sacculations or diverticula of the entire thickness of the intestinal wall. In contrast, in disorders of the myenteric plexus, it is possible that uncoordinated activity by hypertrophied muscle creates areas of increased intraluminal pressure, with protrusion of the mucosa and submucosa along defects created at the points of blood vessel penetration within the intestinal wall, usually along the mesenteric border.

Conclusion

In conclusion, neuromuscular disorders of the gastrointestinal tract result from a variety of pathologic abnormalities of either the smooth muscle or myenteric plexus. There is no reason to believe that any more than the tip of an iceberg has been uncovered so far and it is probable that the pathology of other types of neuromuscular disorders will be described.

Acknowledgements

Parts of this manuscript were originally published in syllabus form by the American Society of Clinical Pathologists and permission was obtained to use this material. This research was supported by Grant DK28180 from the NIDDKD of the National Institute of Health.

References

1 Smith B. *The Neuropathology of the Alimentary Tract*. Edward Arnold: London 1972.
2 Dyer NH, Dawson A, Smith BF, Todd IP. Obstruction of bowel due to lesion in the myenteric plexus. *Br Med J* 1969; **i**: 685–9.
3 Schuffler MD, Jonak Z. Chronic idiopathic intestinal pseudo-obstruction caused by a degenerative disorder of the myenteric plexus: the use of Smith's method to define the neuropathology. *Gastroenterology* 1982; **82**: 476–86.
4 Schuffler MD, Leon SH, Krishnamurthy S. Intestinal pseudo-obstruction caused by a new form of visceral neuropathy: palliation by radical small bowel resection. *Gastroenterology* 1985; **89**: 1152–6.

5 Lhermitte F, Gray F, Lyon-Caen O, Pertuiset BF, Bernard P. Paralysis of digestive tract with lesions of myenteric plexus. A new paraneoplastic syndrome. *Rev Neurol (Paris)* 1980; **136**: 825–36.

6 Schuffler MD, Baird HW, Fleming CR *et al*. Intestinal pseudo-obstruction as the presenting manifestation of small cell carcinoma of the lung: a paraneoplastic neuropathy of the gastrointestinal tract. *Ann Intern Med* 1983; **98**: 129–34.

7 Krishnamurthy S, Schuffler MD, Belic L, Schweid A. An inflammatory axonopathy of the myenteric plexus causing rapidly progressive intestinal pseudo-obstruction. *Gastroenterology* 1986; **90**: 754–8.

8 Schuffler MD, Bird TD, Sumi SM, Cooke A. A familial neuronal disease presenting as intestinal pseudo-obstruction. *Gastroenterology* 1978; **75**: 889–98.

9 Cockel R, Hill EE, Rushton DI, Smith BF, Hawkins CF. Familial steatorrhea with calcification of the basal ganglia and mental retardation. *Quart J Med* 1973; **42**: 771–83.

10 Mayer EA, Schuffler MD, Rotter JI, Hanna P. A familial visceral neuropathy with autosomal dominant transmission. *Gastroenterology* 1986; **91**: 1528–35.

11 Krishnamurthy S, Schuffler MD, Rohrmann CA, Pope CE. Severe idiopathic constipation is associated with a distinctive abnormality of the colonic myenteric plexus. *Gastroenterology* 1985; **88**: 26–34.

12 Smith B. Pathology of cathartic colon. *Proc R Soc Med* 1972; **65**: 288–92.

13 Schuffler MD, Lowe MC, Bill AH. Studies of idiopathic intestinal pseudo-obstruction. I. Hereditary hollow visceral myopathy: clinical and pathological studies. *Gastroenterology* 1977; **73**: 327–38.

14 Schuffler MD, Pope CE. Studies of idiopathic intestinal pseudo-obstruction. II. Hereditary hollow visceral myopathy: family studies. *Gastroenterology* 1977; **73**: 339–44.

15 Faulk DL, Anuras S, Gardner GD, Mitros FA, Summers RW, Christensen J. A familial visceral myopathy. *Ann Intern Med* 1978; **89**: 600–6.

16 Shaw A, Shaffer H, Teja K, Kelly T, Grogan E, Bruni C. A perspective for pediatric surgeons: chronic idiopathic pseudo-obstruction. *J Pediatr Surg* 1979; **14**: 719–27.

17 Schuffler MD, Rohrmann CA, Chaffee RG, Brand DL, Delaney JH, Young JH. Chronic intestinal pseudo-obstruction: a report of 27 cases and review of the literature. *Medicine* 1981; **60**: 173–96.

18 Schuffler MD, Beegle RG. Progressive systemic sclerosis of the gastrointestinal tract and hereditary hollow visceral myopathy: two distinguishable disorders of intestinal smooth muscle. *Gastroenterology* 1979; **77**: 664–71.

19 Mitros FA, Schuffler MD, Teja K, Anuras S. Pathology of familial visceral myopathy. *Hum Path* 1982; **13**: 825–33.

20 Leon SH, Schuffler MD. A visceral myopathy of the colon mimicking Hirschsprung's disease. Diagnosis by deep rectal biopsy. *Dig Dis Sci* 1986; **31**: 1381–6.

21 Hoskins LC, Norris HT, Gottlieb LS *et al*. Functional and morphologic alterations of the gastrointestinal tract in progressive systemic sclerosis (scleroderma). *Am J Med* 1962; **33**: 459–70.

22 Nowak TV, Ionasescu V, Anuras S. Gastrointestinal manifestations of the muscular dystrophies. *Gastroenterology* 1982; **82**: 800–10.

23 Leon SH, Schuffler MD. Intestinal pseudo-obstruction as a complication of Duchenne's muscular dystrophy. *Gastroenterology* 1986; **90**: 455–9.

24 McDonald GB, Schuffler MD, Kadin ME, Tytgat GNJ. Intestinal pseudo-obstruction caused by diffuse lymphoid infiltration of the small intestine. *Gastroenterology* 1985; **89**: 882–9.

25 Krishnamurthy S, Kelly MM, Rohrmann CA, Schuffler MD. Jejunal diverticulosis: a heterogeneous disorder caused by a variety of abnormalities of smooth muscle or myenteric plexus. *Gastroenterology* 1983; **85**: 538–47.

26 Friedman LS, Platika D, Thistlethwaite JR, Kirkham SE, Kolodny EH, Schuffler MD. Jejunal diverticulosis with perforation as a complication of Fabry's disease. *Gastroenterology* 1984; **86**: 558–63.

Gastrointestinal motility disorders — the psychologist's perspective

W E Whitehead

Three critical questions can be asked about the relationship of psychological factors to the etiology and course of gastrointestinal motility disorders:
• Are there psychological traits or psychiatric disorders which are *specific* to gastrointestinal motility disorders? If so, what are the mediating mechanisms?
• Does psychological stress alter gastrointestinal motility? If so, what is the mechanism?
• Might psychological traits be irrelevant to gastrointestinal motility but influence which of the spectrum of people with gastrointestinal motility disorders will seek treatment?

The answers to these questions will determine the kind of psychological assessment gastroenterologists will want to provide for their patients and the role of psychological therapy in the management of patients. The answers to these questions also have implications for preventing gastrointestinal motility disorders and reducing health care costs associated with them through patient education.

Psychopathology associated with gastrointestinal motility disorders

Psychopathology is measured in two distinct ways. One approach is to make a yes/no decision about the presence of a psychiatric disorder such as depression on the assumption that depression, like measles, is present or absent. The second approach is to measure psychological traits on a severity continuum (eg mildly depressed, moderately depressed) on the assumption that depression, like fatness, is a continuous dimension along which people may vary; it may be useful to know how fat or depressed a patient is even though they do not qualify for the diagnosis of morbid obesity or major affective disorder.

Adopting the first strategy, Clouse and Lustman used a well-recognized psychiatric interview technique (Diagnostic Interview Schedule) to assign psychiatric diagnoses to 25 patients with esophageal motility disorders.[1] Eighty-four percent of those with nonspecific motility disorders received psychiatric diagnoses compared to only 31% of patients with normal manometric findings and 33% of patients with other specific, esophageal motility disorders. These psychiatric diagnoses were depression in 13/25, anxiety disorder in 9/25, somatization disorder in 5/25 and phobias in 7/25.

Three published studies have used a similar technique to assign psychiatric diagnoses to patients with irritable bowel syndrome (IBS).[2-4] When these patient samples are pooled (*Table 1*), the leading diagnoses are: hysteria or somatization disorder (20%); depression (20%); and anxiety disorder (14%). Using the Diagnostic Interview

	Nonspecific esophageal motility disorder (%)	IBS (%)	IBS (Hopkins) (%)	General population (%)
Major depression	52	20	37	3.7
Generalized anxiety disorder	36	14	21	25.1
Phobia	38	0	21	23.3
Somatization or hysteria	20	20	0	0.1

Table 1 Psychiatric diagnoses in gastrointestinal motility disorders. Based on pooled data.[1-5] IBS = irritable bowel syndrome.

Schedule, it was found that 9 of 19 IBS patients had psychiatric diagnoses (W E Whitehead *et al*, unpublished observations). This included major depression in 7/19, generalized anxiety disorder in 4/19 and agoraphobia in 4/19.

The studies reviewed above suggest an excess incidence of psychopathology in patients with gastrointestinal motility disorders but do not identify any specific psychiatric disorder which is strongly associated with gastrointestinal motility. Anxiety disorders, phobias and depression are the most common diagnoses (with the exception of substance abuse) made in the general population, and most patients with these diagnoses do not complain of gastrointestinal motility disorders. Somatization disorders (or hysteria) and depression do occur at an unusually high incidence in samples of patients with gastrointestinal motility disorders as compared to general population samples, but not as compared to clinic samples of patients with other physical complaints such as back pain and headaches.[6]

Studies which have used psychometric tests to measure psychological symptoms or personality traits present a similar picture. West reported that patients with IBS showed significant elevations on the Minnesota Multiphasic Personality Inventory (MMPI) scales for hysteria, hypochondriasis and depression,[7] a pattern which is also seen in chronic pain patients.[6] Two studies employing the Hopkins Symptom Checklist found IBS patients to have significant elevations on the subscales for depression, anxiety, interpersonal sensitivity, somatization and hostility.[8,9] Four studies using the Eysenck Personality Inventory found IBS patients to be more neurotic (i.e. to exhibit greater emotional lability) than normal subjects[4,10-12] and a recent study using the Beck Depression Inventory found a higher prevalence of depression in patients with functional gastrointestinal disorders as compared to patients seen in a surgery clinic.[13] Taken as a whole, these and other psychometric tests depict IBS patients as more psychologically distressed than the general population, but less distressed or symptomatic than outpatients seen in a psychiatric clinic. It is particularly important that these studies do not identify a specific pattern of psychological traits which is unique to any gastrointestinal motility disorder.

Psychological stress and gastrointestinal disorders

The stress hypothesis is distinct from the hypothesis that psychological symptoms such as depression and anxiety contribute to bowel symptoms. Normal events such as driving in traffic or interviewing for a job cause some degree of stress to everyone, although individuals differ in how strongly they react to such events. Psychological stress could alter gastrointestinal motility and thereby exacerbate gastrointestinal symptoms, even in patients who are psychologically healthy.

Experimental studies in which a laboratory stressor is introduced while gastrointestinal motility is being recorded make it clear that psychological stress can alter gastrointestinal motility (*Table 2*). Faulkner provided a dramatic example of the effects of psychological stress or emotion on esophageal motility.[14] He performed esophagoscopy with a rigid instrument in a destitute young man in whom he could repeatedly provoke and inhibit vigorous esophageal contractions by alternating mental images of financial hardship with images of financial security. With images of hardship, the instrument was gripped so tightly that it could not be removed.

The studies summarized in *Table 2* provide compelling evidence that experimental stressors do alter gastrointestinal motility. However, there appear to be marked differences between individuals in the direction and magnitude of the changes in motility.[4] These individual differences have not been adequately explained. Almy suggested that the type of motility response provoked in the colon was determined by the nature of the emotion evoked in the patient.[27] However, this hypothesis has not been addressed by subsequent research, in part because it is technically difficult to control the qualitative aspects of a subject's emotional experience. Subjects react to the same experimental situation with different and often with mixed emotional responses.

In several of the studies summarized in *Table 2*, normal subjects (i.e. subjects without identified motility disorders) were found to alter their gastrointestinal motility in response to psychological stress. It is important to determine whether patients with

Esophagus	Stress interview elicits secondary contractions[14-17]
	Loud noises elicit tertiary contractions[18] or increased amplitude of peristaltic contractions[19]
Stomach	Cold stress or electric shock to skin inhibit antral motility, delay emptying[20]
Small intestine	Loud noise stress and dichotic listening decrease transit time[21,22]
	Traffic, arcade games and delayed auditory feedback suppress migrating motor complex, increase irregular contractions[23,24]
Colon	Stress interview or experimental pain increase motility[4,25-27]
	Frustrating cognitive task or cold stress increase motility[26-28]

Table 2 Effects of laboratory stressors on gastrointestinal motility.

identified motility disorders show a qualitatively different motility response from normal. Indirect evidence summarized below suggests that they do.

The motility responses of IBS patients were compared to those of normal controls when a balloon was inflated in the rectosigmoid area.[9] It was found that patients had no more contractile activity than normal subjects prior to balloon distension, but following balloon distension, patients with IBS showed a significantly greater increase in motility. These observations were subsequently replicated in a different group of patients and the motility response to a standard dose (0.1 mg given intramuscularly) of cholecystokinin (CCK) was also tested. IBS patients showed a greater response to CCK than normal subjects and the magnitude of this response to CCK was significantly correlated ($r = 0.65$) with the magnitude of the response to balloon distension. This suggested that the reactivity of the colon to any provocative stimulus differed in IBS patients when compared to normal subjects. It is speculated that this nonspecific hyperreactivity of the colon to stimulation will also characterize the motility response to psychological stress, leading IBS patients to show an exaggerated motility response to stressors as compared to normal subjects.

Recent reports suggest that this hyperreactivity to stimuli occurs in other parts of the gastrointestinal tract as well. Richter and colleagues showed that patients with noncardiac chest pain had a lower threshold for reporting pain when a balloon was inflated in the esophagus.[30] Kellow and Phillips (personal communication) found that IBS patients had an exaggerated motor response and a lower pain threshold when a balloon was inflated in the small intestine.

One approach to investigating the stress hypothesis outside the laboratory is to ask patients if psychological stress causes a change in their bowel symptoms. From 50–85% of IBS patients report such a correlation.[11,31-33] The most frequently mentioned stressors in men are worries about career or finances and in women worries about family or interpersonal relationships.[11,31] These are commonplace worries. The only suggestion of a specific stressor is the report that the death of a parent[11] or loss of a parent through marital dissolution[34] were associated with the onset of IBS in approximately 30% of cases.

Although these retrospective data provide persuasive evidence that psychological stress may cause exacerbations of gastrointestinal motility disorders, the high frequency with which psychological stress precipitates altered bowel habits in normal subjects must be taken into account. Drossman and co-workers found that 68% of a large population sample without symptoms of IBS reported that psychological stressors caused constipation or diarrhea, and 47% reported that psychological stressors caused abdominal pain.[32] IBS patients were significantly more likely to report stress-related changes in bowel patterns (85%) and abdominal pain (69%), but the base rate of such reports among 'normals' suggests that this is not a distinguishing characteristic of IBS patients.

A different approach to studying the association of stress with bowel symptoms is for patients to keep a daily diary in which they rate the intensity of psychological stress and abdominal pain and the frequency and consistency of bowel movements four times each day. This technique was used to study 157 adult women seen in the community. The restrictive criteria listed in *Table 3* to diagnose IBS were applied in this study. These criteria are similar to diagnostic criteria developed by Manning and colleagues[36] and later used by Drossman and co-workers,[32] Thompson and Heaton,[37] and Welch and co-workers.[38] They differ from the conventional criteria used to diagnose IBS by including items which help to establish that the pain is of colonic origin. This is achieved by requiring that the pain be relieved by defecation or by passing flatus and that the onset of pain be associated with a change in bowel pattern. The term functional bowel disorder (FBD) was applied to patients who

1 Abdominal pain that is:

- relieved by a bowel movement, often
- occurs at least 6 times per year
- lasts at least 3 weeks per occurrence

2 Satisfies at least two of the Manning criteria:

- loose stools at the onset of pain
- more frequent bowel movements with the onset of pain
- distension of abdomen
- mucus passed by rectum
- feeling of incomplete emptying, often

3 Exclusion of physical diseases as a cause of symptoms:

- no weight loss greater than 5% in the preceding year
- no gastrointestinal blood loss except from local anal lesions (eg fissures)
- negative lactose tolerance test or negative response to a lactose-free diet
- no evidence of inflammatory bowel disease on barium enema
- no evidence of intestinal parasites

Table 3 Diagnostic criteria for irritable bowel syndrome.

satisfied the conventional criteria of abdominal pain plus constipation or diarrhea in the presence of a negative physical evaluation but who failed to satisfy the more restrictive criteria given in *Table 3*.

As shown in *Figure 1*, on daily symptom logs patients with IBS described themselves as having average amounts of psychological stress which were similar to normal subjects and lactose malabsorbers (LMA). Patients with FBD, however, described themselves as experiencing significantly more stress than normal subjects or patients with LMA or IBS.

With respect to pain (*Figure 1*), patients with IBS as well as patients with FBD and LMA described experiencing more pain than normal subjects. However, patients with FBD were again significantly higher than patients with IBS on symptom log ratings of pain.

The average frequency of bowel movements was similar in the four groups. However, the proportion of each group who reported having at least one bowel movement of an abnormal consistency ('hard' or 'watery') was significantly higher than normal only for the IBS group (*Figure 1*).

The correlation between stress ratings and pain ratings was calculated for each subject separately, and the groups were compared with respect to the proportion of subjects who exhibited statistically significant ($p \geq 0.38$) positive correlations. Only 15% of IBS patients demonstrated significant positive correlations as compared to 22% of normal subjects, 19% of patients with FBD and 27% of patients with LMA. Thus, neither patients with IBS nor patients with FBD showed a greater tendency than normal subjects for stress to covary with abdominal pain.

The correlation between the maximum stress ratings each day and the total number of bowel movements per day was also calculated. The number of pairs of observations used to form these correlations was typically 7, so statistical significance could not be assessed. However, the proportion of each group showing absolute correlations of 0.50 or greater was 18% for IBS, 32% for FBD, 21% for LMA and 20% for normal

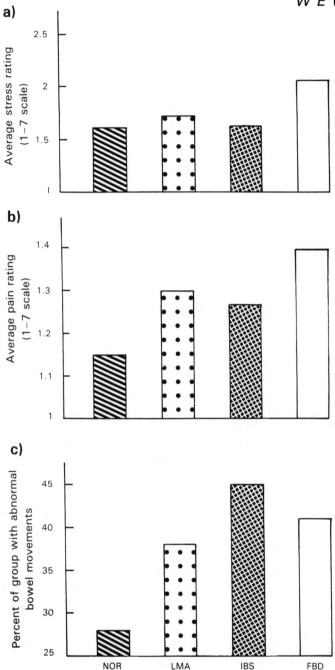

Figure 1 Average ratings for (a) stress and (b) pain, and (c) proportion of subjects reporting abnormal (hard or watery) bowel movements on at least 1 day, in a community study in which participants recorded their symptoms in a daily log over a 7-day period. Subjects rated their most intense experience of stress or pain on a scale from 1 (none) to 7 (very intense). These ratings were made four times a day: on awakening, at noon time, at dinner time, and at bedtime. NOR = normal subjects; LMA = lactose malabsorbers; IBS = subjects with irritable bowel syndrome; FBD = subjects with functional bowel disorder. See text for diagnostic criteria.

subjects. Thus, patients with IBS were no more likely than normal subjects to report that stress covaried with changes in stool frequency, although patients with FBD showed a tendency to report such a covariation at greater than expected frequencies. The proportion of subjects who reported having abnormal bowel movements was insufficient to allow an assessment of the relationship between stress and abnormal stool consistency.

Studies of the effects of laboratory stressors and of naturally occurring stressors generally agree in suggesting that psychological stress does alter gastrointestinal motility and may exacerbate symptoms of gastrointestinal motility disorders. However, these stress-mediated changes occur in normal subjects as well as in patients. There is indirect evidence which suggests that patients with IBS[9] show a greater reactivity to psychological and physical stressors than normal subjects, but the overlap with normal subjects is substantial.[35]

The physiologic mechanisms which mediate the effects of psychological stress on gastrointestinal motility are not as yet known. Such stress effects appear to be paradoxical since the autonomic nervous system response to psychological stressors is usually found to be an increase in sympathetic activation and a decrease in parasympathetic activity. The gastrointestinal motility and secretory responses to stress are parasympathetically mediated, however.[35]

Effects of psychopathology on medical clinic attendance

Patients with IBS exhibit more psychopathology than the general population, but no specific pattern of psychological traits is observed. This lack of specificity makes it unlikely that psychopathology plays an etiologic role in IBS or other gastrointestinal disorders, but the association between psychopathology and the diagnosis of IBS still requires explanation. Two hypotheses which could account for this have been investigated. The first hypothesis is that psychological symptoms might be a consequence of having chronic bowel symptoms rather than their cause. This is sometimes referred to as the somatopsychic hypothesis. To test this, LMA patients were used as a control group because they have bowel symptoms, presumed to be adequately explained by an enzyme deficiency, which are indistinguishable from IBS[39] and which have been present since childhood. If psychological symptoms are a result of chronic bowel symptoms, LMA and IBS patients should show similar, elevated levels of psychopathology.

The second hypothesis is that psychological symptoms may be irrelevant to gastrointestinal motility but may influence which of several patients with gastrointestinal motility disorders will seek medical treatment. There are precedents for this in other areas of medicine.[40,41] To test this hypothesis, women in the community identified as having bowel symptoms indicative of IBS or LMA but not attending medical clinics were compared to women with the same symptoms who were identified through their medical clinic attendance. If psychopathology is unrelated to gastrointestinal motility but has an influence on who will come to the medical clinic, more psychopathology would be expected in the clinic sample than in the community sample for the same diagnoses.

Recruitment methods
The community sample was recruited by contacting the heads of church women's societies and charities and asking them to recruit subjects from among their members in exchange for a financial contribution to the organization's treasury for each woman

completing the study. Subjects were briefed at their first visit and completed a bowel symptom questionnaire which was used to classify them as having IBS or FBD as defined above. At their first visit, subjects were given the Hopkins Symptom Checklist and a brief version of the Neuroticism-Extroversion-Openness Inventory,[42] and they were instructed how to keep a diary of bowel symptoms and psychological stress. At their return visit 1 week later, these subjects were tested for lactose malabsorption by the breath hydrogen method (50 g lactose meal).

The medical clinic sample was drawn from a consecutive series of 209 patients referred for lactose tolerance testing over a 2-year period. Patients were included if they were female, at least 18 years old, and had completed a Hopkins Symptom Checklist and bowel symptom questionnaire when initially evaluated. Medical charts were reviewed in order to exclude patients who had spinal cord injury, diabetes or inflammatory bowel disease. A total of 54 patients remained of whom 23 were classified as LMA, 10 were diagnosed IBS by criteria given above, and 12 were classified as FBD.

Results

When the clinic sample and the community sample were compared on the Hopkins Symptom Checklist, two overall findings were obtained.

First, medical clinic attenders scored significantly higher than the community sample on the psychopathology scales regardless of diagnosis, for each gastrointestinal disorder — IBS, LMA and FBD. This is shown for the global symptom index (an overall measure of psychopathology) in *Figure 2* and for each of the clinical subscales on the Hopkins Symptom Checklist in *Table 4*. This supports the hypothesis that

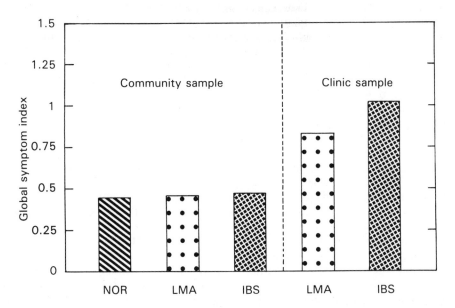

Figure 2 Comparison of a community sample of subjects with bowel symptoms who had not sought medical care to a sample of subjects with similar symptoms seen in a medical clinic. The dependent measure is the Global Symptom Index on the Hopkins Symptom Checklist. This is a measure of overall psychopathology reported on this 90-item inventory. See text for diagnostic criteria. NOR = normal subjects; LMA = lactose malabsorbers; IBS = subjects with irritable bowel syndrome.

	Community				Clinic			
	Normal	LMA	IBS	FBD	LMA	IBS	FBD	Significance
Global Sx index	0.23	0.46	0.41	0.69	0.87	1.01	1.08	S
Somatization	0.43	0.55	0.34	0.73	1.22	1.34	1.27	S
Obsessive compulsive	0.67	0.73	0.55	0.92	1.00	1.32	1.08	S
Interp sensitivity	0.57	0.49	0.60	0.73	0.66	0.93	1.13	S
Depression	0.64	0.59	0.56	0.94	1.21	1.15	1.85	S/Dx
Anxiety	0.36	0.38	0.46	0.67	0.87	0.95	1.03	S
Hostility	0.30	0.36	0.30	0.71	0.65	1.05	1.25	S/Dx
Phobia	0.07	0.13	0.09	0.23	0.38	0.51	0.69	S
Paranoid	0.36	0.32	0.25	0.50	0.52	0.83	0.83	S
Psychoticism	0.25	0.13	0.17	0.35	0.27	0.32	0.78	S/Dx

Table 4 Comparison of clinic and community SCL-90 raw scores. LMA = lactose malabsorbers; IBS = irritable bowel syndrome; FBD = functional bowel syndrome; S = significant difference between community and clinic samples; Dx = significant differences between diagnostic groups.

psychopathology influences who will attend a medical clinic for bowel complaints.

Secondly, in the community sample, patients with IBS and patients with LMA were similar to normal subjects on psychological scales, suggesting that psychopathology is not related to the development of IBS. These data also suggest that the psychopathology seen in IBS patients who are recruited through medical clinics is not a consequence of having chronic bowel symptoms since patients with LMA and patients with IBS were similar to each other in both samples.

Diagnostic criteria are important. When strict research diagnostic criteria are used to diagnose IBS, no relationship between IBS and psychopathology is seen. However, the loose clinical criteria used here to define functional bowel disorder are sometimes used to define IBS, and this resulted in an apparent association with psychopathology even in the community sample. This occurred because abdominal pain is significantly correlated with psychopathology whether or not the abdominal pain is associated with altered bowel function.

These findings are in general agreement with a study reported by Drossman and co-workers,[43] in which 72 patients with IBS who were identified through a medical clinic were compared to 82 persons with IBS symptoms who had not sought treatment and 84 asymptomatic controls. The principal measures of psychopathology were the MMPI and the Illness Behavior Questionnaire.[44] It was found that IBS patients from the medical clinic exhibited significantly more abnormal personalities and more illness behaviour than nonpatients with IBS symptoms or normal subjects, and nonpatients with IBS symptoms were similar to asymptomatic controls on these measures.[43]

Welch and co-workers obtained discrepant findings, however.[38] They used the Hopkins Symptom Checklist to compare IBS patients to nonpatients with IBS symptoms recruited from blood donors and asymptomatic controls. In their study, IBS patients and nonpatients with IBS symptoms were similar to normal subjects on all psychological measures except somatization (hypochondriasis). On this scale, patients and nonpatients were similar to each other but scored significantly higher than normal controls. This discrepancy may be due to differences in the cultural setting (New Zealand vs USA) in which the data were collected.

Role of psychological factors in gastrointestinal disorders

From the results of the studies described here, it can be concluded that psychological traits are unrelated to the development of gastrointestinal motility disorders, but psychological symptoms influence whether or not patients consult a physician. In addition, psychological stress may, independently of psychopathology, alter gastrointestinal motility and produce bowel symptoms. This occurs in normal subjects as well as in patients with gastrointestinal motility disorders.

Implications for psychological assessment and treatment

Psychological disorders should be thought of as independent disorders which have a high probability of being present in patients with gastrointestinal motility disorders. The high prevalence of psychopathology occurs because psychologically-distressed individuals are more likely to attend medical clinics for treatment of benign physical complaints which psychologically better-adjusted individuals ignore or manage themselves.

Because the base rate of psychopathology is high in this population, gastroenterologists should routinely screen new patients for psychopathology by giving a brief, self-administered psychological test. The Hopkins Symptom Checklist is well suited for this purpose because it can be completed in 10–15 minutes and scored either manually or by computer before interviewing the patient.[45] Even if it is not formally scored, the format of the answer sheet allows the physician to rapidly identify those symptoms which the patient checks as 'quite a bit' or 'extremely' distressing and to screen for suicidal thoughts.

An alternative psychometric test which can be recommended is the Millon Behavioral Health Inventory.[46] This 150-item inventory was developed specifically for assessment of psychological symptoms in medical clinic patients. It is scored for 8 scales reflecting the patient's style of coping with problems, 6 scales dealing with psychogenic attitudes (eg future despair, social alienation), 3 psychosomatic scales (including gastrointestinal susceptibility), and 3 prognostic scales. The Millon inventory has appeal to clinical researchers because of its inclusion of a gastrointestinal susceptibility subscale. However, the significance of scores on the other scales is not readily apparent to the nonpsychologist, and the test must be scored and interpreted by the company marketing the test. This limits its usefulness in screening patients for referral to a psychiatrist.

When psychometric testing and discussions with the patient indicate that the patient has a psychiatric disorder severe enough to warrant treatment, the patient should be referred to a psychologist or psychiatrist. Most gastroenterologists do not have the time or the training to provide such treatment, and inept psychotherapy, like inept endoscopy, may be harmful. However, a few gastroenterologists have psychiatric training, and they are ideally suited to manage these patients.

Stress management training may be useful in reducing the frequency and severity of gastrointestinal symptoms associated with motility disorders even in patients who are psychologically well-adjusted. Stress management training involves identifying what causes stress for this patient and teaching a relaxation technique to enable the patient to cope with those stressors which are not avoidable. By making use of commercially available cassette tapes which teach relaxation, the gastroenterologist or his/her nurse can often provide this training without referral to a psychologist.

Psychological treatments for gastrointestinal disorders

Supportive therapy

The most common recommendation made to gastroenterologists for the psychological management of patients with IBS is that they provide supportive therapy. The elements of such treatment are:

• reassurance that the symptoms are not life-threatening
• explanation of the possible role of stress in precipitating exacerbations of symptoms
• sympathy — the communication of concern for the patient's predicament.

Only one controlled study has attempted to evaluate the benefits of supportive therapy. Apley and Hale compared the outcome of treatment after 6–20 years in 30 individuals whom they had treated for recurrent abdominal pain with reassurance and explanation, to the outcome in 30 individuals whom they had evaluated but not treated.[47] There were no differences between the two groups; one-third of each group had bowel symptoms suggestive of IBS at follow-up and another third in each group had other chronic pain complaints such as headaches. Thus, the value of supportive therapy has not been established, although it can be argued that it is an intrinsic aspect of good patient care.

Psychotherapy

Svedlund and co-workers reported the only controlled study of the effects of psychotherapy.[48] They compared a group of 51 IBS patients who received bulk agents, anticholinergics and tranquilizers (medical management) to a second group of 50 IBS patients who received the same medical management plus up to 10 hours (average of 7.4 hours) of psychotherapy. The psychotherapy was described as dynamically oriented. It "aimed at modifying maladaptive behaviour and finding new solutions to problems. The focus was on means of coping with stress and emotional problems". The psychotherapy group showed a significantly greater reduction in abdominal pain and bowel dysfunction than the control group, and results were well-maintained at 15 months follow-up.

An uncontrolled study was reported by Hislop in which 60 IBS patients were treated with insight-oriented psychotherapy.[49] The aim of therapy was "progression towards increasing insight and self-reliance, with genuine reassurance and an understanding of the relationship between the emotional reaction and its somatic expression". Therapy was provided for an average of 2.2 1-hour sessions. After treatment, 46% of patients reported themselves to be asymptomatic or greatly improved, and another 32% reported moderate improvement.

Both these studies obtained surprisingly good results for psychotherapy despite the fact that the amount of therapy provided was very brief. In insight-oriented psychotherapy, 20 contact hours are considered brief treatment, and 60 hours or more are typical.

Stress-management training

Stress-management training refers to a variety of different techniques all of which share the following features.

Arousal reduction training: the patient is taught a method of relaxing which effectively lowers autonomic arousal and subjective tension or anxiety. The commonest techniques are progressive muscle relaxation exercises and nonspecific biofeedback. Progressive muscle relaxation training involves tensing and relaxing different muscle groups in a systematic fashion for 20–30 minutes twice a day. Biofeedback involves using electronic sensors to learn to warm the hands, relax the muscles in the forehead and reduce the number of skin resistance responses associated with sweating.

An emphasis on self-control or coping: the patient is taught to recognize the onset of tension and to use his/her relaxation technique to prevent or reduce arousal in stressful situations.

Cognitive change: patients whose symptoms are triggered by situations that are not actually threatening may be desensitized to those situations by gradual re-exposure. Patients who express a hopeless attitude concerning their bowel symptoms may be encouraged to change those attitudes.

Stress-management training is the simplest and, based on a review of the research literature given above, the most appropriate psychological treatment for patients with gastrointestinal motility disorders. There are many case reports[17,50,51] and uncontrolled studies[8,52,53] which support the efficacy of stress-management training for these disorders, but there are no controlled studies.

Of the psychological treatments which have been proposed for the treatment of esophageal or colonic motility disorders, psychotherapy is the best supported by research evidence. The psychotherapy provided could best be described as superficial since it was limited to 2–10 hours and had as its goal teaching patients more effective ways of coping with stressful situations or emotional conflicts. This type of psychotherapy is similar to stress management training, which also seeks to teach a more effective coping strategy, usually in the form of prescribed relaxation exercises. Such therapy has been shown to have specific value over dietary and pharmacologic therapy in patients with IBS. It may also benefit patients with upper gastrointestinal motility disorders.

References

1 Clouse RE, Lustman PJ. Psychiatric illness and contraction abnormalities of the esophagus. *N Engl J Med* 1983; **309**: 1337–42.
2 Liss JL, Alpers D, Woodruff RA Jr. The irritable colon syndrome and psychiatric illness. *Dis Nerv Syst* 1973; **34**: 151–7.
3 Young SJ, Alpers D, Norland CC, Woodruff RA Jr. Psychiatric illness and the irritable bowel syndrome: practical implications for the primary-care physician. *Gastroenterology* 1976; **70**: 162–6.
4 Latimer P, Sarna S, Campbell D, Latimer M, Waterfall W, Daniel EE. Colonic motor and myoelectrical activity: a comparative study of normal subjects, psychoneurotic patients, and patients with irritable bowel syndrome. *Gastroenterology* 1981; **80**: 893–901.
5 Robins LN, Helzer JE, Weissman MM, Orvaschel H, Gruenberg E, Burke JD Jr, Reiger DA. Lifetime prevalence of specific psychiatric disorders in three sites. *Arch Gen Psych* 1984; **41**: 949–58.
6 Sternbach RA. *Pain Patients: Traits and Treatment.* New York: Academic Press 1974.
7 West KL. MMPI correlates of ulcerative colitis. *J Clin Psychol* 1970; **26**: 214–29.
8 Wise TM, Cooper JN, Ahmed S. The efficacy of group therapy for patients with irritable bowel syndrome. *Psychosomatics* 1982; **23**: 465–9.
9 Whitehead WE, Engel BT, Schuster MM. Irritable bowel syndrome: physiological and psychological differences between diarrhea-predominant and constipation-predominant patients. *Dig Dis Sci* 1980; **25**: 404–13.
10 Esler MD, Goulston KJ. Levels of anxiety in colonic disorders. *N Engl J Med* 1973; **288**: 16–20.
11 Hill OW, Blendis L. Physical and psychological evaluation of "non-organic" abdominal pain. *Gut* 1967; **8**: 221–9.
12 Palmer RL, Stonehill E, Crisp AH, Waller SL, Misiewicz JJ. Psychological characteristics of patients with the irritable bowel syndrome. *Post Grad Med J* 1974; **50**: 416–9.
13 Rose JDR, Thoughton AH, Harvey JS, Smith PM. Depression and functional bowel

disorders in gastrointestinal out-patients. *Gut* 1986; **27**: 1025-8.

14 Faulkner WB Jr. Severe esophageal spasm: an evaluation of suggestion-therapy as determined by means of esophagoscopy. *Psychosom Med* 1940; **2**: 139-40.

15 Rubin J, Nagler R, Spiro HM, Pilot ML. Measuring the effect of emotions on esophageal motility. *Psychosom Med* 1962; **24**: 170-6.

16 Wolf S, Almy TP. Experimental observations on cardiospasm in man. *Gastroenterology* 1949; **13**: 401-21.

17 Jacobson E. Spastic esophagus and mucous colitis: etiology and treatment by progressive relaxation. *Arch Intern Med* 1927; **39**: 433-5.

18 Stacher G, Steinringer H, Blau A, Landgraf M. Acoustically evoked esophageal contractions and defense reaction. *Psychophysiology* 1979; **16**: 234-41.

19 Young LD, Richter JE, Anderson KO *et al*. The effects of psychological and environmental stressors on peristaltic esophageal contractions in healthy volunteers. *Psychophysiology* (In press).

20 Thompson DG, Richelson E, Malagelada J-R. Perturbation of upper gastrointestinal function by cold stress. *Gut* 1983; **24**: 277-83.

21 Cann PA, Read NW, Kammack J *et al*. Psychological stress in the passage of a standard reel through the stomach and small intestine in man. *Gut* 1983; **24**: 236-40.

22 Erckenbrecht JF, Ziemer B, Lesch M *et al*. The effect of longterm mental stress by noise on transit of a meal through the small and large bowel. Paper presented at the European Behavior Therapy Association Meeting. Munich, West Germany, June, 1985.

23 Kumar D, Wingate DL. Irritable bowel syndrome: a paroxysmal motor disorder. *Lancet* 1985; **ii**: 973-7.

24 Valori RM, Kumar D, Wingate DL. Effects of different types of stress and of "prokinetic" drugs on the control of the fasting motor complex in humans. *Gastroenterology* 1986; **90**: 1890-900.

25 Wangel AG, Deller DJ. Intestinal motility in man. III. Mechanisms of constipation and diarrhea with particular reference to the irritable colon syndrome. *Gastroenterology* 1965; **48**: 69-84.

26 Welgan P, Meshkinpour H, Hoehler F. The effect of stress on colon motor and electrical activity in irritable bowel syndrome. *Psychosom Med* 1985; **47**: 139-49.

27 Almy TP. Experimental studies on the irritable colon. *Am J Med* 1951; **9**: 60-7.

28 Narducci F, Snape WJ Jr, Battle WN, London RL, Cohen S. Increased colonic motility during exposure to a stressful situation. *Dig Dis Sci* 1985; **30**: 40-4.

29 Chasen R, Tucker H, Palmer D, Whitehead WE, Schuster M. Colonic motility in irritable bowel syndrome and diverticular disease. *Gastroenterology* 1982; **82**: 1031 (abstr).

30 Richter JE, Barish CF, Castell DO. Abnormal sensory perception in patients with esophageal chest pain. *Gastroenterology* 1986; **91**: 845-52.

31 Chaudhary NA, Truelove SC. The irritable colon syndrome: a study of the clinical features, predisposing causes and prognosis in 130 cases. *Quart J Med* 1962; **31**: 307-23.

32 Drossman DA, Sandler RS, McKee DC, Lovitz AJ. Bowel patterns among subjects not seeking health care. *Gastroenterology* 1982; **83**: 529-34.

33 Hislop IG. Psychological significance of the irritable colon syndrome. *Gut* 1971; **12**: 452-7.

34 Hislop IG. Childhood deprivation: an antecedent of the irritable bowel syndrome. *Med J Aust* 1979; **i**: 372-4.

35 Whitehead WE, Schuster MM. *Gastrointestinal Disorders: Behavioral and Physiological Basis for Treatment*. New York: Academic Press 1985.

36 Manning AP, Thompson WG, Heaton KW, Morris AF. Towards positive diagnosis of the irritable bowel. *Br Med J* 1978; **ii**: 653-4.

37 Thompson WG, Heaton KW. Functional bowel disorders in apparently healthy people. *Gastroenterology* 1980; **79**: 283-8.

38 Welch GW, Hillman LC, Pomare EW. Psychoneurotic symptomatology in the irritable bowel syndrome: a study of reporters and non-reporters. *Br Med J* 1985; **291**: 1382-4.

39 Enck P, Mellibruda L, Wright E, Whitehead WE, Tucker H, Schuster MN. Manning criteria failed to distinguish IBS from lactose intolerance. *Gastroenterology* 1984; **86**: 1070 (abstr).

40 Cochrane R. Hostility and neuroticism among unselected essential hypertensions. *J Psychosom Res* 1973; **17**: 215-8.

41 Davies M. Blood pressure and personality. *J Psychosom Res* 1970; **14**: 89–104.
42 Costa PT Jr, McCrae RR. *The NEO Personality Inventory Manual*. Odessa, Florida: Psychological Assessment Resources 1985.
43 Drossman DA, McKee DC, Sandler RS *et al*. Psychosocial factors in irritable bowel syndrome: a multivariate study. *Gastroenterology* 1987; **91**: xxx.
44 Pilowski N, Spence MD. *Manual for the Illness Behavior Questionnaire (IBQ)*, 2nd ed. Adelaide, Australia: University of Adelaide 1983.
45 Derogatis LI. *The SCL-90 R. Administration, Scoring and Procedures Manual II*. Towson, Maryland: Clinical Psychometric Research 1983.
46 Millon T, Green CJ, Meagher RB. *Millon Behavioral Health Inventory Manual,* 3rd ed. Minneapolis, Minnesota: National Computer Systems 1982.
47 Apley J, Hale B. Children with recurrent abdominal pain: how do they grow up? *Br Med J* 1973; **3**: 7–9.
48 Svedlund J, Sjodin I, Ottosson J-O, Dotevall G. Controlled study of psychotherapy in irritable bowel syndrome. *Lancet* 1983; **ii**: 589–92.
49 Hislop IG. Effect of very brief psychotherapy on the irritable bowel syndrome. *Med J Aust* 1980; **ii**: 620–3.
50 Youell KJ, McCullough JP. Behavioral treatment of mucous colitis. *J Consult Clin Psychol* 1975; **43**: 740–5.
51 Mitchell KM. Self-management of spastic colitis. *Behav Ther Exp Psych* 1978; **9**: 269–72.
52 Weinstock SA. The re-establishment of intestinal control in functional colitis. *Biofeedback and Self-Regulation* 1976; **1**: 324 (abstr).
53 Hall JR. Relaxation, stress management, and the treatment of irritable bowel syndrome. *Paper presented at the 26th Annual Meeting of the Southeastern Psychological Association.* Washington, DC: March 1980.

III
Treatment

Treatment of esophageal motility disorders

D O Castell

As esophageal motility laboratories have become technically more refined, the approach to primary esophageal motility disorders (EMDs) has been modified to some degree. Achalasia, the prototype primary motility disorder, is usually readily identified by the typical abnormalities on the barium esophagram, and its diagnosis confirmed by equally typical motility abnormalities. Effective therapy for this condition is well established.

Diffuse esophageal spasm (DES), on the other hand, is not so readily identified or defined by either radiographic or manometric modalities. The availability of more up-to-date esophageal motility laboratories has provided a greater number of diagnoses of motility abnormalities and, at the same time, provided some degree of confusion owing to recognition of potential motility defects not previously categorized or readily defined. This is particularly true of esophageal spastic disorders. In addition to the motility abnormalities usually described in the patient with typical DES, other abnormalities such as the so-called 'nutcracker esophagus' or esophageal 'supersqueezer' and the 'hypertensive lower esophageal sphincter' are being recognized.

A great many patients also demonstrate primary motility abnormalities that are still unclassified — the nonspecific esophageal motility disorders.

Treatment of achalasia, diffuse esophageal spasm and the other primary EMDs will be reviewed here. It is important to note that, as opposed to achalasia, the recommended therapy for DES and related abnormalities is often empiric due to poor understanding of primary etiology. In general, therapy of these conditions is much less rewarding than that of achalasia.

Clinical manifestations

The cardinal symptoms of esophageal dysfunction are dysphagia and chest pain, including heartburn. Patients with esophageal motility disorders frequently present with a combination of dysphagia and chest pain.

Dysphagia: typical dysphagia due to an abnormality in the smooth muscle section of the esophagus is characterized by problems in the swallowing of any kind of food, liquid or solid. This is the cardinal symptom of achalasia and may precede the final diagnosis by years. Dysphagia in patients with other primary EMDs is more likely to be intermittent in nature, interspersed by many periods of relatively normal swallowing. It also may be related to swallowing of specific substances, such as large boluses of food, medications or cold liquids. The incidence of dysphagia in patients with primary EMDs is quite high when carefully sought. Not uncommonly, the physician who is unfamiliar with esophageal symptomatology will fail to question the patient carefully about swallowing disorders.

Chest pain: intermittent anterior chest discomfort, often very severe and oppressive, and often associated with other systemic symptoms, may mimic coronary disease. This may cause great anxiety for both the patient and physician. With the increasing recognition of the potential for esophageal motility abnormalities to produce chest pain that may mimic angina, there has been greater attention to potential esophageal causes for this 'noncardiac' chest pain. The types of primary EMDs seen in patients with chest pain at the Bowman Gray School of Medicine, Gastroenterology Section, are shown in *Figure 1*. With the exception of associated dysphagia, it is difficult to identify any specific aspect of the chest pain syndrome that will identify clearly the patient's symptom as being esophageal rather than cardiac in origin.

Therapy

Achalasia
The optimal treatment for achalasia is to restore esophageal peristalsis to normal and cause the lower esophageal sphincter (LES) to relax completely. Since neither of these goals is attainable, current therapies are directed at weakening the LES to allow gravity and any remaining contractile activity to move material into the stomach. This is usually attempted by either instrumental dilatation or surgical esophagomyotomy of the LES muscle.

Pneumatic dilatation: the preferred method of instrumental dilatation of the LES is pneumatic dilatation.[1] This has been a successful form of treatment for achalasia for over 30 years. Results of several large series reveal that excellent results can be expected in 75–85% of patients.[2,3] If poor results are obtained with the first dilatation, good results can be expected in many patients when the procedure is repeated. Gastroesophageal reflux complicating pneumatic dilatation is rare, less than 3% in most series. A more serious complication is perforation of the esophagus, which occurs in less than 5% of dilatations.

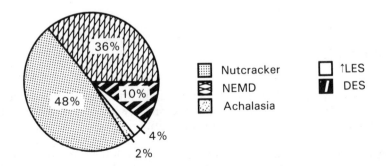

Figure 1 Pie diagram showing frequency of esophageal motility disorders found in 255 of 910 patients referred to the Gastroenterology Section of the Bowman Gray School of Medicine for evaluation of non-cardiac chest pain. NEMD = non-specific esophageal motility disorders; ↑ LES = hypertensive lower esophageal sphincter; DES = diffuse esophageal spasm.

The specific technique for pneumatic dilatation varies considerably. Not only do the dilator bags vary in size and composition but the duration of the actual inflation of the dilator within the LES can range from only a few seconds to as long as 5 minutes. Since no information is available systematically comparing different techniques, the procedure used by most operators is primarily an art taught by those with greatest experience.

Before all pneumatic dilatations are performed, the inflatable bag should be inspected to observe the symmetry of the bag during inflation, the circumference of the centre and outer aspects of the bag should be measured, and checked for leaks by submerging the bag under water.

The patient is fasted overnight and is taken to the radiology suite where the entire procedure is performed. The pneumatic dilator is advanced into the esophagus under fluoroscopic guidance until half of the bag is above the diaphragmatic hiatus and the other half is in the stomach. The bag is distended to its maximal degree as quickly as possible in an attempt to produce the most effective stretch of the LES. The size to which the bag is distended depends on its maximal diameter. Once the predetermined diameter of the bag is reached, the pressure (usually between 12 and 15 pounds per square inch) is maintained for 60 seconds. The pressure is then completely released and the bag is subsequently reinflated for an additional 60 seconds after a rest period of a few minutes. No more than two dilatations are performed at a single session. If the dilatation is successful, the patient experiences considerable pain while the balloon is inflated. The pain should resolve almost immediately following deflation. Persistent pain strongly suggests perforation.

After removal of the dilator, a small amount of barium (15–30 mL) is placed into the distal esophagus via the nasogastric tube with the patient in the semi-upright position. If a small perforation is noted extending beyond the lumen of the esophagus, the patient is restricted from eating or drinking and vital signs are closely observed. If the patient remains relatively asymptomatic but shows a rise in temperature, antibiotics should be given immediately. Conservative treatment is usually sufficient in these patients.[4] On the other hand, if barium is noted to flow freely into the mediastinum and left chest, immediate surgery is indicated. These patients usually exhibit symptoms of shock and develop severe pain within 1–2 hours. A positive Hammon's sign or subcutaneous emphysema indicates the presence of mediastinal air.

Esophagomyotomy: surgical treatment of achalasia with distal esophagomyotomy (Heller procedure) has also been found to be quite effective.[5] Excellent symptomatic improvement following this procedure has been described in 80–90% of patients. The most frequent complications are persistent dysphagia because of an inadequate myotomy or gastroesophageal reflux. Because of the latter, comcomitant antireflux procedures have been advocated to reduce this complication. The necessity for this double procedure is controversial. Suggested indications for surgical therapy of achalasia are:
- several (more than two) unsuccessful attempts at pneumatic dilatation
- esophageal rupture complicating pneumatic dilatation
- difficulty in placing the pneumatic dilator because of extreme esophageal dilatation
- inability to exclude esophageal neoplasm
- achalasia in children under 12 years of age.

Dilatation vs. surgical therapy: both the medical and the surgical treatment of achalasia are effective. Medical treatment is rarely associated with significant reflux; however, the risk of esophageal perforation is ever present. Improvement in dysphagia after dilatation varies among studies, but is probably not as great as that occurring after myotomy. The time spent in the hospital is considerably less in patients who undergo pneumatic dilatation. Optimal results with pneumatic dilatation appear to be obtained in patients over age 45 who have at least moderate esophageal dilatation and dysphagia for longer than 5 years.

An esophagomyotomy, on the other hand, may result in longer, more complete relief of dysphagia. Unfortunately, reflux is a major complication when an overzealous myotomy is performed. Present surgical mortality is very low; however, the morbidity and cost associated with major thoracic surgery are significant. A popular approach is to perform pneumatic dilatation as the initial therapy and reserve myotomy for patients who fail to benefit from dilatation or who have one of the indications for myotomy listed above.

Pharmacologic approaches: efforts to improve esophageal emptying in achalasia through pharmacologic means first began when patients were given amyl nitrite during barium swallow and immediate relaxation of the cardia occurred. Recently, isosorbide dinitrate has been shown to decrease LES pressure and increase radioisotopic esophageal emptying. A clinical trial suggested effective symptomatic improvement with long-term therapy, but many patients experienced headaches from this medication.[6] Attempts to improve esophageal emptying with anticholinergics such as tincture of belladonna, atropine sulfate and dicyclomine have been effective in isolated cases.

An exciting new area of pharmacologic therapy may be developing with the calcium channel antagonists. Nifedipine (10–20 mg *per os*) has recently been found to decrease significantly the LES pressure in patients with mild-to-moderate achalasia and to greatly improve esophageal clearance of a radiolabelled solid meal. In addition, good-to-excellent symptomatic improvement for up to 18 months has been found in some patients when compared to patients receiving a placebo.[6] It has been suggested that this calcium channel blocker may be an effective medical therapy for mild-to-moderate achalasia. Sublingual administration of nifedipine just prior to meals has proved to be effective. The patient can be advised to chew the capsule until the medication is released into the mouth. Absorption is rapid and maximal effects on esophageal pressures occur within 15–30 minutes.

Successful long-term treatment for achalasia usually requires a procedure to alter the abnormal muscular obstructive component at the LES. This can be accomplished with either pneumatic dilatation or a Heller myotomy. It is unlikely that pharmacologic therapy will provide sustained benefit in most patients.

Diffuse esophageal spasm and other motility abnormalities

Treatment of primary esophageal motility disorders other than achalasia includes a variety of medications and manoeuvres. The large number of therapies that have been suggested indicate that a single truly effective treatment is not currently available (*Table 1*). Usual forms of medical therapy include nitrates, anticholinergic drugs and sedative/tranquilizer drugs.

It is generally accepted that esophageal chest pain can be produced by gastroesophageal reflux, an apparent result of the esophageal injury produced by the acid. It is important, therefore, to exclude carefully the presence of reflux-induced symptoms prior to initiating therapy in the patient with a possible EMD. For this reason, during manometric testing to confirm the presence of an EMD, it is advisable to test these patients with intraesophageal acid instillation and to observe the symptom response to this modified Bernstein test. Hydrochloric acid, 0.1N, is instilled into the esophagus at a rate of 7–8 mL/minute for 10 minutes. During the final 5

Treatment modality	Dose	Mode of administration	Complications
Nitrates			
Nitroglycerin	0.4 mg sublingually	Usually prior to meals and prn	Headache
Isosorbide dinitrate	10-30 mg po	30 minutes prior to meals	
Anticholinergics			
Dicyclomine	10-20 mg po	qid	Dry mouth, blurred vision
Psychotropic drugs			
Diazepam	2-5 mg po	qid	Drowsiness
Trazodone	50-100 mg po	bid	Drowsiness
Doxepin	50 mg po	qhs	Impotence
Calcium entry blockers			
Nifedipine	10-20 mg	qid	Dizziness,
Diltiazem	90 mg	qid	headache, edema
Smooth muscle relaxants			
Hydralazine	25-50 mg po	tid	Lupus-like syndrome
Static dilatation	50 French	Repeat as needed	
Pneumatic dilatation	May be indicated if prominent dysphagia		Perforation
Esophagomyotomy	Rarely indicated (intractability)		Thoracotomy, gastroesophageal reflux

Table 1 Possible therapies for primary esophageal motility disorders.

minutes of acid instillation, the patient is studied with manometric recordings of a series of swallows. This allows the combined assessment of both a possible symptom response and a manometric abnormality to intraesophageal acid. If the patient shows a positive response to acid instillation, it is quite likely that gastroesophageal reflux is the inciting cause and therapy should be aimed at resolving this reflux problem. Only after reflux disease has been excluded is it appropriate to proceed with other therapies for a primary EMD. This may even include a trial of therapy (4–8 weeks) with good antireflux treatment. This is particularly important since many of the drugs used to treat motility disorders have the potential to exacerbate reflux. On some occasions, exclusion of reflux may require prolonged 24-hour intraesophageal pH monitoring.

Nitrates: the rationale for the use of the nitrates in the treatment of esophageal motility disorders relates to the pharmacologic action of these compounds in relaxing smooth muscle. The conflicting reports on the effectiveness of these agents in the treatment of spasm has been quite disappointing. Although nitrates have been used for years, the manometric response to nitroglycerin (0.4 mg sublingually) in a patient with diffuse esophageal spasm was first reported in 1973.[7] Occasionally, patients will clearly respond to the use of regular or intermittent sublingual nitroglycerin, particularly when taken just prior to eating. Symptomatic improvement may occasionally occur in response to long-acting nitrates in patients with esophageal spasm. Dosage is often limited by the occurrence of headaches, the major side effect of these drugs.

Unfortunately, therapy with nitrates is not consistently effective in the treatment of esophageal motility disorders, resulting in considerable disappointment in the long-term care of these patients. It must be emphasized that there have been no controlled studies of nitrates in the treatment of esophageal motility disorders other than achalasia.

Anticholinergics: anticholinergic medications have been suggested as therapeutic agents for the treatment of motility disorders for a number of years. Although intravenous atropine sulfate can temporarily relieve a painful esophageal contraction in a patient with diffuse spasm, the effects are much less spectacular when anticholinergics are taken orally. Clinical experience is often quite disappointing and there is no evidence to suggest that any one of the anticholinergics is preferred.

Psychotropic drugs: anecdotal reports have suggested that sedatives, tranquilizers (particularly diazepam) or antidepressants may be effective in patients whose symptomatic esophageal motility abnormalities are precipitated by stress. A recent report seems to substantiate these observations. In a placebo-controlled study, Clouse and co-workers found that low-dose trazodone (100–150 mg/day) can be beneficial in decreasing the symptoms associated with abnormal esophageal contractions.[8] Esophageal pressures, however, were not significantly changed by the trazodone therapy. Behavioural modification programs and biofeedback may also be beneficial in the long-term management of these patients.

Calcium entry blocking agents: drugs that interfere with the entry of calcium into smooth muscle cells have been shown to decrease significantly the contraction pressures in the body of the esophagus in animals. These compounds, including verapamil, nifedipine and diltiazem, have been suggested as potential therapeutic agents for the treatment of esophageal spasm and other primary EMDs.

The most dramatic effect on esophageal contraction pressures in patients with the nutcracker esophagus has been demonstrated with nifedipine. In one study, a reduction in the amplitude of esophageal peristaltic waves of more than 50% occurred following a single oral dose of 30 mg.[9]

In studies with diltiazem, no significant effects were found on esophageal contraction pressures in normal individuals using a variety of doses. However, when the drug was given to patients with nutcracker esophagus, a trend toward decreasing pressures was noted with higher doses (150 mg *per os*). An uncontrolled trial with diltiazem (90 mg qid) in a small group of these patients revealed a dramatic and significant decrease in symptoms of chest pain and dysphagia.[10]

Preliminary reports of recently completed double-blind placebo-controlled studies with calcium entry blockers in patients with recurring noncardiac chest pain have revealed interesting results. In spite of its more dramatic effect on esophageal pressures, nifedipine has been shown to be no more effective than placebo on the overall pain response in a group of 20 patients with nutcracker esophagus.[11] Reports with diltiazem are conflicting and rather preliminary. In one study of 15 patients with chest pain, no significant improvement in symptoms was noted.[12] In a second double-blind crossover study, significant improvement in chest pain for diltiazem compared to placebo was found in 13 patients with the nutcracker esophagus.[13] These studies confirm that decreases in esophageal pressures may not always correlate with pain improvement. Calcium entry blocking agents may be useful in these disorders but may need to be combined with other therapeutic modalities or used in patients with well-defined pain episodes occurring simultaneously with abnormal esophageal contractions.

Hydralazine: one recent study has investigated the manometric effect of the smooth muscle relaxing agent hydralazine in a small group of patients.[14] Although this agent did not affect the resting contraction pressures in the body of the esophagus, it did diminish the pressure response to cholinergic stimulation with bethanechol. In limited experience in three patients with EMDs, regular administration of hydralazine was felt to produce a meaningful degree of symptom improvement.

Other non-invasive methods: evidence that a consistently effective form of medical therapy for motility disorders causing chest pain has not been discovered is provided by the number of other remedies that have been suggested. Because of the potential relationship of spasm to stress, effective treatment with biofeedback has been recorded in an occasional case. This approach depends on teaching the patient to perform double swallows in an attempt to utilize the inhibitory action of the second swallow on the primary peristaltic wave, thus decreasing the potential for an excessively strong contraction.

Esophageal dilatation: many physicians find that the passage of a mercury-filled dilator will promote relief from dysphagia and chest pain in patients with esophageal motility disorders. This form of therapy has evolved primarily from the frustration of many physicians attempting to find appropriate therapy for these conditions and from the observation that some of these patients obtain relief of their symptoms for variable periods of time after the passage of an endoscope. Intermittent dilatation up to a size of approximately 50 French often will provide temporary relief for these patients. The effect is generally minimal, but can be produced with either a large dilator (54 French) or with a much smaller 'placebo' dilator (24 French).[15] It may well be that the effect of dilatation on these patients is primarily a placebo response. At any rate, patients often note some relief for variable periods of time following dilatation.

Pneumatic dilatation: it has been suggested that patients with diffuse esophageal spasm might be treated with pneumatic dilatation of the distal esophagus.[16] This procedure should be considered primarily for those patients with an EMD of which a major component is dysphagia. One must consider the morbidity and risks involved in this procedure, particularly esophageal perforation.

Esophagomyotomy: because of the poor long-term response of many patients to the above measures, some physicians will eventually recommend long myotomy of the smooth muscle esophagus. This consists of a myotomy across the LES (the Heller procedure) with proximal extension of the excision to include the involved area of the spasm. It seems most reasonable to define manometrically the extent of the hypercontracting area and to attempt to extend the incision as far as is necessary to include that section of the esophagus. Experience with esophagomyotomy in the treatment of diffuse spasm and related disorders is considerably limited, although it does seem to be effective in the occasional case.[17] Esophagomyotomy should be reserved for patients with severe symptoms causing significant compromise in their lifestyle who cannot be maintained with the other measures discussed above.[18]

A spectrum of diseases?

In 1967, a single case report indicated that an occasional patient showing the syndrome of diffuse esophageal spasm might eventually make a transition to full-blown achalasia.[19] A subsequent report by Vantrappen and co-workers indicated that this was not an isolated phenomenon, and that transitions of this type might occur occasionally in patients with primary esophageal motility disorders.[20] Subsequently, there have been other cases of this kind reported in the literature. These patients will often present initially with a combination of chest pain and dysphagia and with abnormal motility findings that are at best classified as nonspecific EMDs or possibly diffuse spasm. If followed carefully over a period of 1–2 years, some of these patients will eventually evolve into typical achalasia. This transition is heralded clinically by the loss of the chest pain component of the symptom complex and the predominance of dysphagia. At this stage, the patient has definite achalasia and the treatment should proceed as indicated. This phenomenon probably is not becoming more common, but is being increasingly recognized owing to easier availability of esophageal motility laboratories and the greater opportunity for longitudinal follow-up of patients with primary motility disorders.

Finally, it is important to bear in mind that many of these patients, particularly those with chest pain, will respond well to confident reassurance based on careful diagnostic studies. With the understanding that their symptoms are not due to cardiac disease or another serious malady, and are due to esophageal dysfunction, improvement may be noted.[21] Also, since the symptoms are intermittent and separated by long symptom-free periods in many patients, vigorous therapy may not be warranted. Considering these facts and the observation that current therapies for esophageal motility disorders are often considerably less than satisfactory, we may do well to proceed cautiously, or to follow dictates of the following quotation, attributed to Voltaire: "The art of medicine consists of amusing a patient until nature cures his disease." Or better yet, we should consider the following wise counsel of Sir William Osler: "One should treat as many patients as possible with a new drug while it still has the power to heal."

References

1 Vantrappen G, Janssens J. To dilate or operate? That is the question. *Gut* 1983; **24**: 1013–9.

2 Heitman P, Wienbeck M. The immediate effect of successful pneumatic dilation on esophageal function in achalasia. *Scand J Gastroenterol* 1972; **7**: 197–204.

3 Fellows IW, Ogilvie AL, Atkinson M. Pneumatic dilation in achalasia. *Gut* 1983; **24**: 1020–3.

4 Cameron JL, Kieffer RF, Hendrix TR, Metnigan DG, Baker RR. Selective nonoperative management of contained intrathoracic esophageal disruptions. *Ann Thor Surg* 1979; **27**: 404–8.

5 Ellis FH, Crozier RE, Watkins E. Operation for esophageal achalasia. *J Thorac Cardiovasc Surg* 1984; **88**: 344–51.

6 Gelfond M, Rozen P, Keren S, Gilat T. Isosorbide dinitrate and nifedipine treatment of achalasia: a clinical, manometric and radionuclide evaluation. *Gastroenterology* 1982; **83**: 963–9.

7 Orlando RC, Bozymski EM. Clinical and menometric effects of nitroglycerin in diffuse esophageal spasm. *N Engl J Med* 1973; **289**: 23–5.

8 Clouse RE, Lustman PJ, Eckert TC, Ferney DM, Griffith LS. Low-dose trazodone for symptomatic patients with esophageal contraction abnormalities. A double-blind, placebo-controlled trial. *Gastroenterology* 1987; **92**: 1027–36.

9 Richter JE, Dalton CB, Buice RG, Castell DO. Nifedipine: a potent inhibitor of contractions in the body of the human esophagus. *Gastroenterology* 1985; **89**: 549–54.

10 Richter JE, Spurling TJ, Cordova CM, Castell DO. Effects of oral calcium blocker, diltiazem, on esophageal contractions. *Dig Dis Sci* 1984; **29**: 649–56.

11 Richter JE, Dalton CB, Bradley LA, Castell DO. Oral nifedipine in the treatment of non-cardiac chest pain in patients with the nutrcracker esophagus. *Gastroenterology* (In press).

12 Frachtman RL, Botoman VA, Pope CE. A double-blind crossover trial of diltiazem shows no benefit in patients with dysphagia and/or chest pain of esophageal origin. *Gastroenterology* 1986; **90**: 1420(abstr).

13 Spurling TJ, Cattau EL, Hirszel R. A double-blind crossover study of the efficacy of diltiazem on patients with esophageal motility dysfunction. *Gastroenterology* 1985; **88**: 1596(abstr).

14 Mellow MH. Effect of isosorbide and hydralazine in painful primary esophageal motility disorders. *Gastroenterology* 1982; **83**: 364–70.

15 Winters C, Artnak EJ, Benjamin SB, Castell DO. Esophageal bougienage in symptomatic patients with the nutcracker esophagus. *JAMA* 1984; **252**: 3630–6.

16 Ebert EC, Ouyang A, Wright SH, Cohen S. Pneumatic dilatation in patients with symptomatic diffuse esophageal spasm and lower esophageal sphincter dysfunction. *Dig Dis Sci* 1983; **28**: 481–5.

17 Tummala V, Baue AE, McCallum RW. Surgical myotomy in patients with high-amplitude peristaltic esophageal contractions: manometric and clinical effects. *Dig Dis Sci* 1987; **32**: 16–21.

18 Richter JE, Castell DO. Surgical myotomy for nutcracker esophagus: to be or not to be? *Dig Dis Sci* 1987; **32**: 95–6.

19 Kramer P, Harris LD, Donaldson RM. Transition from symptomatic, diffuse spasm to cardiospasm. *Gut* 1967; **8**: 115–9.

20 Vantrappen G, Janssens J, Hellemans J, Coremans G. Achalasia, diffuse esophageal spasm and related motility disorders. *Gastroenterology* 1979; **76**: 450–7.

21 Ward BW, Wu WC, Richter JE, Hackshaw BT, Castell DO. Long-term follow-up of symptomatic status of patients with non-cardiac chest pain: is diagnosis of esophageal etiology helpful? *Am J Gastroenterol* 1987; **82**: 215–8.

Physiology, diagnosis and treatment of gastroesophageal reflux

R W McCallum, M C Champion

Gastroesophageal reflux (GER) is an extremely common problem. It is endemic in North America and is the major reason for *ad libitum* intake of antacids by the population at large. Its frequency is such that in the largely referral practice of a gastroenterologist, GER and irritable bowel syndrome rank variably as the first and second most commonly seen problems. There is a considerable degree of morbidity associated with GER, the pathophysiology of which has been increasingly elucidated over the past 10 years.

Reflux disease encompasses a wide spectrum of clinical presentations. At one extreme it may present with typical symptoms of heartburn, regurgitation or chest pain and may respond to standard forms of therapy. At the other it may masquerade under the guise of disorders attributed to a cardiac, pulmonary, peptic or gallbladder origin, or it may be resistant to the most aggressive medical therapy.

Since the first description of this entity by Winkelstein in 1935[1] and use of the term 'reflux esophagitis' by Allison in 1946,[2] considerable progress has been made in the pathophysiology and treatment of the entity. Considered synonymous with hiatus hernia at one time, the disease is now recognized as being multifactorial in etiology. The host of factors contributing to this problem may differ from patient to patient.

Several reviews of GER have been published in the literature recently.[3-6] This chapter discusses the pathophysiology and methods of investigation in GER and examines the approaches and outcomes of medical therapy.

Pathophysiology of gastroesophageal reflux

A number of different factors are involved in the mechanisms responsible for GER, all of which are necessary to understand as they form the foundation and rationale upon which medical and surgical therapeutic decisions are based (*Figure 1*).[6]

Pathogenesis

An understanding of the antireflux mechanisms operative in normal subjects is necessary in defining the abnormality present in patients with reflux esophagitis. Recent work has focused mainly on the lower esophageal sphincter (LES), the pinchcock action of the diaphragm, gastric emptying, acid clearance mechanisms in the esophagus, constituents and volume of gastric fluid available for reflux, esophageal mucosal resistance factors and hiatus hernia.

The antireflux mechanisms which form an anatomical barrier to GER may be classified as intrinsic and extrinsic. The intrinsic factor is constituted mainly by the LES, whereas the pinchcock action of the diaphragm, the intra-abdominal segment of the esophagus and other less well-defined structures comprise the extrinsic contributions.

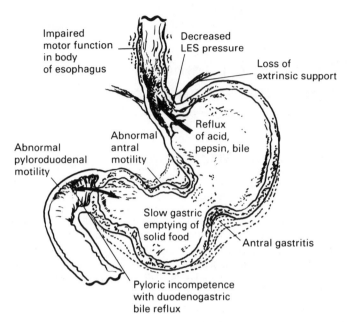

Figure 1   Factors involved in the pathogenesis of gastroesophageal reflux.

Intrinsic factor: the LES has been a subject of extensive study since its first description by Fyke and Code.[7] Even though it is difficult to define the LES morphologically, both *in vivo* and *in vitro* studies have shown it to have distinct functional properties. It maintains a continuous myogenic tone which can be modulated by neural and hormonal influences. Neural excitation either through vagal or intrinsic nerve stimulation causes relaxation of the LES muscle. A vast array of hormones and peptides have been shown to exert an effect on the LES, but their precise physiologic significance is not clear.

There appears to be a general consensus that resting sphincter pressure is vital in prevention of GER. However, the degree of this pressure required for the LES competence has been a matter of considerable debate. Earlier studies showed that the degree of resting LES pressure alone can differentiate between normal asymptomatic subjects and patients with reflux esophagitis, but improvements in esophageal manometric techniques have revealed a marked degree of overlap between these two groups. A high degree of correlation has been found between reflux symptoms and a resting sphincter pressure below 5 mmHg, but for pressures above this level there is a poor correlation if such a pressure is used to define a reflux patient. Data suggest that such a low pressure (<5 mmHg) is not induced by GER itself but is the patient's inherent LES pressure, placing the patient at risk for spontaneous reflux events.

The term 'competence' cannot be equated with the resting sphincter since reflux occurs in normal asymptomatic subjects with a normal sphincter pressure. Recently, this definition has been changed to refer to the frequency of reflux episodes. A greater number of GER episodes account for one of the reasons for occurrence of reflux esophagitis. Furthermore, a number of studies have shown phasic and cyclical variation in the sphincter pressure, therefore casting doubt over the value of resting sphincter pressure as a determinant of the reflux barrier.

This apparent paradox of normal sphincter pressures in reflux patients and occurrence of reflux events in normal subjects has been explained on the basis that dynamic LES events are occurring at the moment of reflux. Prolonged simultaneous manometric and pH studies have shown that acid reflux occurs during periods of transient inhibition or relaxation of the sphincter pressure in normal subjects. Similarly, transient episodes of LES relaxation (TLESR) account for the majority of reflux episodes in reflux patients, although factors such as persistently low basal pressure with feeble LES pressure explain other mechanisms associated with reflux events. Thus, a low sphincter pressure, either persistent or occurring during periods of sphincter relaxation, is central to the GER event. Patients with reflux esophagitis not only have increased numbers of such transient relaxations but also have the higher incidence of reflux associated with TLESRs.

Therefore, what excites or provides the stimulus for these TLESRs? Some may be associated with incomplete peristalsis but the majority are not related to swallowing (*Figure 2*). It is highly unlikely that they represent any pathologic event for a number of reasons: belching and vomiting are associated with a similar relaxation event; they occur in normal subjects; these events have been reported in animal studies.

Sphincteric tone is primarily myogenic in origin and is modulated by hormonal and neural mechanisms. A failure at the myogenic level should result in a persistently low basal tone, as observed in patients with scleroderma and in association with atrophic gastritis. Hormonal factors (cholecystokinin, secretin) may be responsible for the low LES pressure observed after a large and/or fatty meal (*Table 1*). It is highly unlikely that intermittent release of a hormone could account for transient inhibition. Most probably these relaxations are neurally mediated. Vagal cooling has been shown to prevent their occurrence. Equally important is the fact that they do not occur during periods of sleep which might again suggest the central mediation of these relaxations.

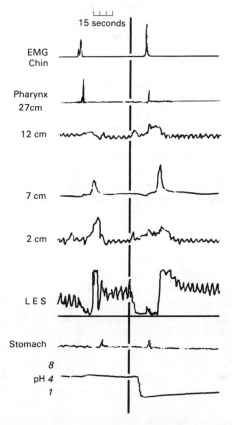

Figure 2 An example of transient relaxation of the LES. To the left of the vertical line are normal swallow-associated events: submental EMG, pharyngeal contraction and esophageal peristaltic contraction. The vertical line represents the onset of the transient relaxation. Note the associated event, i.e. esophageal contractions at the onset of the relaxation. Reflux occurs during transient relaxation of the LES and results in a fall of esophageal pH from 5 to 1.

Foods
Fat
Chocolate

Drugs
Anticholinergics
Nitrates
Theophyllines
Nicotine (smoking)
Alpha-blockers
Calcium channel blockers
Levodopa
Narcotics

Hormones/miscellaneous
Progesterone
Estrogen
Cholecystokinin
Somatostatin
Beta-agonists
Prostaglandins E_1, E_2

Table 1   Agents that decrease LES pressure and/or slow gastric emptying.

Holloway and colleagues have shown that gastric distension could be a stimulus for LES relaxation.[8] With graded distension they were able to elicit an increasing number of LES relaxations in both normal subjects (*Figure 3*) and patients with GER.

Slow or delayed gastric emptying (an observation reported in up to 50% of GER patients) could result in prolonged gastric distension and hence induce transient LES relaxations. A greater gastric volume may also reflux with each relaxation. Recent studies in normal subjects and reflux patients have suggested that gastric distension results in a significant increase in TLESRs and such a reflux may be a major mechanism for the normally observed post-prandial increase in GER.[8,9] In recent studies in normal subjects an increase in LES relaxations was observed after a large meal and a significantly higher percentage had complete relaxation to the gastric baseline, thus promoting more potential for GER (*Figure 4*).[10] The clustering of acid reflux events in the immediate post-prandial period in both normal subjects and GER patients would be consistent with the finding of meal-induced changes in frequency and degree of relaxation of TLESRs. This would also suggest a unifying link for gastric distension which accompanies food ingestion as one provoker of TLESRs.

The explanation of more complete relaxations may rest with the fat content of meals. Larger volumes of food generally contain more fat. The resultant decrease in LES pressure after meals would promote more complete TLESRs (less residual pressure after relaxation). The pathway could involve afferents from stretch receptors in the proximal stomach and fundus travelling to the brain stem and efferent response mediated through the vagus nerve. Any delay in gastric emptying, as reported in some refluxers and states of gastroparesis, may result in prolonged gastric distension, thereby provoking more frequent and complete LES relaxations and more reflux.

Studies on the mechanism of peristalsis have shown that each swallow elicits an initial inhibitory followed by an excitatory stimulus through the vagus nerve to the esophagus.[11] A threshold and subthreshold stimulus always excites both impulses in that sequence. However, a subthreshold pharyngeal stimulus can excite only inhibitory nerves which are responsible for inhibition of any ongoing contraction in the esophagus and relaxations of the LES. Therefore, a subthreshold pharyngeal stimulus could excite an isolated LES relaxation.[9]

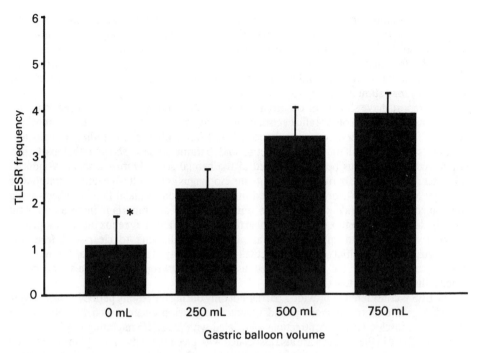

Figure 3 Frequency of TLESR with different gastric balloon volumes. * Indicates all gastric volumes (250–750 mL) induced significantly more TLESR events.

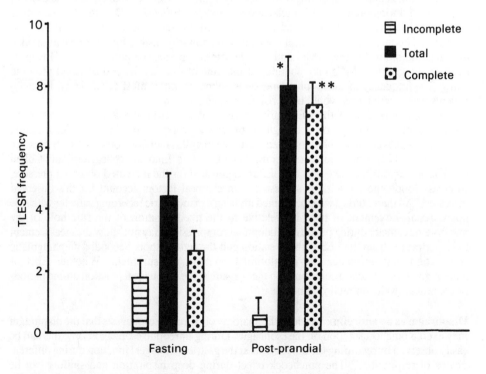

Figure 4 Frequency of TLESR in fasting and post-prandial states.

In support of this hypothesis, Paterson and colleagues have shown that light stroking of the pharynx or low frequency stimulation of the afferent nerve (superior laryngeal nerve) produces isolated episodes of LES relaxation in the opossum.[12] Further support for this concept is borne out by the fact that LES relaxations are absent during sleep.[13] During periods of sleep pharyngeal stimulus is unlikely and during awake periods movement of the buccal structure (i.e. tongue, etc) may stimulate pharyngeal receptors.

A few reports have shown the occurrence of acid reflux during swallow-induced sphincter relaxations. In fact, 50% of the reflux episodes in one study were reported to occur during these periods.[14] Similar observations were reported in 1965 with barium studies. Longhi and colleagues, using simultaneous manometric and barium studies, showed that part of a swallowed barium bolus becomes trapped in the hernial sac.[15] During a swallow-induced sphincter relaxation, the barium refluxes into the esophagus as a result of negative intrathoracic pressure. Mittal and co-workers confirmed this phenomenon in hiatal hernia subjects using simultaneous radionuclide studies.[16] This observation has an important implication. Acid initially cleared after a reflux event can pool in the hernial sac and may reflux into the esophagus during swallow-induced sphincter relaxation. Thus, swallowing to clear acid from the esophagus during the initial reflux event actually leads to delayed acid clearance. This may be a mechanism by which the long-observed association between hiatus hernia and reflux esophagitis can be tied together.

The LES is considered to provide a barrier not only during the resting period but also during periods of gastric contractions and periods of increased gastric pressure caused by contraction of abdominal muscles. Gastric contractions associated with phase III migrating motor complex (MMC) activity in the stomach are also associated with phasic activity in the sphincter, thereby augmenting the pressure of the sphincter. A disorder in this coordination of LES and stomach phasic activity has been cited as the mechanism of reflux in some patients with reflux esophagitis, but this has yet to be confirmed.

Do LES relaxations occur during MMC activity of the stomach? Certainly, MMC activity in the stomach during periods of LES relaxation would promote GER. During LES relaxation periods MMC activity is inhibited, such activity appearing at the same time as the activity in the sphincter. This suggests that the inhibitory phenomenon responsible for LES relaxation also mediates inhibition for the MMC and thus becomes a protective phenomenon. However, occasionally gastric MMCs may continue at the time of the TLESR and so could promote reflux. The frequency of such a phenomenon is unknown, but it must occur rarely. Possibly, patients with scleroderma would be at risk from such an event.

A reflex contraction of the LES during periods of increased gastric pressure caused by abdominal muscle contraction is thought to provide a protective mechanism against reflux. However, there is considerable controversy as to whether this increased observed LES pressure is the result of LES contractions or other mechanical factors. Lind and colleagues[17] and Cohen and Harris[18] favour the view that the LES is responsible for the increased observed pressure, whereas Dodds and co-workers suggest that mechanical factors account for this observed increase.[4,5] All these studies were performed utilizing a manometric recording catheter with side holes. Axial movement of the LES relative to the fixed position of the side hole of the manometric catheter during periods of abdominal compression may not allow the measurement to be performed from the LES with the station pull-through method. Secondly, diaphragmatic contraction may influence the intraluminal pressure measurement. Whether LES or diaphragmatic contraction contributes to the pressure at the esophageal junction during periods of abdominal wall contraction is not clear.

Diaphragm as an antireflux barrier: the anatomy of crural fibres suggests that the diaphragm may exert a pinchcock action on the esophagus. During fibreoptic esophagoscopy, this can be easily observed by recording the movements at the gastric esophageal junction during different phases of respiration.[19] The pinchcock effect during deep inspiration and sniffing can be observed either at the distal esophagus or the stomach (when a hiatus hernia is present). On manometry, two high pressure zones (HPZ) have been described in patients with hiatus hernia; the proximal zone corresponding with the LES and the distal zone with the pinchcock action of the diaphragmatic hiatus. A similar band of HPZ located proximal to the LES has been described in opossums. In this animal the LES is located inside the abdomen.

In the normal anatomical situation in humans, where the diaphragm overlaps the LES, it has been difficult to dissect the individual pressure exerted by these two structures from the pressure monitored at the gastroesophageal junction. Welch and colleagues also observed the diaphragmatic squeeze pressure superimposed on the distal part of the LES.[20] A recent study conducted by Boyle and colleagues in cats has shown that the pinchcock action of the diaphragm does not contribute to the resting pressure observed at the gastroesophageal junction, although a significant increase in this pressure is observed during inspiration and this pressure increases with the depth of inspiration.[21] This effect may be a protective mechanism during inspiration where the pressure gradient between the chest and abdomen increases. A similar pinchcock effect is described during the Valsalva maneuver.

By definition, the sphincter, apart from contributing to the positive intraluminal pressure, should be able to relax or remain inhibited in response to the appropriate stimuli. Indirect evidence suggests that this is true for diaphragmatic squeeze pressure because respiration-induced pressure oscillation does not occur during sphincter relaxation induced by a swallow or esophageal distension. Similarly, a dissociation between the electrical activity of the diaphragmatic costal and crural muscle fibres has been described during esophageal distension, vomiting and eructation. Thus, by augmenting the LES during inspiration, the diaphragmatic pinchcock action may serve as a protective mechanism. However, such a mechanism, if superimposed on the stomach as in patients with hiatus hernia, may be harmful and promote acid reflux because acid secreted in the hernial sac may pool and reflux into the esophagus during swallow-induced sphincter relaxation.

Acid clearance: once acid has refluxed into the esophagus the degree of esophageal mucosal damage can be regarded as a function of the length of time this acid is exposed to the esophageal mucosa. An efficient clearance is thus an important defense mechanism against the development of esophagitis. The esophageal acid clearance mechanism has been investigated in detail in recent years. Helms and colleagues have shown that acid clearance occurs as a two-step process.[22] During the first step (so-called volume clearance) the entire volume of injected acid is cleared by one or two initial esophageal peristaltic contractions. At this time, no radiolabelled acid can be seen in the esophagus, even though the esophageal pH remains low. The effect of gravity on volume clearance, though considered not to be important in normal subjects, may have a marked influence in patients with disorders of peristalsis.

The second step in acid clearance is the neutralization of a small amount of acid coating the walls of the esophagus by saliva traversing with the swallow-associated esophageal contractions. Restoration of the esophageal pH is thus achieved by saliva through its dilution and neutralization effects. Saliva and esophageal contractions amplify each other's effect in restoration of the esophageal pH. In several studies patients with reflux esophagitis have been shown to have delayed acid clearance.[22,23] Two abnormalities which could give rise to such a phenomenon are abnormal esophageal peristalsis and saliva flow, or its neutralization capacity. Marked abnormality in acid clearance has been shown to occur in patients with diffuse esophageal spasm and achalasia. Abnormal peristalsis is observed only occasionally in patients with reflux esophagitis. Patients with chronic strictures in the distal esophagus and/or Barrett's esophagus will have impairments in peristalsis and low amplitude contractions. Sonnenberg and colleagues did not find any difference in the salivary flow and its neutralization capacity in age-matched controls and patients with reflux esophagitis.[24] Interestingly, the incidence of reflux has not been reported to be high in patients with Sjorgren's syndrome, where there is abnormally low salivary flow. Hence only a critically small amount of saliva seems necessary to fulfil its role as 'housekeeper or natural antacid' of the esophagus. The presence of abnormal acid clearance in spite of normal peristalsis and salivary flow deserves further investigation.

The effect of hiatus hernia on acid clearance is controversial. Longhi and Jordan, using simultaneous barium and manometric studies, observed that after an initial swallow of barium, a small amount became trapped in the hiatus hernia.[25] This barium refluxed into the esophagus during swallow-induced sphincter (swallow-induced biphasic phenomenon) relaxation, but came back to the hiatus hernia during aborally-directed peristaltic contraction, thus providing a mechanism of delayed clearance of barium from a normal esophagus.

An acid clearance study in normal subjects showed that each swallow is associated with a stepwise rise in esophageal pH (a monophasic pH response). Long phases of GER were characterized by biphasic pH responses. A study in GER patients with and without hiatus hernia[16] demonstrated that these biphasic pH responses induced by swallowing were present only in hiatal hernia subjects, and that acid clearance was delayed in these patients compared with non-hernia patients, supporting the observations of Longhi and Jordan.[25] An additional mechanism for the delayed acid clearance observed in many patients with reflux may thus be an hiatal hernia.

Sleep and GER
Reflux at night-time or during sleep is considered to be particularly detrimental to the esophageal mucosa. A number of studies have shown that GER patients reflux at night-time during sleep and normal subjects do not. These studies suggest that nocturnal reflux determines the degree of mucosal damage. A study by Dent and colleagues showed that transient periods of sphincter relaxation and GER occur during short periods of arousal from sleep.[26] This is an important observation and probably points toward the mechanism of TLESR.

Subthreshold pharyngeal stimulation or partial swallowing may be the stimulus for TLESR and, since swallowing is markedly depressed during sleep, there is no stimulus for LES relaxation. However, whether GER patients reflux during sleep is not known. This is important because mechanisms other than TLESRs are also operating in GER patients.

Acid clearance during sleep: swallow-induced esophageal contraction and saliva are the two major determinants of acid clearance. Since both swallowing and saliva are inhibited during sleep, acid clearance during sleep is markedly impaired. If a subject goes to sleep just after an episode of GER, acid is not cleared from the esophagus and results in prolonged exposure of the esophageal mucosa to low pH. A study by Orr and colleagues has shown that acid clearance time is a function of wakefulness.[13] The occurrence of GER and clearance of acid therefore seems to be functioning in opposite directions in normal subjects. TLESRs do not occur during sleep, but if GER occurs just before the subject goes to sleep, acid clearance is delayed markedly.

Potency of refluxed material
The composition of the material refluxed into the esophagus is an important factor in determining the presence and severity of GER. Acid and pepsin in small amounts play key roles in generating esophagitis. When patients with Zollinger-Ellison syndrome develop esophagitis, the injury may be so severe as to cause stricture, bleeding or even perforation.[27] Bile and pancreatic secretions (especially following gastric surgery) have an alkaline corrosive effect.[28] At an acid pH, conjugated bile salts can increase the permeability of the esophageal mucosa to hydrogen ions (H^+). However, it has been shown that bile acids do not reflux into the esophagus during reflux episodes in normal subjects and esophagitis patients, and it is suggested that bile does not accompany an acid reflux event.[29] The term 'alkaline reflux' should be reserved for postoperative gastric surgery or pernicious anemia patients.

Gastric volume and emptying
GER occurs more often in the post-prandial state than in the fasting state. One reason for this is that the volume of contents present in the stomach determines the frequency of reflux. The

larger the volume, the more frequent the reflux. In fact, the volume of fluid in the stomach required to produce a GER episode has been used as an index of LES strength. In the post-prandial state the volume of fluid present in the stomach depends upon the following factors:

- volume of food ingested
- volume of gastric secretions
- duodenogastric reflux
- gastric emptying.

Reflux is more common after a large meal. Gastric acid secretion in patients with reflux esophagitis has been studied. GER patients as a group have normal acid secretory parameters, although 5% will be hypersecretors.[30] There is an increased incidence of GER in patients with Zollinger-Ellison syndrome,[31] and this is attributed to an overwhelming effect of hypersecretion of acid. Pyloric incompetence facilitating duodenogastric reflux was proposed as an important contributing factor in a number of ways: a large volume of reflux material would increase the gastric volume and may even slow the gastric emptying rate; bile acid may induce antral gastritis and therefore cause antral hypomotility; bile acids and other alkaline secretions may reflux into the esophagus, damaging the esophageal mucosa directly.

It has been reported that patients with GER disease have higher concentrations of bile acids in the stomach and therefore larger volumes of duodenogastric reflux.[32] However, recent studies using radionuclide methods have shown that duodenogastric reflux is a physiologic phenomenon; concentrations of bile acids in the gastric juice of patients with erosive esophagitis are similar to those of normal subjects.[33] Therefore, the significance of duodenogastric reflux remains controversial.

Gastric retention with accumulation of acid and gastric contents logically may be postulated as a contributory factor in the production of GER. McCallum and colleagues reported delayed gastric emptying in a significant number of patients with GER.[34,35] Behar and Ramsly found that there was an abnormality in the gastric antral motility but that liquid emptying was normal.[36]

Several studies have demonstrated delay of the mean emptying rates for either solids[34,37,38] or liquids[37,39-42] in patients with GER. Other investigators have reported normal solid and liquid emptying in patients with GER.[43-47] It is possible that like the variable LES pressure, patients with GER are a heterogenous population in their severity of reflux and the degree of delayed gastric emptying.

Some patients with GER complain of vomiting that may be related to gastric retention and distension. Certainly, most GER patients complain of bloating, fullness, post-prandial satiety and epigastric discomfort, much of which is explained by delayed gastric emptying. Smoking and high-fat meals also further delay gastric emptying and provoke reflux symptoms (*Table 1*). Gastric distension related to eating could be accentuated by any slowing of gastric emptying. Gastric distension, in turn, promotes more frequent and complete transient relaxations in the LES.[48]

The gastric motility disturbance may be primary (idiopathic) or secondary to an identifiable disease. Because fat delays gastric emptying and lowers LES pressure, it is appropriate to recommend small, soft and semi-solid low-fat meals for reflux patients.

An antireflux operation, fundoplication, is often successful in patients with reflux esophagitis. When gastric emptying studies are performed, surgical failures appear to correlate with slower solid emptying,[49] whereas increased liquid emptying occurs more often. This latter phenomenon is probably attributable to impaired receptive relaxation related to surgical trauma and/or entrapment of the vagus nerve. One of the authors (RWM) has also observed that a population of post-fundoplication patients presenting with increasing symptoms of GER (and therefore termed relative or absolute failure) had an accompanying delay in gastric emptying. This delay may have been present in this patient group from the onset; thus there would be no reason to suppose that a fundoplication would have any real effect on improving the rate of solid gastric emptying in these patients. Interestingly, the literature indicates that symptoms tend to recur over a period of 3–5 years, such that after 5 years there is significant documentation of reflux by esophageal pH studies. It may be indicative that the continued delay in gastric emptying in some patients slowly weakens the efficacy of the antireflux procedure.

Fink and colleagues have reported that the slow gastric emptying of solids in patients with GER can be correlated with the degree and severity of antral gastritis.[30] Presumably this antral gastritis continues after surgery. The cause of the gastritis is not clear. Is it possible that gastric stasis itself could promote gastritis, or could gastritis induce a smooth muscle impairment? In the latter case, the cause of the gastritis could be bile reflux, which raises questions about the competence of the pylorus and the status of duodenal motility in GER.

Another possibility is that at the time of fundoplication, vagal damage occurs as a result of an accidental vagotomy or possibly entrapment of the vagus nerve in the fundoplication wrap. It is estimated that accidental vagotomies or vagal nerve damage may occur in up to 30% of patients undergoing fundoplication, particularly in the setting of a second antireflux operation. Such vagal damage would certainly explain both the more rapid gastric emptying of liquids found in such postoperative settings[50] and the possibility that impaired antral innervation could result in delayed gastric emptying of solids.

Research into the relationship between gastric emptying and GER has highlighted the fact that GER is much more than a disease of the distal 3 cm of the esophagus (the LES). More importantly, it may be a diffuse motility disturbance of the upper GI tract, with events occurring distal to the LES contributing to the reflux events, and the LES the 'victim'.

Tissue resistance

The esophageal epithelium has a capacity to resist injury from refluxed gastric material, and this varies among individuals. Normal squamous epithelium is impermeable, but back diffusion of H^+ and subsequent protein denaturization is potentiated by bile, pepsin and alcohol.[51] Some workers believe that nerve endings in elongated papillae that are present as manifestations of chronic inflammation are brought closer to the lumen by desquamation of the surface epithelial cells and thereby elicit heartburn. The prostaglandins and sucralfate, with their proven mucosal protective actions in the stomach and duodenum, may have a theoretical role in maintaining esophageal mucosal integrity, but this is yet to be proven. Current studies evaluating sucralfate and the prostaglandins indicate no improvement in healing. In addition, there may be other factors that promote healing or delay fibrosis and stricture formation, as well as possibly preventing Barrett's epithelium and its consequences.

In summary, reflux esophagitis is a multifactorial process dependent upon a combination of factors — LES incompetence, gastric volume and emptying, esophageal acid clearance and tissue resistance. Therapy should be directed toward decreasing transient LES relaxations, increasing LES pressure, improving gastric emptying, suppressing gastric acidity, enhancing esophageal clearance or promoting salivation. These observations emphasize the need to regard patients with GER as a heterogeneous group. Although they may present with heartburn and degrees of regurgitation, their individual predominant pathophysiologic changes will vary. This must be appreciated in order to instigate appropriate tests to identify the abnormalities in each individual and initiate 'tailor-made' therapy.

Diagnostic approach to gastroesophageal reflux

The diagnosis of GER is usually based on clinical findings. However, in a small number of patients, the judicious use of a few diagnostic tests may be necessary. Clinically, GER patients present with heartburn, regurgitation and, in many cases, chest pain. This chest pain can be substernal and associated with diaphoresis, shortness of breath and anginal-type radiation. Dysphagia or odynophagia may indicate a stricture, severe mucosal inflammation or an associated esophageal motility problem. Concordant with disordered gastric emptying in some refluxers, post-prandial nausea, bloating and emesis may also occur.

The barium swallow is helpful in defining strictures, ulcers with reflux or Barrett's and can be used initially to evaluate dysphagia and to rule out other GI disease. The majority of symptomatic GER patients (80–90%) will have a hiatal hernia, and evidence suggests that at least 40% of patients asymptomatic for GER and aged over 50 will also have a hiatal hernia. Cine-esophagography has a sensitivity of only 40% for GER, and reflux damage to esophageal mucosa is rarely detected by standard radiographic techniques.[52] In the presence of a hiatal hernia, it is very difficult to evaluate LES competency.

Since Fyke's description of the LES manometrically, there has been much controversy about the value of the measurement technique.[7] It is clear that a single LES pressure recording, unless extreme (e.g. <5 mmHg), is insufficiently discriminatory to suggest reflux. However, manometric demonstration of esophageal spasm, 'nutcracker' or hypercontracting esophagus, or disruption of normal peristalsis may be helpful in explaining the occurrence of atypical chest pain or dysphagia in the absence of mechanical obstruction.

The Bernstein acid perfusion test represents a safe, simple, reproducible and quite sensitive technique for identifying an esophagus sensitive to acid.[53] Even so, a negative test result does not exclude the esophagus as the cause of pain. The reproduction of pain correlates best with symptoms. Positive tests are seen in approximately 85% of patients with symptoms but in up to 15% of asymptomatic subjects. It appears that relief of pain from acid infusion by saline is not a sensitive indicator of a positive Bernstein test. In one study up to 52% of patients failed to obtain relief following saline instillation, and elevation of esophageal pH above 4 or the use of antacids did not influence the outcome of pain relief in refluxers.[54] In the setting of chest pain, which is a combination of heartburn and/or pressure and squeezing, and a negative cardiac evaluation, the Bernstein test may be invaluable if it reproduces the patient's presenting pain. Some centres have not found the test to be as useful.[55]

Up to 50% of patients with objective criteria for GER have no macroscopic evidence of esophagitis upon endoscopy.[56] Characteristic changes seen with esophagitis include erythema, friability, erosions, exudate, ulceration, stricture and, in some cases, Barrett's columnar-lined esophagus. With the aid of the Crosby capsule or Quinton suction biopsy, specimens from 2.5–10 cm above the manometrically determined LES can be obtained easily. Suction biopsies in normal subjects will show GER changes in only 5% of cases; therefore, finding biopsy changes in symptomatic patients is very significant.[57] Routine endoscopic biopsies do not include the lamina propria, and they are also smaller, more fragmented and difficult to orientate. However, the endoscopic biopsy specimens from the newer endoscopes with large biopsy channels (10 F) are adequate and will replace the more arduous suction biopsy technique. Although neutrophils can be observed, the lack of a true esophagitis in biopsies is one of the reasons behind the changes in terminology from reflux esophagitis to GER disease. Finally, intraepithelial eosinophils reported to be helpful in the diagnosis of GER in infants do not seem to suggest GER in adults. Intraepithelial eosinophils were present in 30% of biopsies from pH-proven refluxers and 33% of biopsies from asymptomatic normal control subjects.[58]

The standard acid reflux test (SART), introduced by Tuttle and Grossman in 1958, is a nonphysiologic technique that requires intragastric instillations of acid followed by various artificial maneuvers to raise intragastric pressure.[59] The false positive rate may be as high as 40% and, consequently, the method has lost favour as a means of measuring esophageal pH.

The acid clearance test introduced by Booth and colleagues in 1968 is based on the concept that acid-induced changes in the esophagus lead to disordered peristalsis which in turn results in impaired clearance of refluxed acid.[60] Esophageal pH is measured 5 cm above the manometrically defined LES and, following ingestion of 15 mL of 0.1 N hydrochloric acid, the number of swallows required to raise the esophageal pH to 5 or above is determined. Normally, less than 12 swallows are required. The rate of positive tests in symptomatic patients ranges from 53–100%. Patients with esophageal motility disorders will have false positive results, and manometry should be performed on all study subjects.

The most recent application of esophageal pH measurements, 24-hour monitoring, has emphasized the importance of night-time reflux with episodes of long duration and the concept of upright and supine GER. However, night-time reflux only occurs in 70% of all GER patients.[61] Despite the sensitivity of prolonged pH monitoring for detecting acid reflux, false negative findings range from 10–20%; some of these findings may be bile reflux or may simply represent the artificial settings of hospitalization, which, until recently, has been the method of studying these patients. Presently, there are several 24-hour ambulatory pH monitoring devices, similar to the Holter monitor, on the market. These devices enable 24-hour pH monitoring of patients while allowing them to follow a normal lifestyle. This allows for a more normal physiologic setting for assessing symptoms and severity of reflux. This methodology is also useful in assessing patients who have chest pain considered to be noncardiac in origin. However the variability in meal type and frequency even in individual patients raises questions as to reproducibility of reflux times. More important is the correlation of a pH event (pH$<$4) with heartburn or chest pain.

An alternative to 24-hour pH recording is post-prandial pH recording. In a study in which episodes where the pH fell below 4.0 for 3 hours after breakfast and lunch, and 4 hours after dinner, were monitored, the sensitivity was 77% and the specificity 96%, yielding a positive predictive value of 79%.[61] When this single post-prandial time period was compared to 24-hour testing as a diagnostic test, sensitivity was 77% and specificity 95%. Every patient refluxed post-prandially whereas 30% of GER patients did not reflux at night. In a recent study, reflux was evaluated basally and post-prandially in both the sitting (1 hour) and lying (2 hours) positions. The mean 3-hour post-prandial reflux time was 44.6 ± 6.7 minutes in refluxers, compared to 4.0 ± 1.2 minutes in normal subjects. The value of this exaggerated reflux time may not be appreciated under basal or in nonphysiologic settings. It is felt that post-prandial pH monitoring may be an accurate method which is attractive to both patient and investigator and easily adapted to community hospital and office setting. Post-prandial pH testing is therefore an alternative to 24-hour monitoring.[62] Twenty-four hour pH monitoring is helpful in confirming diagnosis when other tests have been uncertain.

The role for the radionuclide diagnosis of GER needs to be reviewed. In this procedure, 200–300 μCi^{99m}Tc sulphur colloid is swallowed in the form of an isotope-labelled liquid meal, and interval counts are measured with a gamma camera over the area of the esophagus and stomach.[63] The technique is simple, quick and uniformly sensitive in 75–85% of patients with symptoms. Some data show a strong correlation with severity of GER and endoscopic esophagitis, and studies following medical or surgical therapy have demonstrated a significant reduction in radionuclide activity that corresponds closely to the degree of clinical reflux.[64] However, other researchers have been unable to reproduce these data, the method failing to detect any evidence of esophageal counts at times when a simultaneous pH recording in the distal esophagus has documented acid reflux.[65] Future studies in this field should be directed toward defining the contribution of esophageal scintigraphy when used with other esophageal function studies and to demonstrate this test's reproducibility in a number of research laboratories. While it may diagnose more severe and obvious forms of GER, as does the barium swallow, it is not able to detect milder cases.

Blue and colleagues demonstrated esophageal reflux with a DISIDA scan in a patient with a Billroth II anastomosis, indicating that bile reflux may have been the cause of the esophagitis and epigastric pain.[66] In addition, earlier studies demonstrated that patients with pernicious anemia had delayed solid meal gastric emptying.[67] Orlando and Bozynski found that pernicious anemia patients with betazole-fast achlorhydria may still have bilious heartburn and regurgitation with endoscopic and histologic esophagitis despite the absence of acid.[68]

In summary, the combination of a thorough history, physical examination, endoscopy with biopsy, Bernstein acid perfusion testing and esophageal pH studies provide the most accurate means of investigating the patient with reflux symptoms.

Medical therapy of gastroesophageal reflux

This section of the chapter will discuss the current therapeutic approaches to the treatment of GER, emphasizing that the rationale for choosing an individual treatment is based upon an attempt to correct the underlying pathophysiologic mechanisms of the condition.

Management of GER can be subdivided into three phases:
- Phase 1 — Simple antireflux measures
    — antacids
- Phase 2 — Drugs
    — acid suppression
    — prokinetic agents
- Phase 3 — Surgery

PHASE 1

Simple changes in lifestyle can play a major role in the medical treatment of GER. Refluxers should avoid lying down soon after meals, as reflux is greatly increased during this time period. In patients with heartburn at night, elevation of the head of the bed 6–8 inches may be beneficial.[69] Weight reduction with fatty food avoidance or measures to reduce intra-abdominal pressure may reduce symptoms.[70] Foods that lower LES tone, such as chocolate, fat, carminatives (peppermint, spearmint) and coffee are to be avoided, while cigarettes (with their nicotine receptor effect) must be eliminated. A variety of commonly-used drugs decrease LES pressure and/or slow gastric emptying (*Table 1*). In addition smaller, semi-solid meals may be beneficial in decreasing symptoms.[71] There are no published placebo-controlled trials examining the use of antacids alone in the treatment of GER, and yet antacids neutralize acid, bind bile acids and cause small rises in LES pressure. Behar and colleagues found that only 19% of patients treated with antacids obtained symptomatic relief.[72] Whether antacid control of mild to moderate symptoms of GER is a result of true pharmacologic efficacy or is a placebo response remains to be proven. A controlled study showed them to be no more effective than placebo in controlling episodes of heartburn or pain induced by Bernstein infusion, and symptom relief did not correlate with intraesophageal pH. Adequate relief with either antacid (30 mL) or placebo was obtained.[73]

It appears that relief of heartburn pain (once it has occurred) by antacids is dependent on other factors, such as esophageal acid clearance and lavage of damaged mucosa. Meyer and colleagues showed that 7 oz of antacid per day (doses 30 minutes and 1 hour after meals and before bedtime) was no better than placebo in relieving heartburn and regurgitation, both treatments producing a 30% improvement in symptoms (*Figure 5*).[73]

Although antacids are still regarded as the 'mainstay' of medical therapy for GER, they should be used in the knowledge that, probably, they are no better than placebo and that their effect is merely the result of swallowing a volume of liquid, being erect and having a series of saliva-related swallows associated with peristalsis. However, antacids are safe, relatively nontoxic and nonsystemic. The combination of an antireflux regimen with antacids hs and prn for heartburn can be effective in up to 60% of patients presenting with symptoms of GER. In retrospect, this short-lived relief has probably provided 'false reassurance' and led to delays in patients seeking medical assessment. The pathophysiology and damage may continue despite brief intervals of acid neutralization and symptom relief.

This view of a 'fabled' antacid era is borne with observations that severe peptic stricturing has decreased during the H_2 antagonist era. This is consistent with the clinical impression that sustained acid neutralization has prophylactic properties never present during the antacid era.

Antacid-alginate/alginic acid combinations: the antacid-alginate (Algicon®) and antacid-alginic acid (Gaviscon®) combinations are available in liquid or tablet form. When combined

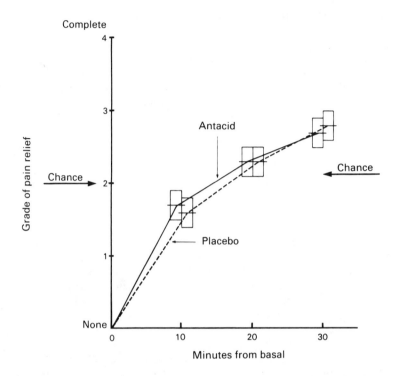

Figure 5   Results of multiple-dose study comparing efficacy of antacids vs. placebo in providing pain relief for patients with gastroesophageal reflux (mean and 95% confidence intervals, n = 240 doses).

with saliva, these compounds form a viscous antacid foam barrier which floats on the stomach contents, serving as a protective barrier for the esophagus against refluxing gastric contents. These agents have not been shown to have any effect on LES pressure. In addition, alginic acid is not an antacid and cannot be represented in this way. Stanciu and Bennett compared the use of antacid with and without the alginate with placebo and found no significant differences in relief of symptoms between the three treatment groups.[74] Graham and colleagues conducted a double-blind trial using prophylactically administered regimens and found symptom relief and healing of esophagitis when antacids were compared with alginate.[75] Their effectiveness in resolving heartburn is probably due to the stimulus of chewing and swallowing which promotes salivation and stimulates peristalsis. This is the same as the 'placebo' effect of swallowing and/or chewing any liquid or substance.

PHASE 2
Should the first phase of therapy prove not to be entirely satisfactory in relieving symptoms, further therapeutic intervention must be considered. Phase 2 therapy can be subdivided into two categories:
- agents which suppress acid production (H$_2$ antagonists [cimetidine, ranitidine, famotidine, nizatidine] and hydrogen-potassium ATPase antagonists [omeprazole])
- prokinetic agents which improve upper GI motility mainly by increasing the LES tone and stimulating gastric emptying (metoclopramide, domperidone, cisapride).
Agents which confer esophageal mucosal protection are also addressed, though to date there are no studies demonstrating their efficacy in GER disease.

Agents which suppress acid production

Gastric acid secretion is not generally increased in GER subjects.[30] The H_2 receptor antagonists and omeprazole have no effect on LES tone, esophageal peristalsis or gastric emptying.

The role of cimetidine and ranitidine in the treatment of GER has been reviewed recently by Richter (*Table 2*).[76]

Cimetidine: in the 10 studies reviewed by Richter on the use of cimetidine in the treatment of approximately 250 patients with GER, all but two of the studies demonstrated that the agent was superior to placebo in decreasing symptoms, but the difference was not usually significant. Significant improvement was documented upon endoscopy in 50% of the studies (*Table 2*).[76] However, only one-third of the studies were able to show healing of esophagitis during therapy. Cimetidine appears to be effective in doses of 300 mg ac meals and hs, 200 mg ac meals and 400 mg hs, or 600 mg bid.

The agent is not approved for the treatment of GER in the USA. Side effects include mental confusion, transaminase and creatinine elevation, gynecomastia and drug interactions with warfarin, beta-blockers, phenytoin, theophyllines and benzodiazepines.

Ranitidine: ranitidine is effective in alleviating symptoms and healing esophagitis in patients with GER. Of the five placebo-controlled trials reviewed by Richter, in which approximately 250 patients received ranitidine, all showed significant improvement in symptoms, with four of the five studies reporting endoscopic improvement of esophagitis (*Table 2*).[76] Ranitidine improved or healed endoscopic esophagitis in 59% of patients, compared with only 34% in the placebo group.

The most recent study is the US multi-centre trial, the largest trial conducted to date on the treatment of GER.[77] One hundred and nineteen ranitidine patients and 118 placebo patients were evaluated for 6 weeks in a double-blind fashion. During this period the severity and frequency of heartburn was significantly inhibited by ranitidine compared with placebo (*Figure 6*). In addition, ranitidine significantly increased the healing rate of those patients with endoscopic esophagitis (60% after 6 weeks for ranitidine vs. 40% for placebo). Symptom improvement was apparent within the first week of therapy, and this effect was sustained with further improvement recorded over the ensuing 6-week period.

	Cimetidine	Ranitidine
Clinical trials	10	5
Number of patients	approx 250	approx 250
Dose	300–400 mg qid	150 mg bid
Duration of study	6–12 weeks	6 weeks
Summary of results		
symptom improvement	8/10	5/5
endoscopy improvement	5/10 60%/30%	4/5 59%/34%
histology improvement	3/3 68%/11%	3/3 67%/38%

Table 2 Cumulative experience with histamine $_2$ antagonists in the acute treatment of GER disease. Reproduced with permission from Richter JE. A critical review of current medical therapy for gastroesophageal reflux disease. *J Clin Gastroenterol* 1986; **8**: 72–80.

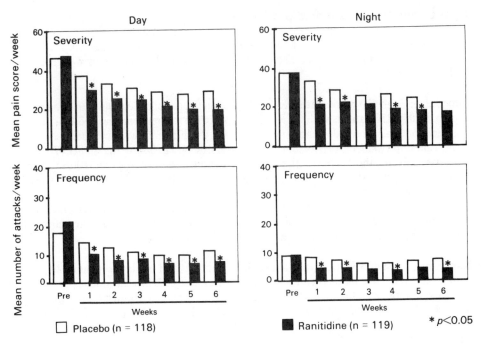

Figure 6   Results of US multi-centre trial comparing use of ranitidine and placebo in the treatment of patients with gastroesophageal reflux.

The study then addressed the question of maintenance therapy for reflux patients with chronic relapsing symptoms. Patients were randomized to placebo or 150 mg ranitidine at night or bid. Only ranitidine bid prevented symptomatic relapse (the point at which the patients discontinued the study). Sixty per cent of patients discontinued with the 150 mg hs dose, while only 10% discontinued on the bid regimen. There was no change in LES pressure after a year, confirming the belief that healing esophagitis in man does not improve LES pressure or influence the underlying pathophysiology of GER disease. Therefore, there appears to be a role for ranitidine in maintenance therapy for GER.

Ranitidine has relatively few side effects, tiredness, headaches and dizziness being the most commonly reported.

In the acute treatment of peptic ulcer disease, therapy is moving toward a single nightly dose regimen. The theory behind this approach is that taking an acid-inhibiting dose at night suppresses nocturnal acid, while during the day intake of food neutralizes the acid. The situation with regard to reflux is different. Eating is detrimental in reflux patients because it distends the stomach and stimulates secretion of acid which can reflux up into the esophagus before it becomes neutralized. Because ranitidine's duration of action is no more than 8–10 hours, a single nightly dose cannot inhibit gastric acid secretion at the time of the next day's evening meal. Therefore, in the case of GER, dose times with ranitidine must be strategically positioned (i.e. twice a day) in order to provide protection for patients when eating large meals, particularly evening meals.

The newer, more potent acid-suppressing drugs such as omeprazole may result in effective single, once-a-day therapy for GER.

Famotidine, nizatidine: famotidine and nizatidine are two recently developed H_2 receptor antagonists which have been released in North America for the treatment of peptic ulcer disease. Their profiles are no better than the experience with ranitidine. Trials on the use of these agents in the treatment of GER are presently being conducted. Preliminary data suggest that both famotidine[78,79] and nizatidine[80] will play a role in the treatment of GER in the future.

Omeprazole: omeprazole is a substituted benzimidazole that specifically inhibits the enzyme hydrogen-potassium adenosine triphosphatase in the parietal cell, the final step in the formation of hydrochloric acid. It is a potent inhibitor of gastric acid secretion and produces long-lasting suppression of basal and stimulated gastric acid secretion.

In a recently published study involving patients with esophagitis, omeprazole treatment over a 4-week period was remarkably effective in healing erosions and ulcers in 81% of patients compared with 6% in the placebo group.[81] Endoscopic healing of esophagitis was accompanied by symptom relief and histologic healing of ulceration.

In the second (dose finding) phase of the study, a further 132 patients were randomly allocated to treatment with 20 mg or 40 mg omeprazole daily, and endoscopic healing was assessed. In patients with the mildest grade of ulcerative esophagitis (grade II–erosions), healing occurred at 4 weeks in 87% of patients receiving 20 mg/day and 97% receiving 40 mg/day. In patients with grade III esophagitis (ulcers), the healing rates were 67% and 88%, respectively. Less than half of those patients with grade IV esophagitis (Barrett's ulcers or confluent ulceration) healed with either the 20 mg (48%) or 40 mg (44%) daily dose of omeprazole.

In the third phase of the study, the rate of endoscopic relapse was determined in 107 endoscopically healed patients after stopping omeprazole therapy. Erosion or ulcerative esophagitis had occurred in 82% of the patients after 6 months.

There is concern about the long-term safety of omeprazole. This is because of raised serum gastrin levels which have been found in both animal and human studies. Animal toxicologic studies with omeprazole have reported localized enterochromaffin-like cell proliferation and in some cases carcinoid tumours in the stomachs of rats after 2 years of treatment with very large doses.[82] These changes in serum gastrin and enterochromaffin-like cells are thought to be species-dependent and unlikely to be clinically important in short-term studies in humans. Considerably more experience on the use of omeprazole will be required before its use can be contemplated for the long-term therapy of GER. However, omeprazole has recently been approved in Canada for the treatment of GER, and it has been approved in the USA for treating reflux esophagitis which has been refractory to standard therapy, including the blockers. Such treatment with omeprazole should be limited to 4–8 weeks. Certainly there is no consideration for this agent in long-term (years) of maintenance therapy in GER. Thus, approval is crucial for long-term symptom relief in this chronically relapsing entity.

Prokinetic agents

The use of prokinetic agents, which increase the LES tone and stimulate gastric emptying, is appealing in the management of GER because it addresses the chronic underlying factors which contribute to the condition. The amount of gastric contents available to reflux into the esophagus and the interrelationship of this delayed gastric emptying in patients with GER has been summarized above (see pathophysiology section — *Figure 1*).

Bethanechol: bethanechol was the first smooth muscle stimulant to be used to treat patients with GER. The agent increases LES pressure and esophageal clearance but it does not augment gastric emptying. It has a negative effect in that it stimulates gastric acid secretion and also decreases the velocity of esophageal peristalsis.

The studies on the use of bethanechol in GER have produced conflicting results. In endoscopically controlled studies it appears to be as effective as cimetidine[83] but no more effective than placebo when bethanechol and antacids were compared to placebo and antacids.[84] Another study demonstrated complete healing of esophagitis in 45% of bethanechol-treated patients compared to 13.6% healing in an antacid/placebo group.[85]

Bethanechol at a dose of 25 mg qid is often not well tolerated. Side effects including abdominal cramps, diarrhea, urinary frequency and blurred vision have limited its acceptance as a treatment for GER.

Metoclopramide: metoclopramide, a procainamide derivative, stimulates GI smooth muscle.[86] It increases both LES pressure and the amplitude of esophageal contractions.[87] It also accelerates gastric emptying in retention states and improves small bowel transit. The exact mechanism which produces these effects on GI smooth muscle has not been precisely defined, but it is partially explained through dopamine antagonism. Although dopamine is regarded as an inhibitory neurotransmitter, the actual existence of dopaminergic neurons in the GI tract has not been clearly established in humans. Metoclopramide also augments acetylcholine release from post-ganglionic cholinergic nerve terminals and sensitizes muscarinic receptors of GI smooth muscle. It may have a direct stimulating effect on smooth muscle, as suggested by its effect on opossum LES, which is not abolished by tetrodotoxin or atropine.[88]

Metoclopramide has the ability to not only stimulate the GI smooth muscle but to coordinate gastric, pyloric and duodenal motor activity, resulting in net aboral movement. This property is incompletely understood, but crucial to the class of prokinetic agents. This differentiates its action from the nonspecific cholinergic effects of bethanechol and explains the observed differences in the effects of metoclopramide and bethanechol on gastric emptying.[89]

Studies showed that metoclopramide, both parenterally and orally, increased the rate of gastric emptying in GER patients in whom emptying was delayed (*Figure 7*).[90] On the other hand, bethanechol did not produce a significant improvement in gastric retention. In the same patients with symptomatic reflux and decreased LES pressure, 20 mg metoclopramide produced a greater increase in sphincter pressure than 25 mg bethanechol, whereas responses to 10 mg metoclopramide and 25 mg bethanechol were similar. Metoclopramide does not increase gastric acid secretion or stimulate endogenous gastrin release, presenting a theoretical advantage over bethanechol.

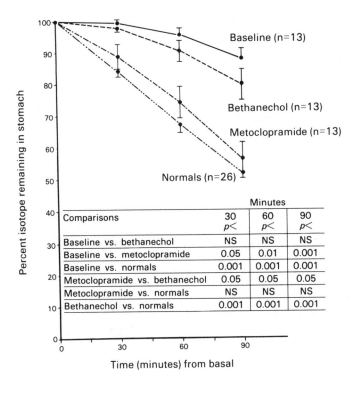

Comparisons	Minutes		
	30 $p<$	60 $p<$	90 $p<$
Baseline vs. bethanechol	NS	NS	NS
Baseline vs. metoclopramide	0.05	0.01	0.001
Baseline vs. normals	0.001	0.001	0.001
Metoclopramide vs. bethanechol	0.05	0.05	0.05
Metoclopramide vs. normals	NS	NS	NS
Bethanechol vs. normals	0.001	0.001	0.001

Figure 7 Comparison of effect of metoclopramide (intramuscularly) and bethanechol (subcutaneously) vs. normals on delayed gastric emptying in patients with gastro-esophageal reflux (mean ± SEM).

Metoclopramide also significantly enhanced gastric emptying in the subgroups of GER patients with slow as well as normal emptying rates.[91] The improvement in the group of esophagitis patients with normal emptying was greater than that reported by Metzger and colleagues in normal volunteers using the same test meal.[92] This result was obtained in a larger population and, although significant, the mean decrement of 10.8%, 90 minutes after the meal, was only half the improvement achieved with metoclopramide in the slow emptying reflux patients (20.3%). For a given patient, this improved emptying rate (although still in the 'normal' range) may be clinically important by reducing the residual gastric volume available to reflux, particularly when combined with the purported reduction in duodenogastric reflux attributed to metoclopramide. These effects, augmented by the accompanying increase in LES pressure, may promote less GER.

A double-blind study showed that metoclopramide significantly reduced day- and night-time heartburn and regurgitation, as well as decreasing the need for antacid use.[93] In addition, the magnitude of increase in LES pressure after metoclopramide did not predict symptomatic response, indicating that the clinical response to this prokinetic compound is more related to enhanced gastric emptying and decreased duodenogastric reflux, thus facilitating acid removal from the region of the proximal stomach and the gastroesophageal junction.

In a follow-up study metoclopramide significantly improved symptoms in a double-blind trial and this symptom improvement was correlated more with increasing gastric emptying and LES pressure than any other parameter.[94]

Guslandi and colleagues randomly treated 45 patients with symptomatic GER and confirmed histologic esophagitis with either metoclopramide (10 mg tid) or ranitidine (150 mg bid).[95] During the 6-week trial, both drugs were effective in producing symptomatic and endoscopic improvement. More recently, metoclopramide with cimetidine was shown to provide symptom relief in patients not already adequately improved by cimetidine alone.[96]

The recommended dose of metoclopramide is 10 mg ac meals and hs. On a physiologic basis it can be recommended that for long-term maintenance therapy a larger single dose of 20 mg either hs or before a large (evening) meal or a known provocative event should be considered.

The major limiting factor with metoclopramide is the high incidence of side effects, which occur in approximately 20% of patients at a dose of 10 mg qid. The most troublesome side effects appear to be restlessness, agitation, somnolence and extrapyramidal symptoms related to intracerebral dopamine antagonism.[87]

Domperidone: domperidone is a peripheral dopamine antagonist which, unlike metoclopramide, does not readily enter the central nervous system. It thus has fewer of the side effects which restrict the use of metoclopramide.

Results of pharmacologic studies on the effects of domperidone on esophageal motility have proved inconsistent. Studies by Brock-Utne and colleagues[97] and Weihrauch and co-workers[98] using domperidone intravenously found increased LES pressure following administration, but other studies have not.[99] Likewise, trials using oral domperidone have produced variable results.[97,99] In addition, pH monitoring[100] found no difference between domperidone and placebo.

Domperidone's prokinetic effect on the stomach and its ability to improve gastric emptying, thereby reducing gastric volume and possibly helping to prevent reflux, have been well documented.[101–105] Therapeutic trials of domperidone in treating GER, however, have also produced equivocal results, and overall have been negative in well-controlled double-blind studies.[106]

Goethals, in a double-blind crossover study comparing domperidone with placebo, found domperidone to be superior in alleviating heartburn and regurgitation.[107] Similarly, Valenzuela found domperidone was significantly more effective than placebo in relieving regurgitation but did not significantly improve heartburn or endoscopic healing.[99]

In a study comparing domperidone and ranitidine alone and in combination, both agents were equally effective in reducing symptoms and promoting healing of esophagitis, but the combination therapy was not significantly superior to either drug alone.[108]

Conversely, in another study comparing domperidone to placebo as add-on therapy to a standard antacid regimen, concomitant domperidone administration did not significantly affect LES pressure, the number of reflux episodes (as recorded by pH meter) or heartburn.[100] However, the domperidone-treated group did show a significant decrease in antacid use over baseline.

These studies suggest that the primary effect which domperidone may have in patients with reflux esophagitis may be due to improved gastric emptying rather than improved esophageal motility. This is consistent with domperidone's dopamine antagonist activity on D_2 receptors in the stomach. Few such dopamine receptors are found in the esophagus and LES.

The recommended dose of domperidone is 10 mg before meals and hs. The overall incidence of side effects with domperidone is less than 7%. Headaches and endocrinological problems related to the hyperprolactinemia (e.g. breast enlargement, nipple tenderness, galactorrhea and amenorrhea), which occur with all dopamine antagonists, appear to be the most troublesome. The dose used in most studies in GER has been 10 mg tid or qid. With less side effects than metoclopramide a higher therapeutic dose can be used. A dose of 20 mg qid has proven effective therapy in a large number of patients with GER (MCC, unpublished data). Consideration should therefore be given to conducting a double-blind investigation into the use of 20 mg or 30 mg qid doses before discarding domperidone in the short-term management of GER. Also, doses of 20 mg or 30 mg before large meals or on an intermittent basis could be an approach for long-term therapy.

Cisapride: cisapride is unique among prokinetic agents because it does not have an antidopaminergic action. Instead, it exerts its effect by increasing the availability of acetylcholine from post-ganglionic nerve endings of the myenteric plexus, leading to improved propulsive motor activity of the esophagus, stomach and small and large bowel. It has no known direct antiemetic properties. Its full pharmacology profile and effects in GER have been extensively reviewed recently.[109]

Cisapride appears to exert its beneficial effects in patients with GER by stimulating esophageal peristalsis, increasing LES tone and stimulating gastric emptying.

These effects have been investigated both in normal subjects and in patients with GER in short-term studies. In healthy volunteers cisapride increased the LES tone and lowered esophageal peristalsis following intravenous and oral administration.[110-112] In GER patients who had an abnormally low LES (<10 mmHg), cisapride raised the amplitude of esophageal peristaltic contractions and normalized the LES.[110]

This effect was confirmed in a study by Collins and Love, in which cisapride 10 mg tid was administered over a 1-month period to patients with symptoms and endoscopic evidence of GER.[113] In this study, radionuclide esophageal transit times were not significantly altered by cisapride. However, the duration of GER, especially at night, was significantly reduced after treatment with cisapride when compared with placebo (p=0.007).

Conversely, Holloway and colleagues in Australia studied 16 patients in a randomized, double-blind, placebo-controlled crossover trial to evaluate post-prandial reflux.[114] Esophageal manometry and pH were monitored after a loading dose of cisapride 10 mg tid for 3 days. The investigators found no significant effect on the rate of reflux, duration of esophageal acid exposure, mechanism of LES incompetence, esophageal peristalsis or basal pH meter pressure.

Comparison of cisapride with placebo: to assess cisapride's efficacy in healing and symptomatic relief, several double-blind randomized trials have been conducted in which the agent was administered in parallel with placebo to patients with grades 0–III esophagitis (Savary Miller classification). Mucosal damage was confirmed by endoscopy at the commencement of the trials, and attempts were made to eliminate placebo responders during an initial run-in period of 1–2 weeks.[115,116]

Cisapride was more effective than placebo in symptomatic and objective findings in patients with endoscopically proven reflux esophagitis. Thus, as assessed objectively and subjectively, these European studies show that cisapride therapy seems to be superior to placebo in patients with reflux esophagitis. Placebo-controlled studies are currently underway in North America and publication of their results are awaited.

Comparison of cisapride with other drugs/combination therapy: cisapride has been compared with ranitidine and metoclopramide in clinical studies. In combination therapy the use of cisapride with or without cimetidine has also been studied.

Cisapride administered in a dose of 10 mg qid tended to affect healing in a higher percentage of patients than ranitidine 150 mg bid after 6–12 weeks of treatment, but the differences were not significant.[117] Similar results were obtained in a study by Manousos and colleagues.[118]

Galmische and colleagues compared the efficacy of cisapride 10 mg qid and cimetidine with placebo and cimetidine in the treatment of 47 patients with erosive or ulcerative esophagitis (Savary Miller grades II–III).[119] The percentage of patients with a good or excellent response in terms of healing rates was significantly higher ($p < 0.025$) in the cisapride/cimetidine group compared with the placebo/cimetidine group.

Further studies are required before the exact role of cisapride, either as an alternative to H_2 receptor antagonists or in combination, is clearly defined. In particular, its role in long-term maintenance therapy could be attractive in view of its good safety profile. Side effects include transient abdominal cramping and some increase in stool frequency.

Cisapride has been approved for the treatment of GER at a dose of 10 mg tid or qid in several European countries, including the UK. It has also been approved in Canada. It remains under experimental investigation in the USA. Based on data from dose-response studies it would appear that an oral dose of 20 mg tid or qid would have greater therapeutic benefit.[120] The results of large multi-centre trials comparing these two dose regimens are awaited. There is a promising role for cisapride in long-term maintenance therapy for reflux, possibly in bid or hs doses. This area requires further investigation.

Esophageal mucosal protection

Sucralfate: sucralfate is an aluminum salt of a sulphated disaccharide used for the treatment of peptic ulcer. It adheres avidly to positively charged proteins in the ulcer base and may also serve as a surface barrier to acid, pepsin and bile at the site of its cytoprotective coagulum. The efficacy of sucralfate in the healing of duodenal ulcer and gastric ulcer vs. placebo and cimetidine is well reported, and a slurry form is often used by endoscopists to heal esophageal ulcers associated with endoscopic scleropathy.

What role does sucralfate play in the treatment of GER mucosal disease? Sucralfate possibly acts to increase tissue electrical resistance and prevent H^+ permeation into damaged mucosa. Schweitzer and colleagues perfused rabbit esophagus with acid, pepsin and hydrochloric acid.[121] When sucralfate was added, a significant reduction in gross and microscopic esophagitis was seen. In addition, mucosal permeability by pepsin was also reduced. Double-blind controlled studies in man, however, have not shown that sucralfate is effective in treating GER.

There does not appear to be any role at present for sucralfate in the treatment of GER. Its very brief contact time with the esophageal mucosa may be a contributing factor.

Prostaglandins: prostaglandins, in particular prostaglandin E_2, have received recent attention. If the concept of mucosal protection is accepted and there is a need for a more resistant esophageal mucosa, then prostaglandins may have a role. Prostaglandins are currently being evaluated in double-blind trials in which doses are both acid-inhibitory and cytoprotective. To date, the results of these trials have all proven negative. Misoprostol, a prostaglandin E_1 derivative, has been the main agent studied.

At one time it was thought that prostaglandins released from the inflamed esophageal tissue might inhibit smooth muscle in the distal esophagus and perpetrate the GER cycle. However, treating GER with indomethacin (a prostaglandin inhibitor) did not gain acceptance. It is now proposed that at least topical prostaglandins in the esophageal lumen may help maintain esophageal mucosal integrity. Any clinical role, however, is not presently apparent.

Combination therapy

The role of combination therapy has not been fully addressed. One possible strategy would be to use a prokinetic agent during the day (to decrease GER by increasing LES tone and also facilitating gastric emptying) and combine this with a long-acting acid-inhibiting drug at night.

In a randomized study the combination of cimetidine and metoclopramide was found to be more efficacious than cimetidine alone in the management of chronic reflux esophagitis.[96] Another study comparing domperidone with ranitidine and a combination of both agents found all three regimens were effective in improving symptoms and healing esophagitis.[108] The combination of cisapride and cimetidine has also been shown to increase esophageal healing rate and significantly improve symptoms compared to cimetidine alone.[117] Candidates for combination therapy include: patients with a long history of recurrent symptoms; patients who develop dysphagia and degrees of structuring; scleroderma patients; patients with Barrett's esophagus, particularly with ulcer and/or stricture.

Maintenance therapy

Once symptoms are under control and the inflamed esophagus has healed, consideration must be given to effective forms of maintenance therapy to reduce the high relapse rate since GER disease is a chronic process with continuing pathophysiology. Some patients may remain asymptomatic on a simple antireflux regimen and antacids on a prn basis. Other patients, however, rapidly relapse upon discontinuation of their therapy. It is for these patients that consideration must be given to some form of maintenance therapy.

The large US multi-centre trial on the use of ranitidine in the treatment of GER is the only study which has examined maintenance therapy.[77] The study compared ranitidine 150 mg hs with 150 mg bid and placebo for 6 months after initial healing of the esophagitis. It was found that the therapeutic dose of 150 mg bid for healing reflux esophagitis was the only effective regimen for preventing relapse.

In a small open study cisapride has proven to be effective in maintenance therapy by preventing relapse of symptoms for up to 1 year in 17 patients treated with doses of 10 mg qid, 10 mg bid and 10 mg hs (MCC, unpublished data).

The same patients as discussed under combination therapy would be leading candidates for maintenance.

PHASE 3

Enthusiasm for surgery for patients with GER has decreased over the last few years. Certainly some patients do require surgery, such as those with intractable symptoms despite full medical therapy and those with significant complications related to GER. Refractory strictures are less common now, possibly because of the H_2 receptor antagonists and other therapies described. Bleeding ulcers with Barrett's esophagus can normally be controlled by single or combination drug therapy.

It is crucial to carry out a thorough diagnostic work-up, including pH monitoring, in order to be sure of the diagnosis. It is even more important to measure LES pressure and esophageal motility. The major complication of fundoplication is too tight a wrap; this is due to a failure to appreciate the peristaltic status and amplitude of contractions in the esophagus and adjust the calibre of the gastroesophageal junction appropriately.

Fundoplication is effective because of two mechanisms:
- Reduction of the hiatus hernia into the abdomen with accompanying improved acid clearance.
- Improvement of the degree of LES transient relaxation that occurs. These relaxations are more incomplete and discourage reflux.

Patients who must be considered as probable candidates for surgery are those who are dissatisfied with their quality of life despite full medical therapy. This can be due to significant symptoms or alternatively significant restrictions in their lifestyle and eating habits because of GER. Obviously, different people have different degrees of tolerance to their heartburn. Economic considerations can also play a role if significant doses of maintenance medications are needed. For such patients, it really is a quality of life decision.

The future

There are several potential improvements in our ability to treat GER on the horizon. Omeprazole has produced impressive results in healing ulcers and erosions over a 4-week period; however, concerns over long-term use make long-term maintenance unattractive.

If anything has been learned from the H_2 antagonist era in the treatment of GER disease, it is that the esophagus is exquisitely sensitive to acid. Larger doses of H_2 antagonists are needed to improve the symptoms of GER and heal esophagitis than are needed to treat peptic ulcer disease. Hypersecretors are rarely being treated here; rather it is becoming increasingly

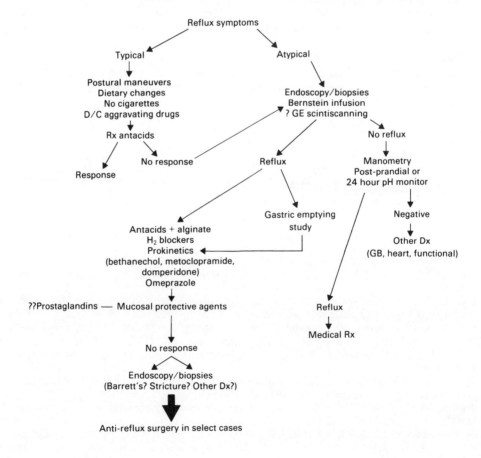

Figure 8   Steps in the diagnosis and treatment of GER.

appreciated that acid secretion must be dramatically inhibited on a sustained basis in order to address symptomatic and objective goals in the treatment of patients with GER. In many cases the endoscopy is normal macroscopically but larger doses of acid-suppressing drugs are needed to reduce symptoms.

Only prokinetic agents address the underlying motility abnormalities responsible for GER disease. Cisapride is a new prokinetic agent in the management of reflux esophagitis. Results of large North American studies using dose regimens of 10 mg and 20 mg qid are awaited.

Further investigations into maintenance therapy are required to determine the minimal dose of an agent which is effective and safe in preventing the high relapse rate which occurs when active therapy in GER patients is discontinued. Different treatment strategies will need to be developed for tailoring of therapy for different subgroups of patients with GER.

Summary
In summary, patients with GER disease are a heterogeneous group (*Figure 8*). Several pathogenic mechanisms may operate in GER, including impaired gastroesophageal junction competence (involving the intrinsic LES as well as the diaphragm or extrinsic LES), decreased esophageal acid clearance, delayed gastric emptying, and impaired esophageal mucosal barrier mechanisms. Essentially, GER can be considered to be a motility disorder of the upper GI tract. Most patients with reflux have symptoms such as heartburn, retrosternal chest pain and regurgitation, although the presentation may involve more epigastric symptoms.

Treatment of GER should start with simple antacid and antireflux measures, including recording of lifestyle, work and eating habits as well as assessment of medications being taken by the patient. If patients fail to respond to these simple Phase 1 measures, then use of acid-suppressing drugs or prokinetic agents individually or, in patients with more severe symptoms, in combination, is advised. A long-term maintenance plan is the goal. Finally, antireflux surgery has a small and decreasing role in the management of refractory or complicated reflux esophagitis.

®Registered trademark

References
1 Winkelstein A. Peptic esophagitis: a new clinical entitity. *JAMA* 1935; **104**: 906–9.
2 Allison PR. Peptic ulcer of the esophagus. *J Thoracic Surg* 1946; **15**: 308–17.
3 Richter JE, Castell DO. Gastroesophageal reflux. *Ann Intern Med* 1982; **97**: 103–7.
4 Dodds WJ, Hogan WJ, Helm JF, Dent J. Pathogenesis of reflux esophagitis. *Gastroenterology* 1981; **81**: 376–94.
5 Dodds WJ, Dent J, Hogan EJ *et al*. Mechanisms of gastroesophageal reflux in patients with reflux esophagitis. *N Engl J Med* 1982; **307**: 1547–52.
6 Holloway RH, Winnan G, McCallum RW. Upper gastrointestinal motility. Part I: the pathophysiologic approach to the management of reflux esophagitis. *Am J Gastroenterol* 1981; **76**: 280–90.
7 Fyke FE Jr, Code CF, Schegal JF. The esophageal sphincter in healthy human beings. *Gastroenterologia* 1956; **86**: 135–50.
8 Holloway RH, Hongo M, Berger K, McCallum RW. Gastric distention: a mechanism for postprandial gastroesophageal reflux. *Gastroenterology* 1985; **89**: 779–84.
9 Mittal RK, McCallum RW. Characteristics of transient lower esophageal sphincter relaxation in humans. *Am J Physiol* 1987; **252**: G636–41.
10 Freidman N, Ren J, Sluss J, McCallum RW. The effect of a large meal and graded intragastric balloon distention or transient lower esophageal sphincter relaxation frequency in normals. *Am J Gastroenterol* 1988; **83**: 1020 (abstr).
11 Gidda JS, Goyal RK. Swallow-evoked potential in vagal preganglionic efferents. *J Neurophysiol* 1984; **52**: 1169–80.

12 Paterson WG, Rattan S, Goyal RK. Experimental induction of isolated lower esophageal sphincter relaxation in anesthetized opossums. *J Clin Invest* 1986; **77**: 1187–93.

13 Orr WC, Johnson LF, Robinson MC. Effect of sleep on swallowing, esophageal peristalsis and acid clearance. *Gastroenterology* 1984; **86**: 814–9.

14 Baldi F, Ferrarini F, Balestra R, Borioni D, Longanesi MM, Barbara L. Oesophageal motor events at the occurrence of the acid reflux and during endogenous acid exposure in healthy subjects and in patients with oesophagitis. *Gut* 1985; **26**: 336–41.

15 Longhi EH, Gordan PH. Pressure relationship responsible for reflux in patients with hiatal hernia. *Surg Gynecol Obstet* 1969; **129**: 734–8.

16 Mittal RK, Lange RC, McCallum RW. Identification and mechanism of delayed esophageal acid clearance in subjects with hiatus hernia. *Gastroenterology* 1987; **92**: 130–5.

17 Lind JF, Warrian WG, Wankling WJ. Response of the gastroesophageal junction zone to increases in abdominal pressure. *Canadian J Surg* 1966; **9**: 32–7

18 Cohen S, Harris LD. The lower esophageal sphincter. *Gastroenterology* 1972; **63**: 1066–73.

19 Mittal RK, Rochester DF, McCallum RW. Sphincteric action of the diaphragm during a relaxed lower esophageal sphincter in humans. *Am J Physiol* 1989; **256**: G139–44.

20 Welch RW, Gray JE. Influence of respiration on recording of LES pressure in humans. *Gastroenterology* 1982; **83**: 590–4.

21 Boyle JT, Altschuler SM, Nixon TE, Tuchman DM, Pack AI, Cohen S. The role of the diaphragm in the genesis of lower esophageal sphincter pressure in the cat. *Gastroenterology* 1985; **88**: 723–30.

22 Helms JF, Dodds WJ, Palmer DW, Hogan WJ, Teeter BC. Effect of esophageal emptying and saliva on clearance of acid from the esophagus. *N Engl J Med* 1984; **310**: 284–8.

23 Stanciu C, Bennett JR. Oesophageal clearings: one factor in the production of reflux esophagitis. *Gut* 1974; **15**: 852–7.

24 Sonnenberg A, Steinkamp U, Weise A *et al.* Salivary secretion in reflux esophagitis. *Gastroenterology* 1981; **83**: 889–95.

25 Longhi EH, Jordan PH. Pressure relationship responsible for reflux in patients with hiatal hernia. *Surg Gynecol Obstet* 1969; **129**: 734–8.

26 Dent J, Dodds WJ, Friendman RH *et al.* Mechanism of gastroesophageal reflux in recumbent symptomatic human subjects. *J Clin Invest* 1980; **65**: 256–67.

27 Dodds WJ, Dehn JG, Hogan WJ *et al.* Severe peptic esophagitis in a patient with Zollinger-Ellison syndrome. *Am J Roentgenol* 1971; **113**: 237–40.

28 Safaie-Shirazi S, Denbesten L, Zike WL. Effect of bile salts on the ionic permeability of the esophageal mucosa and their role in the production of esophagitis. *Gastroenterology* 1975; **68**: 728–33.

29 Mittal RK, Reuben A, Whitney JO, McCallum RW. Do bile acids reflux into the esophagus? A study in normal subjects and patients with gastroesophageal reflux disease. *Gastroenterology* 1987; **92**: 371–5.

30 Fink SM, Barwick K, DeLuca V, Sanders FJ, Kandathil M, McCallum RW. The association of histologic gastritis with gastroesophageal reflux and delayed gastric emptying. *J Clin Gastroenterol* 1984; **6**: 301–5.

31 McCallum RW, Walsh JH. Relationship between lower esophageal sphincter pressure and serum gastrin concentration in Zollinger-Ellison syndrome and other clinical settings. *Gastroenterology* 1979; **76**: 76–81.

32 Kaye MD, Showalter JP. Pyloric incompetence in patients with symptomatic gastroesophageal reflux. *J Lab Clin Med* 1974; **83**: 198–206.

33 Keane FB, Dimagno EP, Malagelada JR. Duodenogastric reflux in humans: its relationship to fasting antroduodenal motility and gastric, pancreatic and biliary secretion. *Gastroenterology* 1981; **81**: 726–31.

34 McCallum RW, Mensh R, Lange R. Definition of gastric emptying abnormalities present in gastroesophageal reflux patients. In: Weinbeck M, ed. *Motility of the Digestive Tract.* New York: Raven Press 1982; 355–62.

35 McCallum RW, Berkowitz DM, Lerner E. Gastric emptying in patients with gastroesophageal reflux. *Gastroenterology* 1981; **80**: 285–91.

36 Behar J, Ramsly G. Gastric emptying and antral motility in reflux esophagitis. *Gastroenterology* 1987; **74**: 253.

37 Maddern GJ, Chatterton BE, Collins PJ, Horowitz M, Shearman DJ, Jamieson GG. Solid and liquid gastric emptying in patients with gastro-oesophageal reflux. *Br J Surg* 1985; **72**: 344–7.

38 McCallum RW. The role of gastric emptying in gastroesophageal reflux disease. In: Dubois A, Castell DO, eds. *Esophageal and Gastric Emptying.* Boca Raton: CRC Press 1984; 121–8.

39 Ippoliti A, McCallum RW, Sturdevant R. Gastric emptying in patients with gastroesophageal reflux.

Clin Res 1976; **24**: 535(abstr).
40 McCallum RW, Berkowitz DM, Lerner E. Gastric emptying in patients with gastroesophageal reflux. *Gastroenterology* 1981; **80**: 285–91.
41 Baldi F, Corinaldesi R, Ferrarini F, Stanghellini V, Miglioli M, Barbara L. Gastric secretion and emptying of liquids in reflux esophagitis. *Dig Dis Sci* 1981; **26**: 886–9.
42 Hillemeier AC, Lange R, McCallum RW, Seashore J, Gryboski J. Delayed gastric emptying in infants with gastroesophageal reflux. *J Pediatr* 1981; **98**: 190–3
43 Kaye MD, Showalter JP. Pyloric incompetence in patients with symptomatic gastroesophageal reflux. *J Lab Clin Med* 1974; **83**: 198–206.
44 Csendes A, Henriques A. Gastric emptying in patients with reflux esophagitis or benign strictures of the esophagus secondary to reflux compared to controls. *Scan J Gastroenterol* 1978; **13**: 205–7.
45 Coleman SL, Rees WDW, Malagelada JR. Normal gastric emptying in reflux esophagitis. *Gastroenterology* 1979; **76**: 1115(abstr).
46 Johnson DA, Winters C, Drane WE *et al.* Solid-phase gastric emptying in patients with Barrett's esophagus. *Dig Dis Sci* 1986; **31**: 1217–20.
47 Shay S, Eggli D, Van Nostrand D, Johnson LF. Gastric emptying of solid food in patients with gastroesophageal reflux. *Gastroenterology* 1985; **88**: 1582(abstr).
48 Holloway RH, Hongo M, Berger K, McCallum RW. Gastric distension: mechanism for post-prandial gastroesophageal reflux. *Gastroenterology* 1985; **89**: 779–84.
49 Maddern GJ, Jamieson GG, Chatterton BE *et al.* Is there an association between failed antireflux procedures and delayed gastric emptying? *Ann Surg* 1985; **202**: 162–5.
50 Brandsborg O, Bransborg M, Loygreen NA *et al.* Influence of parietal cell vagotomy and selective gastric vagotomy on gastric emptying rate and serum gastrin concentrations. *Gastroenterology* 1977; **72**: 212–4.
51 Harmon JW, Johnson LF, Mayodonovitch CL. Effects of acid and bile salts on the rabbit esophageal mucosa. *Dig Dis Sci* 1981; **26**: 65–72.
52 Neumann CH, Forster CF. Gastroesophageal reflux: reassessment of the value of fluoroscopy based on manometric evaluation of the lower esophageal segment. *Am J Gastroenterol* 1983; **78**: 776–9.
53 Bernstein LM, Baker LA. A clinical test for esophagitis. *Gastroenterology* 1958; **34**: 760–81.
54 Winnan GR, Meyer CT, McCallum RW. Interpretation of the Bernstein test: a reappraisal of criteria. *Ann Intern Med* 1982;**96**: 320–2.
55 Hewson EG, Sinclair JW, Dalton CB, Wu WC, Castell DO, Richter JE. The acid perfusion test: is it obsolete? *Am J Gastroenterol* 1988; **83**: 58(abstr).
56 Robinson MG, Orr WC, McCallum RW, Nardi R. Do endoscopic findings influence response to H$_2$ antagonist therapy for gastroesophageal reflux disease. *Am J Gastroenterol* 1987; **82**: 519–22.
57 Knuff TE, Benjamin SB, Worsham F, Castell DO. Histologic evaluation of chronic gastroesophageal reflux: an evaluation of biopsy methods and diagnostic criteria. *Dig Dis Sci* 1984; **29**: 194–202.
58 Tummala V, Sontag S, Vlahcevic R, Barwick K, McCallum RW. Are intraepithelial eosinophils helpful in the histological diagnosis of gastroesophageal reflux? *Am J Clin Path* 1987; **87**: 43–8.
59 Tuttle SG, Grossman MI. Detection of gastroesophageal reflux by simultaneous measurements of intraluminal pressure and pH. *Proc Soc Exp Biol Med* 1958; **98**: 225–7.
60 Booth DJ, Kemmerer WT, Skinner DB. Acid clearing from the distal esophagus. *Arch Surg* 1968; **96**: 731–4.
61 Fink SM, McCallum RW. The role of prolonged pH monitoring in the diagnosis of gastroesophageal reflux. *JAMA* 1984; **252**: 1160–4.
62 Holloway RH, McCallum RW. New diagnostic techniques in esophageal disease. In: Cohen S, Soloway RD (eds). *Diseases of the Esophagus.* New York: Churchill Livingstone 1982; 75–95.
63 Fisher RS, Malmud LS, Robert GS *et al.* Gastroesophageal scintiscanning to detect and quantitate gastroesophageal reflux. *Gastroenterology* 1976; **70**: 301–8.
64 Menin RA, Malmud LS, Robert GS *et al.* Gastroesophageal scintigraphy to assess the severity of gastroesophageal reflux disease. *Ann Surg* 1980; **191**: 66–71.
65 Jenkins AF, Cowan RJ, Richter JE. Gastroesophageal scintigraphy: is it a sensitive clinical test? *Gastroenterology* 1984; **86**: 1125 (abstr).
66 Blue PW, Jackson JW, Ghaed N. Duodenogastroesophageal reflux demonstration with ^{99m}Tc-DISIDA imaging. *Clin Nucl Med* 1984; **9**: 238–9.
67 Frank EB, Lange RC, McCallum RW. Abnormal gastric emptying in patients with atrophic gastritis with or without pernicious anemia. *Gastroenterology* 1981; **80**: 1151(abstr).
68 Orlando RC, Bozynski EM. Heartburn in pernicious anemia: a consequence of bile reflux. *N Engl J*

Med 1973; **289**: 522–3.

69 Johnson LF, De Meester TR. Evaluation of elevation of the head of the bed, bethanechol and antacid foam tablets on gastroesophageal reflux. *Dig Dis Sci* 1981; **26**: 673–80.

70 Price SF, Smithson KW, Castell DO. Food sensitivity in reflux esophagitis. *Gastroenterology* 1978; **75**: 240–3.

71 Holloway RH, McCallum RW. A practical approach to gastroesophageal reflux. *Drug Ther* 1983; **13**: 151–60.

72 Behar J, Sheahan DG, Biancani P, Spiro HM, Storer EH. Medical and surgical management of reflux esophagitis: a 38-month report on a prospective clinical trial. *N Eng J Med* 1975; **293**: 263–8.

73 Meyer CT, Berenzweig H, McCallum RW. A controlled trial of antacid and placebo in the relief of heartburn. *Gastroenterology* 1979; **76**: 1201(abstr).

74 Stanciu C, Bennett JR. Alginate/antacid in the reduction of gastroesophageal reflux. *Lancet* 1974; **i**: 109–11.

75 Graham DY, Lanzar F, Dorsch ER. Symptomatic reflux esophagitis: a double-blind controlled comparison of antacids and alginate. *Curr Ther Res* 1977; **22**: 653–8.

76 Richter JE. A critical review of current medical therapy for gastroesophageal reflux disease. *J Clin Gastroenterol* 1986; **8**: 72–80.

77 Sontag S, Robinson M, McCallum RW, Barwick KW, Nardi R. Ranitidine therapy for gastroesophageal reflux disease: results of a large double-blind trial. *Arch Intern Med* 1987; **147**: 1485–91.

78 Sekiguchi T, Nishioka T, Kogure M *et al*. Once-daily administration of famotidine for reflux esophagitis. *Scan J Gastroenterol* 1987; **22**(134): 51–4.

79 Orr WC, Robinson MG, Humphries TJ, Antonella J, Caliola A. Dose response effects of famotidine on gastroesophageal reflux (GER). *Gastroenterology* 1987; **92**: 1562(abstr).

80 Cloud M, Offen W. Nizatidine 150 mg bid relieves symptoms and decreases severity of esophagitis in gastroesophageal reflux. *Am J Gastroenterol* 1988; **83**: 1019(abstr).

81 Hetzel DJ, Dent J, Reed WD *et al*. Healing and relapse of severe peptic esophagitis after treatment with omeprazole. *Gastroenterology* 1988; **95**: 903–12.

82 Hakanson R, Sundler F, Carlsson E, Mattsson H, Larsson H. Proliferation of enterochromaffin-like (ECL) cells in the rat stomach following omeprazole treatment. *Hepatogastroenterology* 1985; **32**: 48–9.

83 Thanik KD, Chey WY, Shah AN, Hamilton D, Nadelson N. Bethanechol or cimetidine in the treatment of symptomatic reflux esophagitis. *Arch Intern Med* 1982; **142**: 1479–81.

84 Thanik KD, Chey WY, Shah AN, Grutierrez JH. Reflux esophagitis: effect of oral bethanechol on symptoms and endoscopic findings. *Ann Intern Med* 1980; **93**: 805–8.

85 Saco LS, Orlando RC, Levison SL, Bozymski EM, Jones JD, Frakes JT. Double-blind controlled trial of bethanechol and antacid versus placebo and antacid in the treatment of erosive esophagitis. *Gastroenterology* 1982; **82**: 1369–72.

86 Eisner M. Gastrointestinal effects of metoclopramide in man: *in vivo* experiments with human smooth muscle preparation. *Br Med J* 1968; **4**: 679–80.

87 Albibi R, McCallum RW. Metoclopramide: pharmacology and clinical application. *Ann Intern Med* 1983; **98**: 86–95.

88 Cohen S, Di Marino AJ. Mechanism of action of metoclopramide on opossum lower esophageal sphincter muscle. *Gastroenterology* 1976; **71**: 996–8.

89 McCallum RW, Kline MM, Curry N, Sturdevant RAL. Comparative effects of metoclopramide and bethanechol on lower esophageal sphincter pressure in reflux patients. *Gastroenterology* 1975; **68**: 1114–8.

90 McCallum RW, Fink SM, Lerner E, Berkowitz DM. Effects of metoclopramide and bethanechol on delayed gastric emptying present in gastroesophageal reflux patients. *Gastroenterology* 1983; **84**: 1573–7.

91 Fink SM, Lange RC, McCallum RW. Effect of metoclopramide on normal and delayed gastric emptying in gastroesophageal reflux patients. *Dig Dis Sci* 1983; **28**: 1057–61.

92 Metzger WH, Cano R, Sturdevant RAL. Effects of metoclopramide in chronic gastric retention after gastric surgery. *Gastroenterology* 1976; **71**: 30–2.

93 McCallum RW, Ippolitti AF, Cooney C, Sturdevant RAL. A controlled trial of metoclopramide in symptomatic gastroesophageal reflux. *N Engl J Med* 1977; **296**: 354–7.

94 McCallum RW, Fink SM, Winnan GR, Avella J, Callachan C. Metoclopramide in gastroesophageal reflux disease: rationale for its use and results of a double-blind trial. *Am J Gastroenterol* 1984; **79**: 165–172.

95 Guslandi M, Testoni PA, Passaretti S *et al*. Ranitidine vs. metoclopramide in the medical treatment of reflux esophagitis. *Hepatogastroenterology* 1983; **30**: 96–8.

96 Lieberman DA, Keefe EB. Double-blind controlled trial of metoclopramide and cimetidine vs. cimetidine in the treatment of severe reflux esophagitis. *Gastroenterology* 1985; **88**: 1476(abstr).

97 Brock-Utne JG, Downing JW, Dimopoulos GE, Rubin J, Moshal MG. Effect of domperidone on lower esophageal sphincter tone in late pregnancy. *Anesthesiology* 1980; **52**: 321–3.

98 Weihrauch TR, Forster CRF, Krieglstein J. Evaluation of the effect of domperidone on human esophageal and gastroduodenal motility by intraluminal manometry. *Postgrad Med J* 1979; **55**: 7–10.

99 Valenzuela JE. Effects of domperidone on the symptoms of reflux esophagitis. *R Soc Med Int Cong Symp Series* 1981; **36**: 51–6.

100 Blackwell JN, Heading RC, Fettes MR. Effects of domperidone on lower esophageal sphincter pressure and gastroesophageal reflux in patients with peptic esophagitis. *R Soc Med Int Cong Symp Series* 1981; **36**: 57–65.

101 Baeyens R, Reyntjens A, Van de Velde E. Effects of domperidone (R33,812) on the motor function of the stomach and small intestine. *Arzneimittel-Forschung* 1978; **28**: 682–6.

102 Corinaldesi R, Stanghellini V, Zarabini GE *et al.* The effect of domperidone on the gastric emptying of solid and liquid phases of a mixed meal in patients with dyspepsia. *Curr Ther Res* 1983; **34**: 982–6.

103 Del Genio A, Di Martino N, Piccolo S, Maffettone V, Landolfi V, Salvatore M. The effect of domperidone on gastric emptying in reflux esophagitis: a radioisotopic study. *J Nucl Med Allied Sci* 1984; **28**: 251–6.

104 Horowitz M, Maddern GJ, Chatterton BE, Collins PJ, Shearman DJC, Harding P. Acute and chronic effects of domperidone on gastric emptying in diabetic autonomic neuropathy. *Dig Dis Sci* 1985; **30**: 1–9.

105 Champion MC, Gulenchyn KY, O'Leary T, Irving P, Edwards A, Braaten J. Domperidone improves symptoms and solid phase gastric emptying in diabetic gastroparesis. *Am J Gastroenterol* 1987; **82**: 213(abstr).

106 Champion MC. Domperidone: minireview. *Gen Pharm* 1988; **19**: 499–505.

107 Goethals C. Domperidone in the treatment of post-prandial symptoms suggestive of gastroesophageal reflux. *Curr Ther Res* 1979; **26**: 876–80.

108 Masci E, Testoni PA, Passaretti S, Guslandi M, Tihobello A. Comparison of ranitidine, domperidone maleate and ranitidine + domperidone maleate in the short-term treatment of reflux esophagitis. *Drugs Exp Clin Res* 1985; **10**: 1–6.

109 McCallum RW, Prakash C, Campoli-Richards DM, Goa KL. Cisapride: a review. *Drugs* 1988; **36**: 652–81.

110 Janssens J, Ceccatelli P, Vantrappen G. Cisapride restores the decreased lower esophageal sphincter pressure in reflux patients. *Digestion* 1986; **34**: 139.

111 Weiser HF, Holscher A, Zimmerman T. Effect of cisapride and metoclopramide on the lower esophageal motility pressure: a pressure and pH study. *Digestion* 1986; **34**: 142.

112 Wienbeck M, Cuder-Wiesinger E, Berges W. Cisapride acts as a motor stimulator in the human esophagus. *Gastroenterology* 1984; **86**: 1298.

113 Collins BJ, Love AHG. The effect of chronic oral administration of cisapride on the 16 hour pH profile, oesophageal transit and gastric emptying of patients with evidence of gastro-oesophageal reflux: a placebo-controlled trial. *Digestion* 1986; **34**: 142(abstr).

114 Holloway RH, Dent J, Downton J, Mitchell B. Effect of cisapride on post-prandial gastroesophageal reflux. *Digestion* 1986; **34**: 141.

115 Lepoutre L, Bollen J, Vandewalle N *et al.* Therapeutic side effects of cisapride in reflux oesophagitis: a double-blind, placebo-controlled study. In: *Progress in the Treatment of Gastrointestinal Motility Orders.* Excerpta Medica: Amsterdam 1988; 63–5

116 Van Outrye M, Vanderlinden I, Dedullen G, Rutgeerts L. Dose-response study with cisapride in gastroesophageal reflux disease. *Curr Ther Res* 1988; **43**: 408–15.

117 Janisch HD, Huttermann W, Bouzo MH. Cisapride versus ranitidine in the treatment of reflux esophagitis. *Hepatogastroenterology* (In press).

118 Manousos ON, Mandidis A, Michailidis D. Treatment of reflux symptoms in esophagitis patients: comparative trial of cisapride and metoclopramide. *Curr Ther Res* 1987; **42**: 807–13.

119 Galmische JP, Vitaux J, Brandstaetter G *et al.* Benefit of adding cisapride to cimetidine in the treatment of severe reflux esophagitis. *Gastroenterology* 1987; **92**: 1400(abstr).

120 Gilbert *et al.* Effect of cisapride, a new prokinetic agent, on esophageal motor function. *Dig Dis Sci* 1987; **32**: 1331–6.

121 Schweitzer EF, Bass BL, Johnson LF, Harmon JW. Sucralfate blocks pepsin-induced esophageal injury in rabbits. *Gastroenterology* 1984; **86**: 1241.

Treatment of gastric motility disorders

M C Champion

Abnormal gastric motility can result in either delayed or rapid emptying of the stomach, each with attendant symptoms. When treating a gastric motility disorder, three broad areas must be addressed:
- treatment of underlying conditions
- diet
- drug therapy.

Delayed gastric emptying

The causes of delayed gastric emptying, or gastroparesis, are summarized in *Table 1*. The physiology and pathophysiology of the conditions have been reviewed recently.[1] Patients may present with anorexia, post-prandial fullness, bloating, nausea and epigastric pain. In some cases vomiting, often of undigested food eaten hours earlier, may be a problem. Initially, symptoms can be intermittent and may or may not become continuous. Conversely, many patients with gastroparesis may have few or no symptoms and yet an endoscopy will reveal retained food in the stomach (bezoar). Diabetics may also be asymptomatic and present with labile or difficult to control diabetes.

Treatment of underlying condition
There are many potentially correctable conditions which can give rise to gastroparesis. Delayed emptying due to peptic ulcer disease or inflammatory conditions in the stomach will often improve with appropriate treatment. Improvement in metabolic and endocrine abnormalities usually lead to increased stomach motility and a resolution of symptoms. A surgical approach may be necessary to resolve some causes of delayed gastric emptying, e.g. pyloric stenosis caused by previous peptic ulcer disease. Finally, several drugs have been found to cause delayed gastric emptying (*Table 2*). The possibility that a patient's gastroparetic state is the result of medication must always be considered and, whenever possible, these medications should be discontinued.

Diet
Patients with gastroparesis experience difficulty in eating regular sized meals and benefit from having small meals more frequently throughout the day. Furthermore, such patients are prone to bezoar formation. This appears to be due to a decrease or absence of the Phase III cycle of the migrating motor complex, which is responsible for clearing undigested material from the stomach in the fasting state.[2,3] It is therefore appropriate to advise patients to follow a low leguminous diet.

163

Mechanical
- Outlet obstruction due to — carcinoma
                              — peptic ulcer disease
- Hypertrophic pyloric stenosis

Metabolic-endocrine
- Diabetic ketoacidosis
- Diabetic gastroparesis
- Hypothyroidism
- Electrolyte imbalance

Post-gastric surgery
- Vagotomy
- Partial gastrectomy

Acid-peptic disease
- Gastroesophageal reflux
- Gastric ulcer disease

Gastritis
- Atrophic gastritis
- Pernicious anemia
- Viral gastroenteritis (acute)

Collagen vascular disease
- Scleroderma

Pseudo-obstruction
- Idiopathic
- Secondary — amyloidosis
            — muscular dystrophy

Psychiatric disorders
- Anorexia nervosa
- ? Depression

Electrical dysrhythmia
- Tachygastria
- Gastroduodenal dysynchrony

CNS mediated
- Brain tumour
- Bulbar poliomyelitis

Table 1 Causes of delayed gastric emptying (gastroparesis).

Narcotic analgesics
Anticholinergics
Antidepressants
L dopa
Adrenergic agonists (salbutamol)
Loperamide
? Cimetidine
Alcohol

Table 2 Drugs that delay gastric emptying.

A low residue diet may also be beneficial but may exacerbate the problem of constipation when it occurs in conjunction with gastroparesis, such as in patients with diabetic autonomic neuropathy. Patients often find that restricting the fat content of their meals reduces their gastroparetic symptoms. Fat stimulates the release of cholecystokinin which is a potent inhibitor of gastric emptying.

Drug therapy
Initial symptoms of gastroparesis are intermittent and may or may not become continuous, depending on the nature of the underlying condition and its severity. It is becoming increasingly recognized that there is poor correlation between symptoms and the rate of gastric emptying as shown by radionuclide studies. This raises the question of the usefulness of gastric emptying studies in the evaluation of patients with presumed gastroparesis. Symptomatic patients need to be treated regardless of whether such studies reveal abnormal emptying rates. In addition, asymptomatic

patients, particularly diabetics, with evidence of delayed emptying will also benefit from treatment. This can result in better glycemic control and improved nutrition.

Treatment can either take the form of short-term pulse therapy of 2–4 weeks when the patient is symptomatic, or be continuous depending on the underlying condition and the severity of symptoms. Certainly in diabetics long-term therapy is indicated. Several days may lapse between initiation of treatment and clinical improvement, owing to delayed drug absorption in some patients with gastroparesis. In certain conditions such as diabetes and scleroderma, the dose of medication may need to be increased with time as the disease process becomes more severe.

The timing of administration of any gastric prokinetic agent should be such that peak plasma levels and therapeutic activity coincide with eating. This is normally achieved by taking the medication at least 30 minutes pre-prandially. If the patient misses a meal the medication should still be taken to maintain steady state plasma levels.

In addition to mealtime dosing, the evening or hs dose is also important. Gastric prokinetic agents have been shown to improve gastroduodenal coordination and appear to restore a more normal interdigestive myoelectric complex.[2-5] This is particularly important in the overnight fasting state when the stomach clears undigested material in the third phase of the myoelectric cycle. An evening dose of medication seems a logical approach to minimize bezoar formation.

The three gastric prokinetic drugs which will be discussed in detail are metoclopramide, domperidone and cisapride. Other potential prokinetic drugs, both old and new, will also be discussed briefly.

Metoclopramide
Metoclopramide is a procainamide derivative which has both gastric prokinetic and anti-emetic properties. The gastric prokinetic properties result from antagonism of gastric dopamine receptors and augmentation of the release of acetylcholine from the myenteric plexus.[6] The gastric prokinetic effects of dopamine antagonism are summarized in *Figure 1*. Metoclopramide exerts its anti-emetic action on the chemoreceptor trigger zone on the floor of the fourth ventricle and crosses the blood-brain barrier to exert its effect on the intercerebral vomiting centre.[7]

Clinical indications: there have been two recent comprehensive reviews on the pharmacology and clinical application of metoclopramide.[6,7] Metoclopramide has been shown to be effective intravenously in the management of both diabetic[8] and post-vagotomy gastroparesis.[6] Studies have also demonstrated its effectiveness intravenously in shortening the duration of postoperative ileus, in facilitation of tube placement in the stomach and small bowel and in reducing the fluoroscopic time in small bowel x-rays.[7]

The interpretation of studies with oral metoclopramide is more difficult as many of these studies date back to the 1970s and are open studies with small patient numbers. Another difficulty in reviewing studies of that era stems from the many different ways of assessing gastric emptying and the many different methodologies which have evolved over the last 10 years. Certainly, oral metoclopramide appears to be effective in the acute management of many gastroparetic conditions such as those associated with diabetes,[9] following vagotomy and gastric surgery,[10] anorexia nervosa,[11] reflux esophagitis[12] and idiopathic gastroparesis.[13] More recently metoclopramide has been shown to increase delayed emptying in dystrophia myotonica, a progressive wasting disease which affects both skeletal and smooth muscle.[14]

Although prolonged administration of metoclopramide appears to be effective in controlling symptoms, the long-term efficacy of metoclopramide as a gastric prokinetic remains controversial.[6]

Snape, in a double-blind placebo-controlled crossover trial involving 10 diabetics, reported improvement in both symptomatic control and liquid phase gastric emptying after 4 weeks of treatment with metoclopramide 10 mg qid (*Figure 2*).[15]

In a 3-week crossover study involving 20 patients with diabetic gastroparesis, Rici and colleagues found metoclopramide 10 mg tid superior to placebo in improving symptoms. Gastric emptying was improved in 7 patients when compared with the

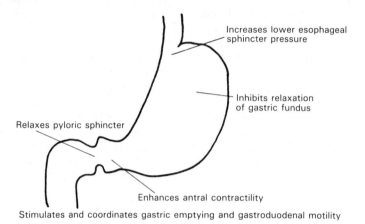

Figure 1 Gastric prokinetic actions of the dopamine antagonists metoclopramide and domperidone.

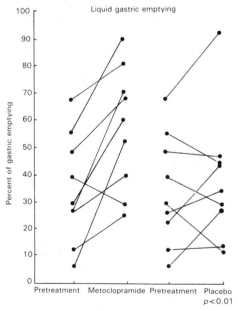

Figure 2 Effects of metoclopramide therapy (10 mg ac meals and hs) on liquid gastric emptying rates in 10 diabetics treated over a 4-week period, compared with placebo. Reproduced with permission from Snape WJ, Battle WM, Schwartz SS *et al*. Metoclopramide to treat gastroparesis due to diabetes mellitus: a double-blind, controlled trial. *Ann Intern Med* 1982; **96**: 444–6.

baseline evaluation; however there was poor correlation between symptoms and improvement in gastric emptying.[9] Gastric emptying was not compared with placebo after long-term treatment.

In another study of gastroparetic patients, Schade reported that, despite symptomatic improvement following 4 weeks of metoclopramide 10 mg before meals, there was no significant improvement in liquid phase gastric emptying when compared to placebo (*Figure 3*).[16]

Long-term symptom improvement may be due to the anti-emetic action on the chemoreceptor trigger zone and the vomiting centre rather than the gastric prokinetic action of metoclopramide.

Side effects: the major limiting factor in the use of metoclopramide is the side effect profile. These side effects are normally dose-related and have been reported in at least 20% of patients,[6] with some studies reporting higher incidences. The most common side effects are neurologic and endocrinologic in nature. Metoclopramide crosses the blood-brain barrier leading to complaints of drowsiness and lassitude. Extrapyramidal side effects due to intracerebral dopamine antagonism have been reported in up to 10% of patients at the recommended dose of 10 mg qid.[17] Hyperprolactinemia can result in mastalgia, gynecomastia, galactorrhea and amenorrhea.

Dose: in acute gastroparesis metoclopramide may be administered parenterally by either the intravenous, intramuscular or subcutaneous route. The subcutaneous route can be useful for self-administration when the patient is unable to tolerate oral metoclopramide. The parenteral dose is 10 mg every 6 hours, but this may vary depending on the indication. The parenteral route can be augmented by oral intake, with tapering of the parenteral dose as symptoms improve.

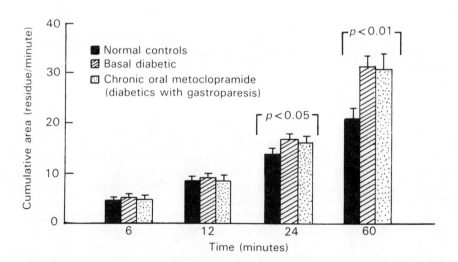

Figure 3 Effects of metoclopramide therapy (10 mg ac meals) on liquid emptying rates in 12 diabetics over a 4-week period, compared with normal controls and basal diabetics. Note lack of significant improvement between basal diabetics and metoclopramide-treated diabetics. Reproduced, with permission, from Schade RR, Dugas MC, Lhotsky DM *et al*. Effect of metoclopramide on gastric liquid emptying in patients with diabetic gastroparesis. *Dig Dis Sci* 1985; **30**: 10–5.

The normal dose of oral metoclopramide in adults is 10 mg at least 30 minutes before the three main meals and at bedtime. The dose can be increased to 20 mg, but this is usually not well tolerated owing to side effects.

A suppository form of metoclopramide is available in Europe but not in North America.

Domperidone

Domperidone, a benzimidazole derivative, is a recently developed dopamine antagonist which does not readily cross the blood-brain barrier. Like metoclopramide, its gastric prokinetic action is by dopamine receptor blockade in the stomach and duodenum (*Figure 1*). Its anti-emetic action occurs only on the chemoreceptor trigger zone which is on the blood side of the blood-brain barrier.[18] The effects of domperidone on gastric emptying rates have not been compared directly in clinical pharmacologic studies with those of metoclopramide or cisapride in humans.

Clinical indications: there have been two recent reviews of the pharmacology and clinical indications of domperidone.[18,19]

Domperidone has been shown to be effective both orally and intravenously in the acute management of gastroparesis associated with diabetes,[20,21] dyspepsia,[22] anorexia nervosa[23] and idiopathic gastroparesis.[24] Domperidone appears to be effective in both controlling symptoms and/or improving gastric emptying under these conditions. In two dose-response studies on the use of parenteral domperidone in the treatment of various gastroparetic conditions, including diabetes, reflux esophagitis, scleroderma, post-surgical and idiopathic gastric stasis, doses of 10 mg did not accelerate gastric emptying significantly whereas 20 mg and 30 mg doses did increase emptying rates.[24,25]

In long-term studies, domperidone has been found to be effective in gastroparesis associated with diabetes (*Figure 4*),[21,26] following vagotomy and gastric surgery[27] and idiopathic gastroparesis.[24] Only two of these studies looked both at symptoms and gastric emptying[21,26] whereas the other studies were either open[24] or crossover[27] with no follow-up gastric emptying tests.

Horowitz studied the effects of acute and chronic administration of domperidone in 12 diabetics in comparison with 22 control patients.[21] In the acute study using 40 mg domperidone orally, both solid and liquid emptying rates were increased significantly when compared with placebo. After chronic administration (35–51 days), domperidone 20 mg ac meals had no significant effect on solid emptying but was still effective in increasing liquid emptying when compared with the 22 controls (*Figure 4*). Symptoms of gastroparesis were also improved after chronic administration.

In a recent randomized, placebo-controlled study, solid phase gastric emptying and symptoms were improved significantly in diabetics treated with domperidone 20 mg ac meals and hs compared with placebo after 4 weeks of therapy.[26]

In 10 out of 12 post-vagotomy patients with evidence of gastroparesis, symptoms such as early satiety and epigastric distress improved or disappeared following administration of domperidone 10 mg tid for up to 4 weeks.[27] Furthermore, nausea and vomiting disappeared in all those patients who had experienced these symptoms at baseline.

In a double-blind crossover study involving patients with idiopathic gastroparesis, symptoms in 5 patients receiving at least 20 mg domperidone qid for 6 weeks were significantly improved when compared with placebo at the end of the study.[24]

Side effects: domperidone has fewer side effects than metoclopramide, the overall incidence reportedly varying from 2–7%, depending on the study.[16,28] The main side effects are dry mouth, headaches and endocrinological problems related to hyperprolactinemia. Like other dopamine antagonists, domperidone stimulates prolactin release from the pituitary by dopamine blockade of receptors on the blood side of the blood-brain barrier. This can result in mastalgia, gynecomastia, galactorrhea or menstrual irregularities. There is no direct correlation between dose and prolactin response, though the increase in prolactin secretion rises with increasing doses of both domperidone and metoclopramide.[29]

Domperidone does not readily cross the blood-brain barrier. Problems such as somnolence and extrapyramidal side effects, which have been reported in up to 10% of patients taking metoclopramide, occur in less than 0.01% of domperidone-treated patients.

The intravenous formulation of domperidone was withdrawn by the manufacturer following the deaths of 9 cancer patients receiving chemotherapy who developed cardiac problems (arrhythmias, sudden death, cardiac arrest) with high bolus doses of up to 100 mg domperidone. Although the manufacturer re-emphasized the appropriate dose regimen,[30] further use of such high doses in oncology practice led to the withdrawal of the parenteral form in 1985.

Dose: initial therapy with oral domperidone is 10 mg before meals and at bedtime. This dose may be increased to 20 mg qid which is well tolerated in most patients and appears to be more effective in the treatment of gastroparesis. Some investigators have found that a dose of 30 mg qid is tolerated in severe gastroparesis.

A suppository form of domperidone (60 mg) is available in Europe but not in North America. The suppository should be administered 2-4 times/day.

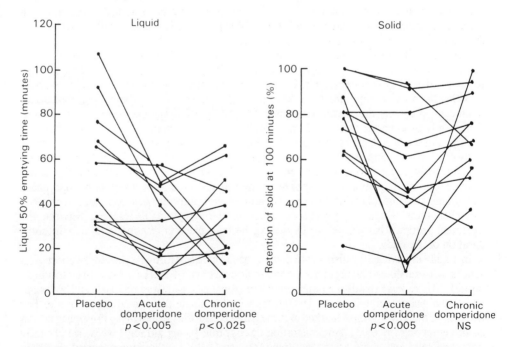

Figure 4   Effects of acute and chronic domperidone therapy (20 mg ac meals) on solid and liquid gastric emptying rates in 12 diabetics compared with controls. Reproduced with permission from Horowitz M, Harding PE, Chatterton BE *et al.* Acute and chronic effects of domperidone on gastric emptying in diabetic autonomic neuropathy. *Dig Dis Sci* 1985; **30**: 1-9.

Cisapride

Cisapride is a new gastric prokinetic agent which is presently undergoing clinical evaluation. It is a benzamide derivative and is noncholinergic and non-antidopaminergic in its action. Cisapride appears to exert its effect throughout the entire gastrointestinal tract by enhancement of the physiologic release of acetylcholine at the myenteric plexus.[31] Cisapride is a potent gastric prokinetic and also stimulates antroduodenal coordination.

Clinical indications: cisapride has been shown to be effective either intravenously or orally in the acute management of many gastroparetic conditions, including diabetes,[32–35] progressive systemic sclerosis,[36] anorexia nervosa,[37] dystrophia myotonica[38] and idiopathic gastroparesis.[39,40] In a combined study, cisapride was also found to be effective in patients with diabetic, postoperative and idiopathic gastroparesis.[41]

In a study of 9 diabetic patients with delayed gastric emptying of indigestible solids (radio-opaque markers), both intravenous cisapride 5 mg and metoclopramide 10 mg accelerated the mean gastric emptying rate of the markers compared with placebo, but the difference was only significant with cisapride.[32]

In a dose-response study involving diabetics with gastroparesis, intravenous cisapride restored prolonged solid phase gastric emptying to normal at doses of 2.5 mg, 5 mg and 10 mg. Cisapride 10 mg produced significantly faster gastric emptying than metoclopramide.[33]

Intravenous cisapride has also been shown to be effective in increasing gastric emptying in patients with progressive systemic sclerosis (at a dose of 10 mg),[36] and in patients with diabetic, postoperative and idiopathic gastroparesis.[41]

Finally, intravenous cisapride 8 mg was effective in accelerating delayed gastric emptying and increasing antral contraction amplitude in 12 patients with anorexia nervosa.[37]

Both acute and chronic administration of oral cisapride has been studied in patients with diabetes mellitus,[34,35] and long-term studies have been performed in patients with scleroderma,[36] dystrophia myotonica[38] and idiopathic gastroparesis.[39,40]

Jian and colleagues compared cisapride 10 mg tid with placebo during a 6-week study involving 27 patients with symptoms of idiopathic dyspepsia.[39] Fifty-nine per cent of these patients had delayed gastric emptying. Gastric emptying rates of both solids and liquids returned to within the normal range after 6 weeks of treatment with cisapride whereas placebo had no significant effect on the gastric emptying. Symptoms of dyspepsia were also improved significantly by cisapride at weeks 3 and 6 of the treatment period.

Corinaldesi and colleagues compared cisapride 10 mg tid to placebo in a 2-week crossover study involving 12 patients with chronic idiopathic dyspepsia and gastroparesis.[40] There was no washout between the two treatment periods. All 12 patients had symptoms of dyspepsia and delayed solid-phase gastric emptying. There was a significant improvement in the solid-phase gastric emptying rate following 2 weeks of treatment with cisapride when compared to placebo. However, there was no significant difference in the symptomatic response between the treatment groups. This was felt to be due to the high placebo response and also the short duration of the study.

In a study involving 20 patients with diabetic gastroparesis, Horowitz studied the effect of an acute single oral dose of 20 mg cisapride and treatment over a 4-week period with cisapride 10 mg qid.[34] There was a significant improvement in esophageal emptying ($p<0.01$) and both solid and liquid gastric emptying rates ($p<0.001$) with the single dose of 20 mg cisapride. The response to therapy was most marked in those patients with the greatest delay in esophageal and gastric emptying ($p<0.05$). Administration of cisapride 10 mg qid for 4 weeks significantly improved solid and liquid gastric emptying rates ($p<0.001$), although esophageal emptying rates did not differ significantly between the treatment and placebo groups (*Figure 5*). However, at the end of the treatment period, there was a significant improvement in the symptoms of patients receiving cisapride (n=8) compared with placebo (n=9).

In a further, recently completed study, 18 symptomatic diabetics with delayed gastric

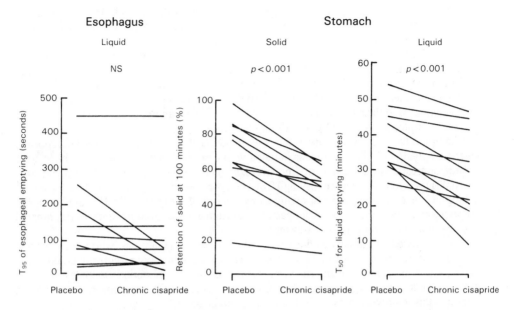

Figure 5 Effects of cisapride therapy (20 mg ac meals and hs) on esophageal and gastric emptying in 20 diabetics over a 6-week period, compared with placebo. Reproduced with permission from Horowitz M, Maddox A, Harding PE *et al*. Acute and chronic effects of cisparide on gastric and esophageal emptying in insulin-dependent diabetes mellitus. *Gastroenterology* 1987; **92**: 1899–907.

emptying were randomized to treatment with either cisapride 10 mg ac meals and hs or placebo.[35] After 4 weeks of treatment, a significant improvement in the solid-phase gastric emptying rate was observed, with improvement in six of seven symptoms of gastroparesis. Nausea, early satiety, anorexia, post-prandial epigastric discomfort, bloating and constipation all improved significantly. There was no apparent significant improvement in vomiting, which was possibly due to the small number of patients in each treatment group who presented with this symptom. Overall, there was a significant improvement in the total symptom score and the global evaluation of the patient both by the investigator and the patient.

Horowitz evaluated 8 patients with progressive systemic sclerosis in a 4-week open study.[36] The patients had had symptoms of progressive systemic sclerosis for at least 12 months before entering into the study. All the patients had delayed solid gastric emptying and in 5 cases liquid emptying was also delayed. There was considerable variation in gastrointestinal symptoms, which were usually only mild in severity. Following 4 weeks of therapy with cisapride 10 mg qid, there was a significant improvement in mean gastric symptoms ($p<0.001$), mean esophageal symptoms ($p<0.025$) and total symptom score ($p<0.001$).

There have been two studies involving a combination of patients with gastroparesis and the results were presented collectively. McCallum studied 22 patients with a variety of gastroparetic conditions.[41] These included diabetics (n=8), patients with idiopathic gastroparesis (n=7) and gastroparesis following gastric surgery (n=7). After a 2-week baseline period to assess the symptoms, patients were allocated to treatment with cisapride 10 mg tid or placebo for 6 weeks in a randomized double-blind crossover trial, with a 2-week washout period in between. A significant improvement in the symptoms of nausea, bloating, vomiting and heartburn was observed in patients following 6 weeks of treatment with cisapride, compared with controls.

In another combined study involving patients with gastroparesis, including diabetics (n=8) and patients with idiopathic (n=5) and chronic idiopathic pseudo-obstruction (n=15),[42] Camilleri compared cisapride 10 mg tid with placebo over a 6-week treatment period. At the end of the study there was a significant improvement ($p<0.05$) in the solid phase gastric emptying rate in the cisapride-treated group compared with placebo. There was also a significant improvement in pain in the cisapride-treated patients. However, there was no significant improvement in the other symptoms of gastroparesis.

Three long-term studies of up to a year, involving a total of 33 patients, have been conducted. McCallum studied 6 patients (5 idiopathic gastroparesis, 1 diabetes) over a 1-year period.[43] The patients received cisapride 20 mg tid for a total mean time of 9 months (range 3–13 months). At the final assessment, gastric emptying was normalized and was significantly improved ($p<0.01$) when compared to the baseline gastric emptying test. The mean frequency and severity of the patients' symptoms improved by 52% during the study.

Champion followed 6 patients over a 1-year period.[44] All the patients had an abnormal gastric emptying rate. Treatment was initiated with cisapride 10 mg ac meals and hs. After 1 month of treatment, a significant improvement in the solid-phase gastric emptying rate ($p<0.001$) was found. Over the ensuing 12 months, the dose of cisapride had to be increased to 20 mg qid in 2 of the 6 patients, owing to recurrence of symptoms. At 12 months, gastric emptying and total symptom score for gastroparesis remained significantly improved compared with baseline and pre-treatment assessment.

Abell followed 21 patients with a variety of gastroparetic conditions, who were receiving cisapride 10 mg tid, for at least 1 year.[45] Compared with baseline, both solid- and liquid-phase gastric emptying rates were improved at the end of the 1-year period ($p<0.05$). In the 9 diabetics in this group there was a significant improvement in the symptoms of gastroparesis, although this improvement was not found in the nondiabetics.

Side effects: cisapride appears to be well tolerated by patients and has fewer side effects than the dopamine antagonists. The overall incidence of side effects in placebo-controlled studies was 13.2% (n=730) for cisapride and 10.6% (n=644) for placebo. The most frequent side effects were transient loosening of stools, abdominal discomfort and headache.[46]

Dose: full dosing specifications of cisapride in the treatment of gastroparesis are still being determined. Orally, 10 mg of cisapride taken 30 minutes before meals and at bedtime is effective in many gastroparetic conditions. This dose can be increased to 20 mg qid in severe gastroparetic patients without any apparent increase in side effects.

Cisapride has been approved for the treatment of gastroparesis in several European countries, including the UK, and Canada. It remains under experimental investigation in the USA.

Other drugs

There are several other therapeutic agents which have prokinetic properties with potential clinical use.

Bethanechol: bethanechol is a cholinomimetic agent which stimulates the parasympathetic nervous system. Gastric motility appears to be improved by increasing gastric tone and restoring a more normal migrating myoelectric complex.[2,3] In a study of patients with gastroparesis and reflux esophagitis it was not effective in improving gastric emptying, whereas metoclopramide was.[12] However, bethanechol appears to be effective as adjunctive therapy with the dopamine antagonists. This could prove helpful with metoclopramide where side effects limit the dose. Unfortunately, bethanechol has side effects resulting from overstimulation of the parasympathetic nervous system; these include abdominal discomfort, excessive salivation, flushing of the skin and excessive sweating.

Naloxone: opiate receptors have been demonstrated throughout the gastrointestinal tract. Opiate peptoids appear to act as neurotransmitters for both gastric motility and secretion. Naloxone, a parenteral opiate antagonist, appears to have an inhibitory effect on gastric emptying when used at a dose of 2 mg intravenously,[47] whereas in larger intravenous doses of

5 mg it accelerates gastric emptying.[48] Further studies are necessary to define the exact role of naloxone or its oral equivalent naltrexone in the therapy of gastroparesis.

Clebopride: clebopride is a new dopamine antagonist. A benzamide derivative, clebopride is a more selective blocker of the dopamine 1 receptors that the dopamine 2 receptors. For this reason, even though it crosses the blood-brain barrier, clebopride does not seem to be associated with the extrapyramidal side effects found with metoclopramide. Clebopride appears to have anti-emetic and gastric prokinetic properties. The agent has been studied in Europe and South America for several years and preliminary tests are underway in North America. Its potential clinical indications are for reflux esophagitis, gastroparesis and as an anti-emetic.[49]

Zacopride: zacopride is another gastric prokinetic agent under preliminary evaluation. It appears to have gastric prokinetic and anti-emetic properties. Its action seems to be as a serotonin antagonist together with some dopamine antagonism and cholinergic activity.

Rapid gastric emptying

Patients with rapid gastric emptying often present with symptoms of either early or late dumping syndrome.

Early dumping symptoms are principally epigastric fullness, pain, nausea, vomiting, diarrhea and a general feeling of lassitude and weakness which normally occurs 10–30 minutes after meals. The etiology of early dumping syndrome is multifactorial with at least one component being hypovolemia; this is caused by fluid shift secondary to hyperosmolar fluid being present in the small bowel.

Symptoms of late dumping syndrome are due to hypoglycemia following an initial rapid rise of glucose post-prandially which stimulates an exaggerated insulin response which results in hypoglycemia 1–3 hours after eating.

Rapid gastric emptying may be a factor in the pathogenesis of duodenal ulcer disease. Early studies showed patients with this disease emptied solids more rapidly than normal[50] although liquid emptying remained unaffected.[51] However, these observations have been challenged by a study which looked at gastric emptying in patients with duodenal ulcer disease before, during and after therapy with cimetidine. Gastric emptying of the solid component of a test meal was more rapid during treatment with cimetidine, resulting in a narrowing of the normal difference between the emptying rates for solids and liquids. This effect was thought to be due to a reduction in gastric volume caused by inhibition of acid secretion by cimetidine. No difference was detected in the rate of gastric emptying between duodenal ulcer patients and controls before or after ulcer healing with cimetidine.[52]

Patients with Zollinger-Ellison syndrome may have symptoms of rapid gastric emptying. The diarrhea which occurs in patients with Zollinger-Ellison syndrome results from a combination of rapid gastric emptying, large gastric output and impaired fat absorption due to the low pH in the duodenum causing inactivation of the pancreatic lipase. Cimetidine does not normalize this rapid gastric emptying, indicating that factors other than acid hypersecretion alone play a role in the rapid emptying of both solids and liquids in patients with Zollinger-Ellison syndrome.[53]

The incidence of dumping syndrome following vagotomy and gastric surgery varies from 1–22%, depending on the type of surgery performed; highly selective gastric vagotomy produces the lowest incidence, truncal vagotomy and antrectomy the highest.[54] Chronic diarrhea may follow any ulcer operation and usually improves with time, although 1% of patients have long-term problems. Diarrhea following gastric surgery appears to result from a combination of vagal denervation of the gut, rapid gastric emptying and increased secretion of bile acids following vagotomy.

Treatment of underlying condition
The symptoms of rapid gastric emptying are rarely problematic in patients with duodenal ulcer disease. In patients with Zollinger-Ellison syndrome, dumping syndrome is rare and diarrhea is often controlled with H_2 receptor antagonism if the gastrin-secreting tumour is not resectable. Further surgery for dumping syndrome following gastric surgery has unpredictable results.

Diet
Attention to diet is an important part of the medical management of dumping syndrome. Patients should eat frequent small meals low in carbohydrate, minimizing fluid intake at the time of eating. The dietary fibre pectin has been demonstrated to cause symptomatic improvement and delay emptying in patients with dumping syndrome.[55]

Drug therapy
Medication may also be useful to decrease gastric emptying rates and slow gastrointestinal transit. Drugs to consider in this condition include probanthine, L dopa, codeine or other opiates. However, these drugs have many side effects and with codeine and other opiates there is risk of addiction with long-term therapy. Therefore, drug therapy should be considered only in severe situations.

The parenteral narcotic antagonist naloxone has also been shown to delay emptying in normal subjects at a dose of 2 mg intravenously.[47] Naloxone, or its oral equivalent natrexone, may have a role in the treatment of patients with rapid gastric emptying although further studies are required.

Conclusion

The management of both rapid and delayed gastric emptying can be subdivided into treatment of the underlying condition, diet and drug therapy.

In patients with delayed gastric emptying, treatment of the underlying condition can often result in improvement in symptoms and gastric motility. Dietary modification is helpful and there are effective gastric prokinetic agents available, with many candidate agents currently being reserved for severe cases only.

The management of patients with rapid gastric emptying is mainly dietary, drug therapy being reserved for severe cases only.

References
1 Minami H, McCallum RW. The physiology and pathophysiology of gastric emptying in humans. *Gastroenterology* 1984; **86**: 1592-610.
2 Malagelada J-R, Rees WDW, Mazzotta LJ, Go VLW. Gastric motor abnormalities in diabetic and post-vagotomy gastroparesis: effect of metoclopramide and bethanechol. *Gastroenterology* 1980; **78**: 286-93.
3 Fox S, Behar J. Pathogenesis of diabetic gastroparesis: a pharmacologic study. *Gastroenterology* 1980; **78**: 757-63.
4 Schuurkes JAJ, Helsen LFM, Van Nueten JM. Improved gastroduodenal coordination by the peripheral dopamine antagonist domperidone. In: *Motility of the Digestive Tract*. Raven Press. 1982; 565-72.
5 Stacher G, Gaupmann G, Mittelbach G, Schneider C, Steinringer H, Langer B. Effects of oral cisapride on interdigestive jejunal motor activity, psychomotor function and side effect profile in healthy man. *Dig Dis Sci* 1987; **32**: 1223-30.
6 Albibi R, McCallum RW. Metoclopramide; pharmacology and clinical application. *Ann Intern Med* 1983; **98**: 86-95.

7 McCallum RW. Review of the current status of prokinetic agents in gastroenterology. *Am J Gastroenterol* 1985; **80**: 1008–16.
8 Wright RA, Clemente R, Wathen R. Diabetic gastroparesis: an abnormality of gastric emptying of solids. *Am J Med Sci* 1985; **289**: 240–2.
9 Ricci DA, Saltzman MB, Meyer C, Callachan C, McCallum RW. Effect of metoclopramide in diabetic gastroparesis. *J Clin Gastroenterol* 1985; **7**: 25–32.
10 McClelland RN, Horton JW. Relief of acute persistent post-vagotomy atony by metoclopramide. *Ann Surg* 1978; **188**: 439–45.
11 Salem JW, Lebwohl T. Metoclopramide-induced gastric emptying in patients with anorexia nervosa. *Am J Gastroenterol* 1980; **74**: 127–32.
12 Fink SM, Lange RC, McCallum RW. Effect of metoclopramide on normal and delayed gastric emptying in gastroesophageal reflux patients. *Dig Dis Sci* 1983; **28**: 1057–61.
13 Perkel MS, Moore C, Hersch T, Davidson ED. Metoclopramide in patients with delayed emptying: a randomized double-blind trial. *Dig Dis Sci* 1979; **24**: 662–6.
14 Horowitz M, Maddox A, Maddern GJ, Wishart J, Collins PJ, Shearman DJC. Gastric and esophageal emptying in dystrophia myotonica: effect of metoclopramide. *Gastroenterology* 1987; **92**: 570–7.
15 Snape WJ, Battle WM, Schwartz SS, Braunstein SN, Goldstein HA, Alavi A. Metoclopramide to treat gastroparesis due to diabetes mellitus: a double-blind controlled trial. *Ann Intern Med* 1982; **96**: 444–6.
16 Schade RR, Dugas MC, Lhotsky DM, Gavaler JS, Van Thiel TH. Effect of metoclopramide on gastric liquid emptying in patients with diabetic gastroparesis. *Dig Dis Sci* 1985; **30**: 10–5.
17 Bateman DN, Rawlins MD, Simpson JM. Extrapyramidal reactions with metoclopramide. *Br Med J* 1985; **291**: 930–2.
18 Champion MC. Domperidone. *Gen Pharmacol* (In press)
19 Champion MC, Hartnett M, Yen M. Domperidone, a new dopamine antagonist. *Can Med Assoc J* 1986; **135**: 457–61.
20 Heer M, Muller-Duysing W, Benes M, Weitzel M, Pirovino M, Altorfer J, Schmid M. Diabetic gastroparesis: treatment with domperidone — a double-blind, placebo-controlled trial. *Digestion* 1983; **27**: 214–7.
21 Horowitz M, Harding PE, Chatterton BE, Collins PJ, Shearman DJC. Acute and chronic effects of domperidone on gastric emptying in diabetic autonomic neuropathy. *Dig Dis Sci* 1985; **30**: 1–9.
22 Corinaldesi R, Stanghellini V, Zarabini GE et al. Effect of domperidone on the gastric emptying of solid and liquid phases of a mixed meal in patients with dyspepsia. *Curr Ther Res* 1983; **34**: 982–6.
23 Stacher G, Kis A, Wiesnagrotzki S, Bergman H, Hobart J, Schneider C. Oesophageal and gastric motility disorders in patients categorized as having primary anorexia nervosa. *Gut* 1986; **27**: 1120–6.
24 McCallum RW, Ricci D, DuBovik S et al. Effect of domperidone on gastric emptying and symptoms in patients with idiopathic gastric stasis. *Gastroenterology* 1984; **5**: 1179 (abstr).
25 Albibi R, DuBovik S, Lange RC, McCallum RW. A dose response study of the effects of domperidone and gastric retention in man. *Am J Gastroenterol* 1983; **78**: 679 (abstr).
26 Champion MC, Gulenchyn K, O'Leary T, Irving P, Edwards A, Braaten J. Domperidone improves symptoms and solid phase gastric emptying in diabetic gastroparesis. *Am J Gastroenterol* 1987; **82**: 213 (abstr).
27 Molino D, Mosca S, Angrisani G, Magliacano V. Symptomatic effects of domperidone in post-vagotomy gastric stasis. *Curr Ther Res* 1987; **41**(1): 13–6.
28 Miederer SE. A German multicentre trial with domperidone in dyspeptic disorders. *Therapeutics Today* 1987; **6**: 43–8.
29 Brogden RN, Carmine AA, Heel RC et al. Domperidone: a review of its pharmacological activity, pharmacokinetics and therapeutic efficacy in the symptomatic treatment of chronic dyspepsia and as an anti-emetic. *Drugs* 1982; **24**: 360–400.
30 Cameron HA, Reyntjens AJ, Lake-Bakaar G. Cardiac arrest after treatment with intravenous domperidone. *Br Med J* 1985; **290**: 160.
31 Reyntjens A, Verlinden M, Aerts T. Development and clinical use of the new gastrointestinal prokinetic drug cisapride (R51 619). *Drug Dev Res* 1986; **8**: 251–65.
32 Feldman M, Smith HJ. Effect of cisapride on gastric emptying of undigested solids in patients with

gastroparesis diabeticorum: a comparison with metoclopramide and placebo. *Gastroenterology* 1987; **92**: 171–4.

33 McHugh S, Lico S, Meindok H, Diamant NE. Intravenous cisapride in diabetic gastroparesis. *Gastroenterology* 1986; **90**: 1545 (abstr).

34 Horowitz M, Maddox A, Harding PE *et al*. Acute and chronic effects of cisapride on gastric esophageal emptying in insulin-dependent diabetes mellitus. *Gastroenterology* 1987; **92**: 1899–907.

35 Champion MC, Gulenchyn K, Braaten J *et al*. Cisapride improves symptoms and solid phase gastric emptying in diabetic gastroparesis (DGP). *Diabetes* 1988; **37**(Suppl 1):84 (abstr).

36 Horowitz M, Maddern GJ, Maddox A, Wishart J, Chatterton BE, Shearman DJ. Effects of cisapride on gastric and esophageal emptying in progressive systemic sclerosis. *Gastroenterology* 1987; **93**: 311–5.

37 Stacher G, Bergmann H, Weisnagrotzki S *et al*. Intravenous cisapride accelerates delayed gastric emptying and increases antral contraction amplitude in patients with primary anorexia nervosa. *Gastroenterology* 1987; **92**: 1000–6.

38 Horowitz M, Maddox A, Wishart J, Collins PJ, Shearman DJ. The effects of cisapride on gastric and esophageal emptying in dystrophia myotonica. *J Gastro Hepat* 1987; **2**: 285–93.

39 Jian R, Ruskone A, Ducrot S, Chaussade S, Rambaud JC, Bernier JJ. Radionuclide and therapeutic assessment of chronic idiopathic dyspepsia (CID). *Gastroenterology* 1986; **90**: 1477 (abstr).

40 Corinaldesi R, Stanghellini V, Raiti C, Rea E, Salgemini R, Barbara L. Effect of chronic administration of cisapride on gastric emptying of a solid meal and on dyspeptic symptoms in patients with idiopathic gastroparesis. *Gut* 1987; **28**: 300–5.

41 McCallum RW, Peterson J, Dubovik S. The effect of cisapride on gastric emptying and the symptoms associated with gastroparesis. *Gastroenterology* 1986; **90**: 1541.

42 Camilleri M, Abell TL, Brown ML, Hench VS, Zinsmeister AR, Malagelada JR. Motor transit and symptomatic effects of cisapride in patients with upper gut dysmotility. *Gastroenterology* 1987; **92**: 1337.

43 McCallum RW, Plankey MW, Fisher KL. Chronic oral cisapride therapy increases solid meal gastric emptying and improves symptoms in patients with gastric stasis. *Gastroenterology* 1987; **92**: 1525 (abstr).

44 Champion MC. Management of idiopathic, diabetic and miscellaneous gastroparesis with cisapride. *Scand J Gastroenterol* 1989 (In press).

45 Abell TL, Camilleri M, DiMagno EP, Hench VS, Malagelada JR. Cisapride is effective in the long-term treatment of gastric motor disorders. *Gastroenterology* 1987; **92**: 1287.

46 Reyntjens A, Verlinden M, Schuermans V. Safety of cisapride: clinical and laboratory findings. *Prog Med* 1987; **43**: 19–26.

47 Champion MC, Sullivan SN, Chamberlain M, Vezina W. Naloxone and morphine inhibit gastric emptying of solids. *Can J Physiol Pharmacol* 1982; **60**: 732–4.

48 Mittel KR, Frank EB, Lang R, McCallum RW. Effect of morphine and naloxone on lower esophageal sphincter pressure and gastric emptying in man. *Dig Dis Sci* 1986; **31**: 936–42.

49 Bavestrello L *et al*. A double-blind comparison of clebopride and placebo in dyspepsia secondary to delayed gastric emptying. *Clin Ther* 1985; **7**: 468–73.

50 Fordtran JS, Walsh JH. Gastric acid secretion rate and buffer content of the stomach after eating: results in normal subjects and in patients with duodenal ulcer. *J Clin Invest* 1973; **52**: 645–57.

51 Cobb JS, Bank S, Marks IN *et al*. Gastric emptying after vagotomy and pyloroplasty: relation to some post-operative sequelae. *Am J Dig Dis* 1971; **16**: 207–15.

52 Holt F, Heading RC, Taylor TV, Forrest JA, Tothill P. Gastric emptying abnormal in duodenal ulcer disease? *Dig Dis Sci* 1986; **31**: 685–92.

53 Harrison A, Ippoliti A, Cullison R. Rapid gastric emptying in Zollinger-Ellison Syndrome. *Gastroenterology* 1980; **78**: 1180.

54 Champion MC. Complications of upper gastrointestinal surgery. *Med N Am* 1984 (2nd series); **17**: 2220–7.

55 Leeds AR, Ralphs DNL, Ebied F *et al*. Pectin in the dumping syndrome: reduction of symptoms and plasma volume changes. *Lancet* 1981; **ii**: 1075–8.

Treatment of functional diseases of the small intestine

J R Mathias

Although the term 'functional diseases of the small intestine' implies that such diseases are without an organic basis, emerging evidence indicates that these diseases of the gastrointestinal tract do have a recognized organic cause. The problem is that conventional diagnostic techniques do not pinpoint or perhaps do not even suggest the underlying disease. The patient with functional disease therefore becomes frustrating to the physician. But the frustration of the physician is usually exceeded by that of the patient, who is often classified as psychoneurotic and told "the problem is all in your head and you must just learn to live with it", when in fact the patient has organic disease that is difficult to diagnose.

This discussion of the current knowledge of the recognized syndromes of functional bowel disease of the small intestine will review: (1) the symptoms and physical diagnostic findings; (2) the objective findings that may be obtained by conventional testing techniques; and (3) current therapeutic considerations and experimental pharmacologic drugs that may become available.

Because the term 'functional bowel disease' suggests, inaccurately, that the pathophysiology of the disease has been identified and treatment for the symptom complex is known, the use of this term should be discouraged. It would be preferable either to define the symptom complex as the specific disease is currently understood or to refer to the problem as 'motility disorders of undefined etiology'. These diseases may either involve the muscle of the gastrointestinal tract or be disorders of the enteric nervous system. They might even be referred to in the future as neurotransmitter diseases involving specific potential putative neuroactive substances found within the intestinal wall.

Gastroduodenal motor dysfunction

Gastroduodenal motor dysfunction is a newly defined entity that occurs primarily in young women (mean age 32.8 years, ratio 15 women to 1 man).[1] The presenting symptoms typically are unexplained chronic nausea, abdominal pain and intermittent episodic vomiting. The symptoms may cycle and worsen in the post-luteal phase of the menstrual cycle and subside or lessen after the onset of menses. The physical findings are always normal.

Clinical evaluation usually includes a complete blood count, serum chemistries, x-ray studies that include an upper gastrointestinal x-ray examination with a small bowel series, a barium enema, endoscopic retrograde cholangiopancreatography, ultrasound of the gallbladder and computed tomography (CT) of the abdomen. The results of these tests are always normal even though they may have been repeated on numerous occasions.[2,3] Endoscopic procedures, including esophagogastroduodenoscopy and colonoscopy, also show normal results.[2,3]

Radiolabelled meals, on the other hand, may provide objective evidence of some abnormality in the functioning of the stomach and upper small intestine.[4] Approximately one-third of patients with gastroduodenal motor dysfunction have prolonged gastric emptying. Since receptors for osmolality, distension, pH, fat, carbohydrate and protein are in the duodenum and upper jejunum, it is not surprising that delayed emptying may be a factor in this disease.[5-10]

Additional objective evidence may be obtained through recording of intestinal pressure changes that show abnormal motility patterns. A semiconductor recording probe that is easily passed by nasal intubation (*Figure 1*) has been developed.[11] Because of the small size of the probe (8F or 2.7 mm in diameter), prolonged recording periods may be obtained with minimal discomfort to the patient.

The migrating motor complex (MMC) — a broad front of slow, propagating ring contractions — cycles the intestinal tract in animals[12] and in humans.[13,14] In human control subjects this complex cycles the intestine about every 80–100 minutes (mean ± SEM 92.7 ± 5.6 minutes) and only when a person is fasting. The MMC is thought to act as an 'intestinal housekeeper', clearing unwanted debris from within the lumen of the tract.[15] The MMC helps to differentiate normal from abnormal motor patterns in patients with unexplained symptoms that have been presumed to be either functional or motility disorders.[14,16-18]

Characteristics of gastroduodenal motor dysfunction have been obtained from recordings of the stomach and upper small intestine (*Figure 2*). The characteristics include: first, the presence of antral dysfunction, which is defined either as an in-

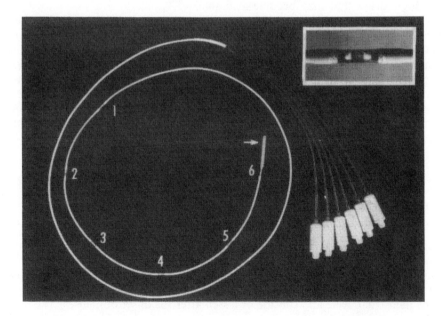

Figure 1 Semiconductor recording probe consisting of six ultraminiature strain gauges spaced 10 cm apart. The end of the probe is covered with a flexible rubber tip. Reproduced with permission from Mathias JR *et al*. Development of an improved multi-pressure-sensor probe for recording muscle contraction in human intestine. *Dig Dis Sci* 1985; **30**: 119–23.

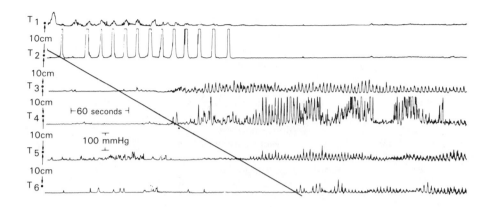

Figure 2 A disrupted migrating motor complex (MMC) with antral dysfunction. Transducer placement is illustrated schematically on the left, and time and pressure calibrations are also shown. T_1 and T_2 represent activity from the body and antrum of the stomach, respectively; T_{3-6} represent activity from the duodenum and upper jejunum. Antral activity is irregularly increased in frequency (to approximately 6/minute), and amplitude is low (<100 mmHg). In addition, the activity front in the small intestine shows that disruption does not propagate smoothly and has high-amplitude contractions (>100 mmHg; T_4 and T_6). Reproduced with permission from Mathias JR, Finelli DS. Functional diseases of the small intestine. In: Cohen S, Soloway R, eds. *Functional Disorders of the Gastrointestinal Tract*. New York: 1987, Churchill Livingstone 1987.

crease in the number of antral contractions (more than 3.5 contractions/minute) or as contractions that are low in amplitude (less than 100 mmHg); and second, dysfunction in the duodenum and jejunum as shown by high-amplitude contractions (more than 100 mmHg) or the presence of disorganized, retrograde MMCs.

Other investigators have used electrical techniques to assess the integrity of the antrum. You and co-workers described a young woman who had a variable frequency of, and an increase in, the slow wave (or pacemaker) rhythm of the antrum; they called this phenomenon 'tachygastria with tachyarrhythmia'.[19] Telander and co-workers demonstrated a similar condition in a young child with recurrent vomiting.[20]

Stern and co-workers have demonstrated experimentally tachygastria with tachyarrhythmia in subjects who were placed in a drum that was painted with black and white stripes and could be rotated at varying frequencies to simulate motion.[21] When the drum was rotated, most subjects became nauseated and began vomiting. The electrical rhythms of their stomachs were simultaneously recorded by cutaneous electrodes; the resultant enterogastrogram showed a change in gastric electrical rhythm. Whether the enterogastrogram will provide a simple noninvasive technique for diagnosing this disorder remains the subject for continued investigation.[22]

Therapy for gastroduodenal motor dysfunction remains as challenging as establishing the diagnosis (*Table 1*). Unfortunately, although metoclopramide, a first-generation gastric prokinetic drug, has been useful in the therapy for many of these patients, numerous adverse side effects limit its usefulness in many of these patients.

Several new drugs are currently under investigation for gastroduodenal motor dysfunction. One of the most promising is domperidone, which, like metoclopramide, is also a dopamine antagonist but rarely crosses the blood-brain barrier and thus

Gastric prokinetic drugs

Metoclopramide
Domperidone
Cisapride

Adrenergic agonists

Alpha$_1$-agonist
— Ephedrine sulfate

Alpha$_2$-agonist
— Lidamidine HCl (or metabolites)

Fibre

Psyllium seed preparations
Methyl cellulose
Bran

Table 1 Therapy for patients with gastroduodenal motor dysfunction.

has fewer side effects.[23] Since both metoclopramide and domperidone stimulate the release of prolactin from the posterior pituitary, the problem of breast enlargement with lactation remains the most common side effect with either compound. Both of these prokinetic drugs may be effective in controlling the nausea and vomiting of many patients with gastroduodenal motor dysfunction, but they do not affect the pain component.

A second drug that may have excellent therapeutic effects is cisapride, which is thought to coordinate the mechanical contractions between the stomach and upper small intestine.[24] Current studies are under way to assess the effectiveness of this compound.

One of the mechanisms of this disorder may be a lack of inhibitory control of the intestine, resulting in an increase in contractile activity. Use of ephedrine sulfate, an adrenergic agonist, in very small doses (8.5–11.5 mg tid) has met with reasonable success in some patients. In addition, semiconductor probe recordings before and after therapy showed that the patients had significantly decreased activity of the intestine. The problems with ephedrine sulfate, however, are the adverse side effects such as tremor, nervousness and insomnia that it causes in these subjects, even when the ephedrine sulfate is administered in small doses.

An experimental drug, lidamidine hydrochloride (a proposed alpha$_2$-adrenergic agonist), has also been studied by probe recordings of patients with gastroduodenal motor dysfunction before and after treatment.[25] The decrease in intestinal activity with lidamidine is similar to the effects of ephedrine but without the unwanted side effects. This drug (or its future metabolites) appears to have a promising future for controlling abdominal pain in these patients.

Bulk in the form of psyllium seed or methyl cellulose preparations is also helpful in controlling the symptoms, as well as constipation, which may or may not be a problem in these patients. Doses in the range of 2–4 tablespoonfuls twice daily may be needed for effective therapeutic control. The patient must be encouraged to take these medications; nausea may increase and abdominal bloating may occur initially, but usually subsides within a short time.

Intestinal pseudo-obstruction

Intestinal pseudo-obstruction comprises several diseases.[26] The usual complaint of a patient with this disorder is frequent and intermittent episodes of abdominal distension. An x-ray film of the abdomen discloses air/fluid levels suggestive of a mechanical obstruction. Exploratory laparotomy is often performed on these patients without finding a cause for the distension. More importantly, full-thickness biopsy specimens of the bowel wall (small intestine and colon) are not taken; thus, the abdomen has been explored without a resultant diagnosis.

The four main categories for known pseudo-obstruction are: collagen-vascular diseases, such as scleroderma; endocrine disorders, such as diabetes mellitus, myxedema and hypoparathyroidism; drugs, including the tricyclic antidepressants, opiates and clonidine; and neurologic disorders, such as Parkinson's disease (*Table 2*).

Acute intestinal pseudo-obstruction (Ogilvie's syndrome)

Acute intestinal pseudo-obstruction was first described in 1948.[27] It involves massive dilatation of the colon and usually occurs in older people secondary to metabolic derangements such as potassium, magnesium or calcium deficiencies or to post-operative (especially for orthopedic or urologic conditions) or post-traumatic states. X-ray examination discloses massive dilatation of the colon, especially the cecum. Distension of the colon of more than 10 cm is critical and if therapy is not initiated, perforation may occur from necrosis.

Abdominal distension is rapid and progressive, usually within 2–3 days after an orthopedic or urologic procedure. Often there are few subjective symptoms such as abdominal pain. Nausea and vomiting may be absent. The abdomen is markedly distended and tympanitic but seldom tender. Bowel sounds are usually present but may vary. Abdominal radiographs show massive dilatation of the cecum and segmental dilatation in the ascending, transverse or descending colon without air/fluid levels.

Management in most cases is conservative, consisting of stopping oral intake, applying decompression by nasogastric and rectal tube, correcting fluid and electrolyte imbalance and minimizing the use of narcotic analgesics, anticholinergics and other medications known to induce bowel hypomotility. Laxatives and therapeutic enemas should be avoided because they can increase the intracolonic pressure and thus increase the likelihood of perforation. Colonic contrast studies should also be avoided if possible, but a radiopaque enema (diatrizoate meglumine/diatrizoate sodium; Gastrografin®) may be considered and performed gently to show that there is no mechanical lesion.

If the cecal diameter is increasing beyond the critical range of about 10 cm or if impending perforation is feared, colonoscopic decompression may be undertaken. The colonic decompression should be performed by an experienced colonoscopist because it may be difficult to reach the right side of the colon through an unprepared bowel or through a colon containing Gastrografin if an enema has already been given

®Registered trademark.

Diseases involving intestinal smooth muscle
Collagen-vascular disease
— Scleroderma
— Systemic lupus erythematosus
— Dermatomyositis
Muscular dystrophies
— Myotonic dystrophy
— Duchenne-Aran muscular dystrophy
Amyloidosis

Endocrine disorders
Diabetes mellitus
Myxedema
Hypoparathyroidism
Pheochromocytoma

Neurologic disorders
Parkinson's disease
Hirschsprung's disease
Chagas' disease
Ganglioneuroma of intestine

Pharmacologic causes
Phenothiazines
Tricyclic antidepressants
Anti-parkinsonian medications
Clonidine (alpha$_2$-adrenergic agonist)
Ephedrine (alpha$_1$-adrenergic agonist)

Miscellaneous
Nontropical sprue
Jejunal diverticulosis
Jejunoileal bypass
Cathartic colon
Psychosis
Radiation enteritis
Eosinophilic gastroenteritis
Porphyria
Paraneoplastic syndromes
— Oat cell carcinoma of the lung
— Carcinoid

Table 2   Known causes of intestinal pseudo-obstruction. Modified, with permission, from Anuras S, Christensen J. Recurrent or chronic intestinal pseudo-obstruction. *Clin Gastroenterol* 1981; **10**: 177.

as a diagnostic procedure. For this reason, decompression by colonoscopy may be considered the procedure of choice and can be safe, with a high degree of success. Colonoscopy is also of diagnostic value when organic obstruction lesions are suspected. Tube cecostomy has been used under similar conditions with varying degrees of success.

If several areas of necrosis or perforation are present or suspected, a right hemicolectomy or subtotal colectomy may be necessary; the mortality ranges from 25–30%. The chance of perforation in Ogilvie's syndrome is approximately 15%. Mortality increases markedly if perforation occurs.

Chronic intermittent intestinal pseudo-obstruction

Chronic intermittent pseudo-obstruction, which may occur at any time during life, not only includes small bowel dilatation and large dilated colon but also may include severe gastric atony.[28] This form of pseudo-obstruction may be acquired or familial.[26,29,30] Normal neural responses to swallowing and intestinal distension may be impaired as a result of a neural transmission defect in the myenteric plexus (enteric nervous system) or degenerative changes in the myenteric plexus neurons, or both.[31-33]

Medical therapy has little success in this form of pseudo-obstruction. Many patients undergo numerous diagnostic procedures, including surgical exploration, but no lesion is found. If surgery is performed and no mechanical lesion is found, full-thickness biopsy specimens of the small intestine and colon should be obtained for histologic examination. Routine hematoxylin and eosin staining is used to examine the muscle, and silver or neuron-specific enolase staining is employed for the myenteric plexus neurons. Once the entity of chronic intermittent intestinal pseudo-obstruction is recognized repeated surgical intervention should be avoided because fibrous tissue causing intra-abdominal adhesions, only complicates the management of these patients.

Medical therapy (*Table 3*) involves prokinetic drugs, such as metoclopramide, domperidone, cisapride and/or bethanechol; pseudocholinesterase inhibitors, such as edrophonium hydrochloride; and oral liquid diets that are chemically defined. Parenteral hyperalimentation, either for short intervals or on a long-term basis, may be the only form of therapy that is effective and life-saving for these patients. Since this form of therapy is very costly, the decision to initiate it must be considered carefully. It is hoped that effective medical therapy will be developed as the pathophysiology of this disorder is defined. The pathophysiology is probably multifactorial and therefore therapy will require numerous medications, based on specific defects as they are defined by future research.

Idiopathic intestinal hollow visceral myopathy neuropathy

The term 'hollow visceral myopathy' suggests that this form of pseudo-obstruction is primarily a myopathy in which fibrous tissue replaces predominantly the longitudinal muscle layer of the intestine.[34,35] However, the disease has been found to involve the neurons of the myenteric plexus, indicating that the disorder may be a myopathy or a neuropathy, or both.[36] The presence of damaged neurons is the most common underlying pathophysiologic event (J R Mathias, unpublished observations).

This disease affects hollow viscera, such as the alimentary tract, ureters, bladder and urethra.[37] For unexplained reasons, fibrosis of the lens of the eye and the presence of hepatic portal fibrosis may also be associated with the condition. Because of the frequent occurrence of lower quadrant pain, fallopian tube dysfunction may also be a part of the syndrome, but this remains speculation at this time.

Symptoms usually appear after the first 10 years of life and consist of recurrent post-prandial abdominal pain, distension and intermittent vomiting. Bacterial overgrowth in the small intestine may cause diarrhea. Urinary complaints are seldom present, but if a careful history is obtained, it may show the patient has vague urinary symptoms that have been overshadowed by the gastrointestinal tract problems. Some patients may also state that they urinate only once or twice daily, which they consider normal.

Radiographic studies usually show dilatation of the stomach and small intestine, most often in the duodenum. The findings may be obvious and show mega-duodenum,[26] but usually they are likely to be more subtle and be overlooked or

Stop oral intake during exacerbations

Nasogastric and rectal decompression

Correct fluid and electrolyte imbalance

Decompressive colonoscopy

Gastric prokinetic drugs

   — Metoclopramide
   — Domperidone
   — Cisapride
   — Bethanechol

Liquid diet (chemically defined supplements)

Avoid drugs that inhibit motility (anticholinergics, antiadrenergics, opiates)

Total parenteral hyperalimentation (short- or long-term)

Surgery (exploration — obtain full-thickness biopsy specimens if
   no obstruction is found)

Avoid fibre

Good dental hygiene

Antibiotics when indicated for bacterial overgrowth

Psychological evaluation

Table 3   Therapy for chronic intermittent intestinal pseudo-obstruction.

interpreted as the superior mesenteric artery syndrome. Multiple segmental dilatations of the small intestine occur less often in hollow visceral myopathy than they do in acute intermittent pseudo-obstruction. A barium enema x-ray study often discloses redundant colon or megacolon. Intravenous pyelography usually shows only an enlarged bladder with the contrast material retained after voiding.[26] A cystometrogram will show increased filling pressures or spasm of the bladder, or both.

Medical therapy (*Table 4*) with gastrointestinal drugs such as metoclopramide, bethanechol or edrophonium hydrochloride has been problematic. Antibiotics may be of value if diarrhea is present and is caused by bacterial overgrowth. In general, however, patients with intestinal hollow visceral myopathy may require long-term parenteral hyperalimentation to manage their nutrition. Many surgical procedures for localized dilatation of the small intestine have been performed on some patients. The results from surgery are mixed, but generally surgery should be avoided because of the diffuse involvement of the intestine and the increased formation of adhesions from each laparotomy. If it is a major problem, the urinary tract disease may be managed with an indwelling Foley catheter or by training patients to catheterize themselves several times daily.

Intestinal visceral hollow myopathy (see *Table 3*)
  Urinary tract care
    Catheterization—indwelling Foley catheter
    Catheterization—in/out every 6 hours
    Antibiotics, eg, trimethoprim-sulfamethoxazole
    Opiates

Severe intestinal constipation (see *Table 3*)
  Anal manometry
  Consider 95% colectomy if anal manometry excludes short-segment
  Hirschsprung's disease

Roux-en-Y syndrome (see *Table 3*)
  Consider a jejunostomy feeding tube below the end-to-side anastomosis of
    the Roux limb
  Avoid truncal vagotomy if possible
  Opiates

Table 4 Therapy for intestinal visceral hollow myopathy, severe intestinal constipation and Roux-en-Y syndrome.

Severe intestinal constipation

Severe intestinal constipation, a recently described entity, was recognized in a group of patients complaining of chronic nausea with post-prandial bloating, accompanied by long-standing severe constipation (obstipation) refractory to currently available medical therapy.[38] These patients often do not pass a stool for 10–14 days without enemas or manual disimpaction.

A total of 26 such patients (25 women, 1 man; mean age, 42 years) were investigated in one study.[39] Semiconductor probe recordings of the upper gastrointestinal tract disclosed abnormalities in motor function consistent with neuromuscular dysfunction. All of the patients then underwent a subtotal (95%) colectomy with biopsy of the ileum. The tissue samples from the colon and small intestine were examined by routine histologic techniques with hematoxylin and eosin stains and silver-staining techniques. Histologic studies showed normal muscle in all the tissue samples. The predominant abnormality was moderate-to-severe neurologic damage to the argyrophilic neurons of the myenteric plexus. This type of damage is thought to be characteristic of severe intestinal constipation, which is probably a subtype of idiopathic intestinal pseudo-obstruction. Argyrophilic neurons of the myenteric plexus are believed to be involved in nerve-to-nerve transmission; therefore, their loss because of neurologic injury may result in the loss of effective muscle contraction.

Physical examination of patients with severe intestinal constipation shows no objective abnormalities except abdominal distension. Laboratory findings are also normal. A barium enema x-ray study, however, usually shows a redundant colon with loss of the haustral folds. Because these patients have usually been taking laxatives for prolonged periods, there is always the question of which came first — constipation requiring medication for evacuation or neurologic damage from long-term laxative usage? Medical histories generally indicate that constipation precedes the use of laxatives to achieve normal evacuation.

Effective therapy for severe intestinal constipation remains unclear (*Table 4*). In the study involving 26 patients, subtotal (95%) colectomies were performed in the hope of eliminating the storage function of their colons.[39] Thus far, results have been encouraging, but long-term follow-up (more than 5 years) will be necessary for a more definitive determination of the effect of surgery on this disorder. In addition, the prokinetic drug cisapride, which stimulates the release of acetylcholine at the myenteric plexus ganglion, may offer effective medical therapy. Double-blind trials are ongoing to assess the effectiveness of this prokinetic pharmacologic agent for treatment of this disorder.

As in all forms of pseudo-obstruction, bulk therapy of any type should be avoided because the bulk only aggravates the inability of the colon to evacuate itself. Usually, low-residue diets offer some relief of the symptoms.

Since the human intestinal tract contains 1×10^8 neurons and many different neurotransmitters,[40] the magnitude of this disease, as well as of pseudo-obstruction in general, almost certainly will require creative and imaginative investigation and a multidisciplinary approach for a solution.

Pseudo-obstruction secondary to neoplastic disease

Schuffler and co-workers have described several patients who have a pseudo-obstruction complex both clinically and by histologic examination of the enteric plexus.[41] Tumour cells are absent, but there is extensive neurologic damage similar to that in severe intestinal constipation. Oat cell carcinoma of the lung and carcinoid are the two tumours associated with this paraneoplastic syndrome. The mechanism remains unknown.

Sequelae from abdominal surgery

Certain surgical therapeutic techniques that were accepted in the past now need to be reassessed. With the medication presently available to control gastric acid secretion (H_2 agonists), truncal vagotomy should be considered a potential form of serious iatrogenic disease in some patients — those with compromised enteric nervous systems that cannot yet be diagnosed. Subjects who have undergone truncal vagotomy combined with a Billroth I or II operation may find their clinical problem much worse after surgery than before. Several well-defined post-gastrectomy syndromes have been described. In addition, surgical attempts to correct some post-gastrectomy syndromes, such as post-vagotomy diarrhea or alkaline gastritis/esophagitis, with loop reversals or a Roux-en-Y anastomosis, respectively, may induce clinical problems that are at least as debilitating as those the patient had before the 'corrective' surgery.

It has to be recognized that, by correcting intractable ulcer disease with surgery, more difficult and iatrogenic problems may be subsequently induced. Less extensive operative procedures, such as selective vagotomy, preserving the vagal fibres to the antrum and small intestine, should be considered in patients who need surgery. This is especially important for young women of childbearing age, who seem most vulnerable to these types of post-gastrectomy problems.

Roux-en-Y syndrome

The Roux-en-Y procedure for bile reflux gastritis or esophagitis or both has been used to reverse the unwanted complications of bile reflux after truncal vagotomy and drainage procedure (pyloroplasty, gastroduodenostomy or gastrojejunostomy). The reversal of the bile salt-induced disease is often replaced in time by a different syndrome consisting of a constellation of symptoms that include chronic nausea, vomiting and abdominal pain aggravated by eating.[16] The medical therapy for this disorder is both challenging and frustrating (*Table 4*). Nutritional balance and pain control are the major problems. Radiolabelled meals have demonstrated extreme delay in emptying of both solids and liquids. The Roux limb often fails to convert to a fed state, and high-amplitude contractions of more than 200 mmHg occur below the end-to-side jejunal anastomosis. The key issue is not to perform the Roux-en-Y but to avoid having to do the procedure because of the initial truncal vagotomy.

Conclusion

The so-called 'functional' diseases such as those described here are emerging as organic diseases of the gastrointestinal tract involving alterations of both the muscle of the intestinal wall and the nerves of the myenteric plexus. The challenge lies ahead in discovering which specific neurotransmitters are deficient, or perhaps are interacting in a nonphysiologic way because of the altered function of nerve or muscle. The first step is to recognize that these clinical symptom complexes, heretofore called functional, do indeed have an organic basis. Future research will improve understanding of the basic mechanism, or mechanisms, causing these symptoms and should lead to the development of pharmacologic substances that can be applied effectively because they are based on specific pathophysiology. Understanding the diseases that are now grouped under this classification will expand with better understanding of the physiology and with improved technology. One fact, however, is incontrovertible: the diseases that constitute what are now conceptually thought of as functional diseases are perhaps the most important, difficult and common of all the problems that gastroenterologists encounter.

Acknowledgements
The author wishes to thank Alice Cullu and Mary Clench for their editorial assistance.

References
1 Way LW. Abdominal pain and the acute abdomen. In: Sleisenger MH, Fordtran JS eds, *Gastrointestinal Disease*. Philadelphia: WB Saunders 1978; 394.
2 Edwards FC, Coghill NF. Clinical manifestations in patients with chronic atrophic gastritis, gastric ulcer and duodenal ulcer. *Q J Med* 1968; **37**: 337.
3 Ingram PW, Evans G. Right iliac fossa pain in young women. *Br Med J* 1965; **2**: 149–51.
4 Martin JL, Beck WJ, McDonald AP, Carlson GM, Mathias JR. ^{99m}Tc-labeled solid-phase meal: a quantitative clinical measurement of human gastric emptying. *J Clin Gastroenterol* 1983; **5**: 315–9.
5 Hunt JN, Pathak JD. The osmotic effects of some simple molecules and ions on gastric emptying. *J Physiol (Lond)* 1960; **154**: 254–69.
6 Hunt JN, Spurrell WR. The pattern of emptying of the human stomach. *J Physiol (Lond)* 1951; **113**: 157–68.
7 Hunt JN, Knox MT. The slowing of gastric emptying by four strong acids and three weak acids. *J Physiol (Lond)* 1972; **22**: 187.
8 Hunt JN, Knox MT. A relationship between the chain length of fatty acids and the slowing of gastric emptying. *J Physiol (Lond)* 1968; **194**: 327–36.
9 Minami H, McCallum RW. The physiology and pathophysiology of gastric emptying in humans. *Gastroenterology* 1984; **86**: 1592.

10 Stephens JR, Woolson RF, Cooke AR. Effects of essential and nonessential amino acids on gastric emptying in the dog. *Gastroenterology* 1975; **69**: 920-7.

11 Mathias JR, Sninsky CA, Millar HD, Clench MH, Davis RH. Development of an improved multi-pressure-sensor probe for recording muscle contraction in human intestine. *Dig Dis Sci* 1985; **30**: 119-23.

12 Szurszewski JH. A migrating electric complex of the canine small intestine. *Am J Physiol* 1969; **217**: 1757-63.

13 Vantrappen G, Janssens J, Hellemans J, Choos Y. The interdigestive motor complex of normal subjects and patients with bacterial overgrowth of the small intestine. *J Clin Invest* 1977; **59**: 1158-66.

14 Sninsky CA, Cottrell CR, Martin JL, Fernandez A, Mathias JR. Gastroduodenal dysfunction by small intestinal recording probe in patients with unexplained abdominal pain, nausea and vomiting. *Gastroenterology* 1982; **82**: 1183 (abstr).

15 Code CF, Marlett JA. The interdigestive myoelectric complex of the stomach and small bowel of dogs. *J Physiol (Lond)* 1975; **246**: 289-309.

16 Mathias JR, Fernandez A, Sninsky CA, Clench MH, Davis RH. Nausea, vomiting and abdominal pain after Roux-en-Y anastomosis: motility of the jejunal limb. *Gastroenterology* 1985; **88**: 101-7.

17 Malagelada JR, Stanghellini V. Manometric evaluation of functional upper gut symptoms. *Gastroenterology* 1985; **88**: 1223-31.

18 Summers RW, Anuras S, Green J. Jejunal manometry patterns in health, partial intestinal obstruction and pseudo-obstruction. *Gastroenterology* 1985; **88**: 1290.

19 You CH, Chey WY, Lee KY. Gastric and small intestinal myoelectric dysrhythmia associated with chronic intractable nausea and vomiting. *Ann Intern Med* 1981; **95**: 449.

20 Telander RL, Morgan KG, Kreulen DL *et al.* Human gastric atony with tachygastria and gastric retention. *Gastroenterology* 1978; **75**: 497-501.

21 Stern RM, Koch KL, Stewart WR, Linblad I. Spectral analysis of tachygastria recorded during motion sickness. *Gastroenterology* 1987; **92**: 92-7.

22 Stern RM, Koch KL. *Electrogastrography: Methodology, Validation and Applications.* New York: Praeger Publishers 1985.

23 Davis RH, Sninsky CA, Clench MH, Mathias JR. Effects of domperidone on gastroduodenal motor activity in patients with gastroduodenal dysfunction. *Gastroenterology* 1984; **86**: 1058 (abstr).

24 Camilleri M, Malagelada J-R. GI motility disturbances in patients with orthostatic hypotension. *Gastroenterology* 1985; **88**: 1852-9.

25 Sninsky CA, Martin JL, Mathias JR. Effect of lidamidine hydrochloride, a proposed alpha$_2$-adrenergic agonist, in patients with gastroduodenal motor dysfunction. *Gastroenterology* 1983; **84**: 1315 (abstr).

26 Anuras S, Christensen J. Recurrent or chronic intestinal pseudo-obstruction. *Clin Gastroenterol* 1981; **10**: 177.

27 Ogilvie H. Large intestine colic due to sympathetic deprivation. A new clinical syndrome. *Br Med J* 1948; **ii**: 671-73.

28 Dudley HAF, Sinclair ISR, McLaren IF *et al.* Intestinal pseudo-obstruction. *J R Coll Surg Edin* 1958; **3**: 206.

29 Falk DL, Anuras S, Christensen J. Chronic intestinal pseudo-obstruction. *Gastroenterology* 1978; **74**: 922.

30 Maldonado JE, Gregg JA, Green PA, Brown AL Jr. Chronic idiopathic intestinal pseudo-obstruction. *Am J Med* 1970; **49**: 203-12.

31 Sarna SK, Daniel EE, Waterfall WE *et al.* Postoperative gastrointestinal electrical and mechanical activities in a patient with idiopathic intestinal pseudo-obstruction. *Gastroenterology* 1978; **74**: 112-20.

32 Schuffler MD, Pope CE. Studies of idiopathic intestinal pseudo-obstruction II. Hereditary hollow visceral myopathy: family studies. *Gastroenterology* 1977; **73**: 339-44.

33 Schuffler MD, Jonak Z. Chronic idiopathic pseudo-obstruction caused by a degenerative disorder of the myenteric plexus: the use of Smith's method to define the neuropathy. *Gastroenterology* 1982; **82**: 476-86.

34 Falk DL, Anuras S, Gardner GD *et al.* A familial visceral myopathy. *Ann Intern Med* 1978; **89**: 600-6.

35 Jacobs E, Ardichvili D, Perissino A *et al.* A case of familial visceral myopathy with atrophy and fibrosis of the longitudinal muscle layer of the entire small bowel. *Gastroenterology* 1979; **77**: 745–50.

36 Smout AJPN, DeWilde K, Kooyman CD, Ten Thije OJ. Chronic idiopathic intestinal pseudo-obstruction, coexistence of smooth muscle and neuronal abnormalities. *Dig Dis Sci* 1985; **30**: 282–7.

37 Law DH, Ten Eyck EA. Familial megaduodenum and megacystitis. *Am J Med* 1962; **33**: 911.

38 Krishnamurthy S, Schuffler MD, Rohrmann CA, Pope CE. Severe idiopathic constipation is associated with a distinctive abnormality of the colonic myenteric plexus. *Gastroenterology* 1985; **88**: 26–34.

39 Sninsky CA, Davis RH, Clench MH, Howard RJ, Schuffler MD, Jonak Z, Mathias JR. Severe idiopathic intestinal constipation: comparison of histology and gastrointestinal tracing in human subjects. *Gastroenterology* 1984; **86**: 1259 (abstr).

40 Gershon MD, Erde SM. The nervous system of the gut. *Gastroenterology* 1981; **80**: 1571–94.

41 Schuffler MD, Baird HW, Fleming CR *et al.* Intestinal pseudo-obstruction as the presenting manifestation of small cell carcinoma of the lung: a paraneoplastic neuropathy of the gastrointestinal tract. *Ann Intern Med* 1983; **98**: 129–34.

Surgical treatment of gastric and small intestinal motility disorders

K A Kelly

Functional motor disturbances of the stomach and small intestine are characterized by the absence of any mechanical lesions of the gastrointestinal tract to account for these disorders. For the most part, the lumen is open and unobstructed but the stomach and small intestine either do not propel content forward at a sufficiently fast rate or else they propel content forward too rapidly. The stasis or the rapid transit results in symptoms that ultimately require treatment.

Gastric atony

General principles

Symptoms: disorders of gastric atony produce a feeling of pain and fullness in the upper abdomen with bloating, flatulence and eructation. The patient may feel nauseated and also may vomit food and sometimes bile. Vomiting of food ingested over 24 hours before is a strong indication of prolonged gastric stasis. Because of their inability to eat, patients feel poorly, have a loss of appetite and develop malnutrition and weight loss. The lack of passage of content from the stomach into the small intestine leads to constipation.

Diagnosis: the condition can often be diagnosed on the basis of the history and the physical findings of the dilated stomach in the left upper quadrant of the abdomen. A large gastric chamber can be suspected by percussion, and a succussion splash can be elicited on shaking the patient.

Nasogastric aspiration of a gastric residua greater than 100 mL 8 hours after a meal is suggestive of slow gastric emptying, as is the aspiration of food particles or debris that have been ingested more than 8 hours before the test. Gastroscopy will also show the large gastric residua, the retained food and bezoars should they be present. Radiology will confirm the presence of residual fluid, retained food and bezoars, and show the dilatation of the stomach that usually ensues in conditions of gastric atony. In addition, the contrast media will empty slowly from the stomach. The quantitation of rate of emptying using contrast media is difficult but a qualitative assessment is usually possible. The radiologist will usually be able to state that gastric emptying is slower than for control, healthy patients.

The quantitation of the rate of gastric emptying is best accomplished using isotopic techniques. Liquids, such as water, can be labelled with ^{111}In-DTPA and solids can be labelled with ^{99m}Tc attached to proteins, such as those present in egg white or liver. After ingestion, the rate of disappearance of these substances from the stomach can then be quantitated using external scintigraphic counting techniques. The rate of disappearance of the radioactive markers is plotted against time. Data obtained from patients can be compared to data from healthy individuals and gastric stasis confirmed.

In addition, special diagnostic techniques are sometimes of use in states of gastric atony. The electrical pattern of the tunica muscularis of the stomach can be documented using cutaneous or intragastric electrodes to monitor the pacesetter potentials generated by the gastric wall. The pacesetter potentials normally are generated by the gastric pacemaker which is located in the mid-gastric corpus along the greater curvature.[1] The pacemaker generates an electrical signal, called the pacesetter potential or slow wave, which propagates from its site of origin in a distal or caudad direction to the pylorus at a frequency of about 3 cycles/minute. The velocity of propagation increases as the cycles move from the pacemaker toward the pylorus. The cycles phase the onset of action potentials and hence of contractions in the gastric smooth muscle. Deviations from this pattern, such as tachygastria (more frequent pacesetter potentials) or bradygastria (less frequent pacesetter potentials) are sometimes associated with gastric atony.

The pattern of gastric contractions can also be documented using open-tipped, perfused, pressure-sensitive catheters or small balloons passed into the distal stomach. These catheters or balloons will usually show contractions of lesser frequency and amplitude than those present in healthy individuals and, when there is a disturbance in the pacemaker rhythms, they may show abnormal rhythmic sequences as well.

Acute postoperative gastric atony

Cause: the most common functional motor disorder of the stomach is acute postoperative ileus. Most authorities believe that this condition is caused by the release of excessive quantities of adrenaline and noradrenaline brought about by the operation.[2] The excess catecholamines, in turn, inhibit the contractile activity of the stomach and the intestinal tract. The stomach and intestine dilate, secretions and gas collect within their lumens, and forward propulsion is greatly slowed. The condition results in anorexia, nausea, distension and vomiting. There is a failure to pass flatus or stool and a general feeling of ill health. No specific tests are usually required to achieve a diagnosis as it is seen to some degree after every operation and is obvious to both patient and physician.

Treatment: the usual treatment is to give nil *per os*, place the patient on intravenous nutrition, aspirate the gastrointestinal content with a nasogastric tube and wait for spontaneous resolution.

The condition is usually self-limiting. The small intestine resolves its postoperative ileus within 24–36 hours, while the stomach takes somewhat longer to resolve, usually about 2–3 days. No specific treatment is usually necessary because of the spontaneous resolution of the condition. In particular, surgery is not indicated because it is the operation itself which has led to the problem.

When the condition is more severe than usual, oxygen inhalation will sometimes cause an exchange of oxygen for nitrogen in the bowel lumen if the partial pressure of oxygen in the bloodstream can be increased sufficiently. With the diffusion of nitrogen from the gut lumen into the blood, the oxygen left in the lumen will then be metabolized. The net result will be a decrease in the amount of gas within the intestinal lumen. Other treatments include blockade of the sympathetic discharge using spinal anesthesia, regional blockade with local anesthetics or generalized ether anesthesia. There may also be a role for pharmacotherapy with sympathetic beta-blockers, such as propranolol. However, no controlled clinical trials of modern beta-blocker therapy have thus far been reported.

Prolonged postoperative gastric atony

Cause: occasionally, and especially after gastric operations performed upon older individuals who have had a long-standing obstruction of the stomach, a state of prolonged postoperative gastric atony ensues after corrective gastric surgery. This usually occurs in an older person with an obstructing duodenal ulcer or gastric outlet obstruction secondary to a peptic ulcer and massive gastric dilatation. The obstruction and the ulcer are treated by vagotomy and drainage procedure or gastrectomy. Following the operation, the patient develops a prolonged postoperative gastric atony which may last for 2–3 weeks or even longer.

The cause of this condition is thought to be similar to that of acute postoperative ileus, but the stomach that has been obstructed seems to be unusually sensitive to the condition. The condition becomes persistent and does not readily resolve.

Treatment: gastroscopy should be performed to ensure that the gastric anastomosis, the gastroenterostomy or the pyloroplasty is patent. Almost always, the gastroscope can be passed from the stomach through the stoma into the small intestine, demonstrating that there is no clear-cut mechanical obstruction.

The treatment for the condition is similar to that for cases of acute postoperative ileus — nil *per os*, nasogastric aspiration and intravenous fluid therapy. The patient is encouraged to ambulate. After a week or so, intermittent clamping of the nasogastric tube can be attempted or the tube can be removed and passed in the morning and in the evening to aspirate the gastric content. Also, trials of food by mouth can be given, although they usually are not tolerated.

Medical therapy with metoclopramide, urecholine or both may be attempted. Metoclopramide should be given intravenously, 10 mg every 2–4 hours, and urecholine subcutaneously, 10 mg, again every 2–4 hours. An increase in the rate of gastric emptying may or may not result following such therapy.

Reoperation should be avoided if at all possible. A period up to 4–6 weeks of intravenous therapy should be pursued. However, if at the end of this time gastric emptying has not resumed, reoperation may be required. At the reoperation, a distal hemigastrectomy and a gastrojejunostomy should be performed. The end of the gastric remnant should be anastomosed to the side of the jejunum in the antecolic position with an isoperistaltic orientation (*Table 1*).

Primary gastric atony

Cause: primary gastric atony is rare and most often seen in young or middle-aged women. The condition is characterized by a gastric stasis with resulting gastric distension, bloating, pain, nausea and vomiting of ingested food. Weight loss ensues because of the inability to eat. Constipation is often seen because of the failure of food to pass through the small intestine into the colon.

The cause of this condition is unknown. Studies of the electrical and motor activity of the stomach have sometimes shown a disorganized pattern of gastric electrical pacesetter potentials. In tachygastrias or gastric dysrhythmias, the pattern of the pacesetter potentials is not regular and rhythmic. Ectopic pacemakers may appear at various sites in the distal gastric tunica muscularis where they generate gastric pacesetter potentials that have either slow or rapid frequencies.

Condition	Operation
Gastric atony	
• Acute postoperative	• None
• Prolonged postoperative	• Billroth gastrectomy
• Chronic, primary or secondary	• Roux gastrectomy
• Roux-stasis syndrome	• Near-total, Roux gastrectomy
Rapid gastric emptying	Roux gastrectomy
Reflux alkaline gastritis	Roux gastrectomy
Small intestinal stasis	None
Small intestinal rapid transit	Reversed intestinal segment

Table 1   Surgical treatment of gastrointestinal functional motor disorders.

Treatment: no medical treatment has yet been devised for this condition. In some instances, the ectopic pacemakers can be resected by a near-total gastrectomy, and gastrointestinal continuity restored, either with an end-to-side gastrojejunostomy or a Roux gastrojejunostomy, sewing the end of the stomach to the side of the proximal end of a Roux limb.[3] The resection of the ectopic pacemakers allows the stomach to empty more expeditiously and the patient can subsequently eat.

Secondary gastric atony

Cause: gastric atony can be secondary to previous gastric operations, such as truncal vagotomy, or to medical conditions such as diabetes mellitus. The signs and symptoms of secondary gastric atony are similar to those of primary gastric atony and the diagnosis is usually obvious from the history of operation or the presence of diabetes mellitus.

Treatment: the condition is usually poorly responsive to dietary or medical therapy and surgery may be necessary. The operation recommended is an extensive hemigastrectomy or a near-total gastrectomy with a Roux-en-Y gastrojejunostomy. The Roux operation will usually speed up the slow gastric emptying and allow the patient to resume eating satisfactorily. The Roux procedure also prevents reflux of small intestinal content into the stomach. Should small intestinal content reach the stomach, alkaline reflux gastritis and its attendant symptoms may result, especially when gastric stasis is present.

The Roux limb should be constructed from the proximal jejunum and made approximately 40 cm in length. The proximal end of the Roux limb is closed and the distal cut end of the gastric remnant sewn to the side of the proximal end of the Roux limb in an end-to-side manner. This allows an anastomosis that has a diameter of about 4 cm. The jejunojejunostomy, made to restore intestinal continuity, is fashioned at a site 40 cm distal to the gastrojejunostomy.[3] A feeding jejunostomy should usually be placed at the time of the Roux gastrectomy to facilitate feeding in the postoperative period and to obviate a period of prolonged parenteral nutrition while the gastric anastomosis heals.

Roux-stasis syndrome

Cause: some patients with a Roux-en-Y gastrojejunostomy will develop upper gastrointestinal stasis following this operation. The incidence of the Roux-stasis syndrome in a series of patients who have had the Roux operation at the Mayo Clinic is about 25–30%.[4]

It is not clear whether the stasis results from a failure of gastric content to empty from the stomach into the Roux limb or whether there is a component of stasis within the limb itself. It seems likely that both stasis in the gastric remnant and stasis in the Roux limb can contribute to this condition. In a review of over 200 patients, the syndrome was more common in individuals who had gastrojejunostomy Roux-en-Y than in those who had esophagojejunostomy Roux-en-Y.[4] Also, diversion of chyme to the exterior from a cannula placed at the distal end of a canine Roux loop markedly increased the speed of emptying from the stomach and the loop, showing that rapid transit through a Roux loop is possible. These data point to the stomach, rather than the Roux limb itself, as a cause of stasis. On the other hand, the Roux-stasis syndrome can occur in individuals with esophagojejunostomy. Also, ectopic pacemakers can appear in Roux limbs that drive the limbs in a reverse or orad direction.[5] Mathias and colleagues have shown abnormal motor patterns in Roux limbs in patients with stasis.[6] Thus, both the gastric remnant and the Roux limb itself seem likely to contribute to the condition.

The symptoms and diagnosis of the condition are similar to those produced by other causes of gastric atony.

Treatment: the treatment for the Roux-stasis syndrome usually has two components. The first is a resection of most of the remaining gastric remnant, resulting in a near-total gastrectomy. Only 1–2 cm of proximal stomach are left, the remainder being resected. The near-total gastrectomy is followed by a reconstruction of gastrointestinal continuity, again using the Roux technique. The small gastric stump is sewn end-to-side to the proximal end of the Roux loop. The second feature is to adjust the length of the Roux limb so that it is no greater than 40 cm in length. If the Roux limb is longer than 40 cm, it should be shortened. Long Roux limbs predispose to stasis.[4]

Rapid gastric emptying

General principles

Symptoms: conditions of rapid gastric emptying usually result in both gastrointestinal and cardiovascular symptoms. The condition is called the 'dumping syndrome'. When chyme is passed prematurely into the small intestine, it distends the small intestine, stimulates peristalsis, causes borborygmi and results in rapid transit and explosive diarrhea. Digestion and absorption are impaired and weight loss ensues.

If the food is hypertonic, upon entering the small intestine it causes fluid to pass from the bloodstream into the enteric lumen, resulting in hypovolemia, tachycardia and a decrease in the blood pressure. These cardiovascular changes in turn produce systemic symptoms such as weakness, faintness, sweatiness and the need to lie down. Thus, both enteric and cardiovascular symptoms result from rapid gastric emptying.

Diagnosis: rapid emptying can be readily diagnosed using scintigraphic tests. In this situation, rapid gastric emptying is found rather than the slower gastric emptying in gastric atony.

In addition, the entry of the chyme prematurely into the small intestine may result in the release of excessive amounts of gastrointestinal hormones, such as gastrointestinal polypeptide, neurotensin, enteroglucagon and peptide PYY.[7] The resulting hyperglycemia also causes release of an excessive amount of insulin. Appearance of these abnormal concentrations of hormones in the bloodstream can be documented by measuring their concentration in the plasma in the post-prandial period after a suitable test meal. Whether these hormonal changes account for some of the symptomatology of the rapid gastric emptying state, or are merely secondary to the rapid gastric emptying, is not clear at this time.

The dumping syndrome is almost always accompanied by rapid gastric emptying, but rapid emptying may be present without causing the dumping syndrome.

Primary rapid gastric emptying

There is no clearly described state of primary rapid gastric emptying. Rapid gastric emptying does sometimes accompany other disorders, such as peptic ulcer, but there are no clear-cut reports of rapid gastric emptying, primary or idiopathic in origin.

Rapid emptying secondary to gastric operations

Cause: rapid emptying of liquids is frequently seen following gastric surgery. Truncal vagotomy results in rapid gastric emptying because the vagal inhibitory innervation to the stomach is divided. This inhibitory innervation is responsible for receptive relaxation of the stomach with swallowing and gastric accommodation and gastric distension. The lack of receptive relaxation and accommodation after vagotomy results in an increase in intragastric pressure with eating which magnifies the gradient in pressure between the stomach and small intestine and results in the rapid emptying, especially of liquids.

When gastrectomy, pyloroplasty or gastroenterostomy accompany the vagotomy, the rapid emptying is magnified because the resistance to outflow from the stomach to the small intestine is decreased by the so-called 'drainage' operations. Thus, the combination of poor receptive relaxation and accommodation and a decrease in gastric outlet resistance results in rapid emptying of both liquids and solids.

Treatment: the rate of emptying can be decreased by several operative techniques. When patients have a pyloroplasty or a gastroenterostomy, the pyloroplasty can be taken down and the pylorus reconstructed or the gastroenterostomy can be taken down and the defects in the stomach and small intestine closed. The procedures will increase resistance to outflow of chyme and slow the rate of gastric emptying, thus combatting the symptoms produced from the rapid emptying. The danger is that the rate of emptying after the reconstruction will be so slow that symptoms of gastric stasis will then ensue.[8]

An alternative approach is to convert to a Roux gastrectomy. The rate of emptying from the gastric remnant into a Roux limb is approximately the same as that from the stomach into the small intestine in healthy individuals. Thus, the symptoms of rapid emptying will usually abate after conversion to a Roux gastrectomy.

Reflux alkaline gastritis

General principles

Symptoms: the reflux of small intestinal contents into the stomach produces pain, nausea and vomiting, especially of bilious content. There may also be traces of blood in the gastric vomitus as well as in the stool. The condition can be suspected endoscopically by the appearance of small intestinal content within the gastric lumen and the secondary changes of hyperemia and ulceration, together with biopsy evidence of mucosal inflammation. The correlation of the histologic and endoscopic features with the severity of the symptoms, however, is poor. The histologic features and endoscopic features do not necessarily indicate that, for example, surgery should be performed.

Diagnosis: the rate of and quantity of reflux can also be documented scintigraphically by using the HIDA technique and looking for the appearance of the radioactively-tagged bile within the gastric lumen. The type of bile acids present in the gastric juice, their concentration and the rate of their appearance have been used to substantiate the diagnosis and provide criteria for surgery.[9] However, the type of bile acids and their rate of appearance in the gastric lumen have not clearly been correlated with symptoms or necessarily with response to the therapy.[10]

Primary reflux alkaline gastritis

Cause: primary reflux alkaline gastritis can occur in individuals who have not undergone gastric surgery or have suffered from gastrointestinal disease. In these individuals, content from the small intestine spontaneously refluxes from the duodenum through the pylorus and into the stomach. The reflux is associated with abdominal pain, nausea and vomiting of food, especially bile. Gastroscopy often shows an inflamed gastric mucosa which is most severe in the distal stomach. The mucosa is friable and easily bleeds and may contain tiny ulcerations. Biopsies may or may not show chronic gastritis.

Treatment: the condition is best treated by resection of the antrum, closure of the proximal duodenum and reconstruction of gastrointestinal continuity using the Roux-en-Y gastrojejunostomy. The length of the Roux limb should be made approximately 40 cm. The end of the gastric remnant should be anastomosed to the side of the proximal portion of the Roux limb, with the Roux limb in the ante-colic position.

Postoperative reflux alkaline gastritis

Cause: alkaline gastritis is much more common following gastric operations that destroy, bypass or resect the gastroduodenal junction. Operations such as pyloroplasty, gastroenterostomy and antrectomy all allow small intestinal content to reflux back into the stomach and bring about the changes in the gastric mucosa and produce the gastric symptoms.

Treatment: Roux gastrojejunostomy should be employed.[8] The operation will prevent the reflux of small intestinal content, especially bile and pancreatic juice, from reaching the gastric remnant. Marked improvement in symptoms should be seen in about 70% of cases.

Small intestinal stasis

General principles

Symptoms: the symptoms produced by small intestinal stasis are abdominal pain, distension, cramping, borborygmi and often constipation which sometimes alternates with diarrhea. The slow passage through the small intestine leads to poor appetite. When food is eaten, nausea and often vomiting of both food and small intestinal contents occur.

Diagnosis: radiography will reveal a pattern of dilated small intestine. The diagnosis is supported by the use of contrast media, which outlines the dilated distended gut and moves slowly through it.

The rate of transit through the small intestine is best quantitated using radioactive markers tagged to liquids or solids. The markers can either be given into the stomach or perhaps preferentially into the small intestine distal to the pylorus. The rate of marker transit through the small intestine from the duodenum to the cecum can then be assessed accurately using external scintigraphy. If both liquids and solids are tagged, the rate of progression of each substance through the small intestine can be quantitated. Usually, however, both liquids and solids move through the small intestine at a similar rate.

The electrical patterns of the small intestine can also be assessed using electrodes, either applied intraluminally or during the operation. The electrodes allow assessment of the pattern of the pacesetter potentials and check for increases or decreases of frequency or alterations in rhythm. The pattern of contractions, both during fasting and with feeding, can also be assessed using open-tipped catheters or small balloons. The fasting pattern of migrating motor complexes beginning in the duodenum and progressing slowly distally from the duodenum to the ileum over a 2-hour period can be documented and the disturbance in the fasting patterns assessed. Also, the suppression of the fasting pattern with feeding and the emergence of the intermittent contractile pattern characteristic of the fed state can be documented. Both of these patterns may be changed in states of small intestinal stasis.

Specific disorders of stasis

Cause: stasis in the small intestine may be primary and idiopathic or secondary to systemic diseases, such as amyloidosis, scleroderma, lymphoma and other conditions. The net result is a failure of transit of content through the small intestine with resulting stasis, collection of food, secretions and gas within the lumen and dilatation of the bowel. Because they are unable to eat, the patients lose weight.

Treatment: an operation is often necessary to rule out a mechanical lesion or an inciting cause. At the time of the operation, the entire gastrointestinal tract should be carefully inspected to rule out a mechanical cause of the stasis. A biopsy should be made from a dilated segment of intestine when one is present. If none is present, a wedge biopsy from the proximal jejunum should be obtained. The biopsy should be generous in size and full-thickness in depth. A feeding jejunostomy should also be done, first, to allow decompression of the small intestine should the postoperative ileus be prolonged and, secondly, to allow a trial of the instillation of nutrients directly into the small intestine in the postoperative period.

Resections of segments of small intestine can also be considered, but they are usually not indicated. The disease is frequently a generalized disorder; resection of one portion of the small intestine will not solve the problem in other portions. Extensive enterectomies have been recommended for this condition to decrease the symptoms produced by the dilated and incompetent bowel. However, the use of extensive enteric resections has not received a careful clinical trial.

Two other techniques can be considered, but both are highly experimental. The first is the use of electrical pacing to drive the pacesetter potentials of the small intestine and hence to drive the contractions.[11] There is no clear-cut evidence, however, that pacing will have a beneficial role in these disorders. The inability of the muscle to respond to endogenous neurohormonal stimuli indicates that it will not respond to exogenous electrical stimuli. A second experimental approach with possible application in the future is the use of intestinal transplantation. Autographs of small intestine will function satisfactorily in terms of digestion and absorption of foodstuffs and the maintenance of a reasonably healthy life.[12] However, the problems of rejection of a homograft and the graft vs. host interaction have not been satisfactorily resolved as yet to allow a recommendation of transplantation for individuals with these disorders. At present, it is safer to treat individuals with intestinal stasis syndromes with total parenteral nutrition.

Small intestinal rapid transit

General principles

Symptoms: rapid transit through the small intestine results in poor digestion and absorption of foodstuffs with resultant diarrhea and weight loss. The early appearance of small intestinal content in the large intestine may overwhelm the ability of the large intestine to absorb water and electrolytes and result in the production of excessive amounts of short chain fatty acids from the malabsorbed carbohydrates. Both of these conditions can lead to diarrhea, which is often explosive and watery.

Diagnosis: scintigraphic and manometric studies are useful aids to the diagnosis of rapid transit. Large amplitude contractions may appear which propagate rapidly through the small intestine, the so-called propulsive propagating contractions. These are normally found only in the distal ileum, but in states of rapid transit they may appear at more proximal sites where they sweep content more rapidly through the small intestine. The electrical counterpoints of the states of rapid transit have not, as yet, been clearly documented.

Specific disorders of rapid transit

Cause: states of small intestinal rapid transit are usually primary or idiopathic in origin or secondary to rapid emptying from the stomach, usually after gastric operations. Vagotomy and extensive gastrectomy, usually in patients with peptic ulcer disease, are likely causes of rapid transit. It is curious, however, that individuals undergoing total gastrectomy, where food enters directly into the small intestine after it passes through the esophagus, are sometimes not greatly troubled by rapid transit and diarrhea. In fact, in one series of patients, the mean transit from the esophagus to the large intestine in patients with total gastrectomy was similar to the mean transit found in healthy controls.

Treatment: surgery to reverse a 10 cm segment of small intestine from its usual oral-aboral orientation to an aboral-oral orientation[13] is the usual course of treatment. The segment should be positioned at a site about 100 cm distal to the stomach or the gastrointestinal or esophageal-intestinal anastomosis. The reversed segment will slow transit through the bowel proximal to its location and, hence, will ameliorate the diarrhea. The segment should not be made longer or shorter than 10 cm. A longer segment will produce intestinal obstruction. Shorter segments have little effect.

An experimental approach to treating states of rapid small intestinal transit has been electrical pacing. In this approach, the pacesetter potentials of the small intestine are driven in a backwards or oral direction by the pacing in an attempt to reverse the pattern of contractions in the small intestine and hence slow the transit.[15-17] This approach has worked satisfactorily in dogs but has not yet been tried in man. While it is possible to pace the small intestine in man with electrical stimuli, the pacesetter potentials of the human small intestine appear to be more resistant to pacing than those of the dog.

References
1 Hinder RA, Kelly KA. Human gastric pacesetter potential: site of origin, spread and response to gastric transection and proximal gastric vagotomy. *Am J Surg* 1977; **133**: 29–33.
2 Smith J, Kelly KA, Weinshilboum RM. Pathophysiology of postoperative ileus. *Arch Surg* 1977; **112**: 203–9.
3 Telander RL, Morgan KG, Kreulen DL, Schmalz PF, Kelly KA, Szurszewski JH. Human gastric atony with tachygastria and gastric retention. *Gastroenterology* 1978; **75**: 497–501.
4 Gustavsson G, Ilstrup DM, Morrison P, Kelly KA. The Roux-stasis syndrome after gastrectomy. *Am J Surg* (In press).
5 Morrison P, Kelly KA, Hocking M. Electrical dysrhythmias in the Roux-en-Y jejunal limb and their correction by pacing. *Gastroenterology* 1985; **88**: 1508.
6 Mathias JR, Fernandez A, Sninsky CA, Clench MH, Davis RH. Nausea, vomiting and abdominal pain after Roux-en-Y anastomosis: motility of the jejunal limb. *Gastroenterology* 1985; **88**: 101–7.
7 Cranley B, Kelly KA, Go VLW, McNichols LA. Enhancing the anti-dumping effect of Roux gastrojejunostomy with intestinal pacing. *Ann Surg* 1983; **198**: 516–24.
8 Kelly KA, Becker JM, van Heerden JA. Reconstructive gastric surgery. *Br J Surg* 1981; **68**: 687–91.
9 Ritchie WP Jr. Alkaline reflux gastritis: an objective assessment of its diagnosis and treatment. *Ann Surg* 1980; **192**: 288–98.
10 Boren CH, Way LH. Alkaline reflux gastritis: a re-evaluation. *Am J Surg* 1980; **140**: 40–6.
11 Richter HM, Kelly KA. Effect of transection and pacing on human jejunal pacesetter potentials. *Gastroenterology* 1986; **91**: 1380–5.
12 Sarr MG, Kelly KA. Myoelectric activity of the autotransplanted canine jejunoileum. *Gastroenterology* 1981; **81**: 303–10.
13 Sawyers JL, Herrington JL Jr, Buckspan GS. Remedial operations for alkaline reflux gastritis and associated postgastrectomy syndromes. *Arch Surg* 1980; **115**: 519–24.
14 Gustavsson S, Kelly KA. Total gastrectomy for benign disease. *Surg Clin N Am* (In press).
15 Gladen HE, Kelly KA. Electrical pacing for short bowel syndrome. *Surg Gynecol Obstet* 1981; **153**: 697–700.
16 O'Connell PR, Kelly KA. Enteric transit and absorption after ileostomy: alteration with jejunal pacing. *Gastroenterology* 1985; **88**: 1521.
17 Hoepfner MT, Kelly KA, Sarr MG. Pacing the canine ileostomy. *Gastroenterology* 1986; **90**: 1462.

A treatment strategy for the irritable bowel

W G Thompson

The irritable bowel syndrome (IBS) may be defined as altered bowel habit and abdominal pain accompanied by gaseousness for which no pathophysiologic or pathologic abnormality can be proven. Distension, relief of pain with defecation, mucus in the stool, rectal dissatisfaction and alternating constipation and diarrhea are frequent accompanying features.[1,2] The commonly accepted explanation for these symptoms is intestinal dysmotility, but despite the sophisticated investigative technology currently available, the exact nature of the dysfunction is unknown. Small bowel motility responses to stressful stimuli are abnormal in IBS patients.[3] A paradoxical increase in motility index in constipation and decrease with diarrhea has been observed.[4] A predominant 3 cycles/minute colonic rhythm is reported in IBS patients.[5,6] These phenomena are of great interest but they are not specific for the IBS and cannot consistently be correlated with IBS symptoms. One reason for this inability to relate physiology to symptoms may be the lack of accurate definition of the IBS.

Since there is no recognizable pathophysiology, there is no diagnostic test and the IBS must be defined by symptoms. There are several different symptom complexes which may represent different dysfunctions. It seems unlikely that disparate syndromes such as spastic constipation, functional diarrhea, nonulcer dyspepsia and the chronic abdomen have a physiologic common denominator.[7] Further, it is unclear whether IBS symptoms result from a normal perception of abnormal gut function rather than an abnormal perception of normal gut function.[8] The reproduction of an IBS patient's pain by balloon distension in the large and small bowel sheds little light on this issue.[9-11] The riddle is succinctly put by Almy: is the IBS "a qualitative or merely quantitative departure from the psycho-physiologic reactions of normal people?".[12] Is diarrhea, like tears, an individual's response to his or her dietary and psychosocial environment?

Before discussing management, one must consider another conundrum. The IBS is very common in Western society.[13] Abnormal bowel habit and abdominal pain occur in a third of apparently healthy adults.[14-20] Less than half of such sufferers see a doctor about their symptoms yet they constitute 17–52% of patients referred to gastroenterologists[1,2,21-25] (Table 1). The reason for the referral to a specialist may be the clue to successful management. Severity of symptoms is unlikely to be the only explanation. Fear of serious disease is undoubtedly important. It seems also that IBS sufferers who do consult physicians are more likely to have an emotional problem or personality disorder than those who do not.[26,27]

Primary care physicians and specialists alike find management of IBS patients to be one of their most demanding tasks. Since the prognosis in terms of life expectancy is good, the cause unknown, the symptoms variable and most treatments unproven, one must take special care to protect the patient from harmful investigations and

Author	Country	Year	Percent functional	Percent that are female
Switz et al [23]	USA	1976	23	—
Ferguson et al [24]	Scotland	1977	31	—
Fielding et al [21]	Ireland	1977	52	66
Manning et al [1]	England	1980	29	—
Sullivan et al [22]	Canada	1983	17	74
Harvey et al [25]	England	1983	48	—
Kruis et al [2]	West Germany	1984	23	—

Table 1 Proportion of gastroenterology referrals that are functional.

therapy. Clearly, an investigation and treatment protocol applied to a benign condition which affects a third of adults must take several factors into consideration. These include the risk of missing serious disease, the cost of tests and drugs, the worries of the patient and the risk of inducing or reinforcing illness behaviour. The following strategy builds on what is known about the IBS and, when science fails, emphasizes the art of medicine.[28] Above all, common sense should prevail. It is not sufficient to tell the IBS patient his or her tests are negative and therefore he or she has no disease. Management is more demanding, for the patient is not imagining his or her symptoms.

The first clinical encounter

When confronted with a patient with IBS, the physician's primary objectives should be:
• to make a positive diagnosis on the basis of accepted criteria while looking for evidence of co-existent organic disease
• to secure the patient's confidence.
These objectives are best achieved by a careful history and physical examination, complete blood count and sigmoidoscopy.

There is ample evidence that a positive diagnosis can be made on the first clinical encounter by careful history alone,[1,2] and that this diagnosis seldom requires revision over time.[29] A physical examination will help exclude organic disease. No signs of the irritable bowel have been agreed upon, although multiple abdominal scars should alert the examining physician's suspicions.[30,31] An abnormal white blood cell count, hemoglobin or erythrocyte sedimentation rate suggests organic disease instead of, or in addition to, the irritable bowel and therefore demands further investigation.

Sigmoidoscopy
Sigmoidoscopy is of marginal benefit in the diagnosis of the IBS. It can reveal local disease such as anal fissures or proctitis. Those secretly abusing anthraquinone

laxatives may have melanosis coli. The spastic colon may demonstrate spasm or scybala and air insufflation may reproduce the patient's pain. However, successful management commences with the first clinical encounter and the most important benefit of sigmoidoscopy may be symbolic. The owner of an irritable bowel has never seen it and may therefore be greatly reassured by one who has. This is analogous to the reassurance of patients with noncardiac chest pain by a negative cardiogram despite its acknowledged diagnostic inefficiency.[32] Since carcinoma of the colon is very common and may co-exist with the irritable bowel, patients over 40 should have an air contrast barium enema even though the symptoms are not those of a carcinoma.

Reassurance

Because only a minority of IBS sufferers report their symptoms to a doctor,[14-20] it is well to establish why the patient has chosen this time to consult. A recent death in the family, fear of cancer, maladaption to stress at home or at work are clues that may be fundamental to management. Reassurance that no serious disease exists, explanation of how the gut muscle might generate symptoms and a sympathetic hearing of emotional conflicts may be the most important services that a physician can render to the IBS patient. It is yet another mystery why in Western countries women are more likely to visit a doctor about their IBS, while in India the opposite is the case.[13] Such a paradox is testimony to the profound effect of culture and environment on the 'illness behaviour' of IBS patients. Whitehead[17] has suggested that this illness behaviour is learned in early life: it should not be needlessly reinforced by an insecure diagnosis and repeated tests.

Those patients with serious mental illness need identification and psychiatric management. Inquiries should be made about drugs that might affect gut function. Excessive use of alcohol, coffee, diet drinks or candies containing sorbitol[33] or fructose[34] may cause diarrhea. In non-Caucasians, lactose intolerance may be important. An irritable bowel may be triggered by an attack of gastroenteritis, often 'traveller's diarrhea'. Post-infection IBS is said to have a better prognosis than the spontaneous syndrome, and reassurance that the offending organism has long since departed may be salutary.

Psychotherapy

Generations of physicians have been indoctrinated in the advantages of supportive psychotherapy. Most agree that it is important to talk to patients, but there is so little time. The therapeutic benefit of doctor/patient communication is difficult to prove, but a report from Sweden lends support to this notion.[36] Compared to controls IBS patients who received eight sessions of "supportive psychotherapy which could be performed in any physician's office" showed greater improvement in IBS and psychological symptoms 3 and 15 months later. It is vital to explore and discuss the patient's hidden agenda. Why has he or she come? Clearly, the stressed, the unloved and the cancerophobic have very special needs.

When taking the patient's history, it is well to subclassify the IBS symptoms as spastic colon, diarrhea, constipation, gas, nonulcer dyspepsia or chronic abdominal pain. Many patients will respond to reassurance and a bulking agent, so drugs have no place initially. Although none have a proven benefit, generally certain drugs may be used to good effect for certain subtypes.

Bran

Although over 90% of gastroenterologists in the USA and Britain recommend bran, the controlled studies extant do not strongly support its efficacy[37-43] (*Table 2*). The main benefit appears to be improvement in constipation, a fact that was established

Author	Year	Number of patients	Agent	Fibre (g)	Study design	Duration (weeks)	Placebo response (%)	Result
Soltoft et al[37]	1976	29	Bran biscuits	14.4	Double-blind	6	65	Nil
Manning et al[38]	1977	13	Bran 20 g/day	7	Single-blind	6	18	Improved pain, bowel habit, mucus
Brodribb*[39]	1977	9	Bran biscuits	6.7	Double-blind	12	NA	Improved symptoms, less pain — especially 3 months
Ornstein et al*[40]	1981	58	Bran biscuits	7	Double-blind crossover	16	NA	Improved constipation, little effect on stool weight
Weinreich*[41]	1982	39	Bran 12 g/day	5	Double-blind crossover	52	56	Improved
Cann et al[42]	1984	38	Bran 20 g/day	9.6	Open	4	NA	Improved constipation
Lucey et al[43]	1987	28	Bran biscuits	12.8	Double-blind crossover	12	71	No change in symptoms or stool-weight
Hodgson*[48]	1977	16	Methylcellulose 1 g/day	—	Blind	12	NA	Nil
Ritchie and Truelove[49]	1979	12	Isbaghula 7 g/day	—	Double-blind	12	NA	Benefit
Ewerth et al*[50]	1980	9	Isbaghula 8 g/day	—	Double-blind crossover	8	NA	Reduced pain and hard stools
Ornstein et al[40]	1981	58	Isbaghula 9 g/day	—	Double-blind crossover	16	NA	Improved constipation, little effect on stool weight
Longstreth et al[51]	1981	26	Psyllium 10.8 g/day	—	Double-blind	8	71	Nil
Prior et al[52]	1986	80	Isbaghula 10.8 g/day	—	Double-blind	12	50	Improved constipation, transit, global response

* Diverticular disease.

Table 2 Placebo-controlled trials using bran and pharmaceutical bulking agents in IBS and symptomatic, uncomplicated diverticular disease.

over 50 years ago.[44] The modern rationale for the use of bran was provided by Cleave and Burkitt.[45,46]

The seven IBS bran studies shown in *Table 2* have used various definitions, doses and durations of treatment.[37-43] Patients with uncomplicated diverticular disease are included since it seems likely that symptoms here are those of a co-existent irritable bowel.[47] These studies may be criticized for their small numbers, faulty study design and imprecise inclusion criteria. In some the dose of bran may have been too small, and in others the treatment period may have been too short (less than 3 months). The most recent study seems to satisfy these criteria yet fails to demonstrate benefit.[43] It should be noted, however, that few subjects were constipated and the bran failed to increase stool weight.[43] There is also the extraordinary 71% placebo response, which provides little room for bran to show a superior effect.[43] Use of artificial bulking agents such as methylcellulose and isbaghula/psyllium have a similar story,[40,47-51] yet a recent report does show some benefit for IBS patients using isbaghula (*Table 2*).[52] An Indian study suggests that the optimum dose of isbaghula/psyllium is 20 g (3 rounded teaspoonsful) per day.[53]

In a practical vein, it is useful to prescribe 1 tablespoonful of bran 3 times a day with meals. Such a regimen can be measured and recorded, so that on the follow-up visit both patient and doctor are clear about compliance. Those unwilling or unable (some are intolerant) to take bran may find psyllium a satisfactory yet expensive substitute. The spastic colon patient, in particular, will notice that the small pellety stools are replaced by ones that are bulky and easily passed. Thus, convinced of benefit, no further cajolling is necessary to convince the patient to work bulk into the diet.

Placebo effect

A great many drugs have been tried in the management of the IBS. Although clinical drug trials usually have many flaws, the one common factor is a very high response to placebo. *Table 3* illustrates a placebo response of 30–60% in several IBS drug trials selected at random.[54-58] The consistency of this high placebo response throws doubt on any studies which report a lower one. No drug has convincingly and repeatedly shown an improvement over placebo in IBS trials and it is probable that none is generally effective. On the basis of one or two successful short-term trials, it is difficult to justify the general use of any systemic agent for the treatment of a benign condition such as IBS which affects so many people over long periods of their lives.

Three important considerations arise from this high short-term therapeutic benefit of placebos in the IBS. First, it demonstrates the known variability of the disease and supports the contention that no drug is justified in the routine treatment of that 10–15% of the population who visit the doctor because of their IBS. Even if efficacy was repeatedly demonstrated, it is necessary to ascertain which symptoms or syndromes are most likely to benefit, weigh the adverse affects of the drug and consider the long-term implications of drug therapy. Many physicians find the deception implied by the use of a deliberate or pure placebo such as a sugar pill repellent.[60] It is said that if a pure placebo is to work, the patient should believe that it will have a pharmacologic effect. Yet clinical trials are effective in spite of informed consent. Further, in neurotic patients a placebo remained effective when the patient knew that the pill he was receiving was inert.[61] It seems that the symbolic giving of pills has therapeutic value. On the other hand, the use of logical or impure placebos (drugs whose action might make sense but whose effects are not due to their pharmacology) risks double deception if both patient and physician accept their efficacy.[62]

Despite such caviats, so-called impure placebos which have a plausible phar-

Author	Year	Drug tested	Placebo response (%)
Lichstein and Mayer[54]	1959	Belladonna	30
Kasich et al[55]	1959	Meprobamate	47
Wayne[56]	1969	Chlordiazepoxide hydrochloride clidinium bromide	38
Page and Dirnberger[57]	1981	Dicyclomine	54
Fielding[58]	1982	Domperidone	57
Kruis et al [59]	1986	Mebeverine	60
Range			30–60

Table 3 The placebo response in IBS.

macologic rationale, yet do no harm, may be useful in certain instances. For example, a drug such as simethicone, whose surfactant activity disperses bubbles without actually dispelling the gas, may exert a placebo effect while passing harmlessly through the gut, inert and unabsorbed.

The third and most important implication of the favourable response to placebos is that it points to the benefits of a successful physician/patient encounter. When a physician explains an illness and makes it more understandable to the patient, when he or she cares and helps the patient feel that something can be done, then a placebo response is more likely.[60] Patients who received postoperative explanation of incisional pain and reassurance that medication was available required less analgesics and had a shorter hospital stay than controls.[63]

Thus, careful consideration of the patient's complaint and those circumstances that led him or her to seek medical attention, reassurance that no serious disease exists, and the use of bran at least for its placebo effect will be of benefit in most patients. Many patients fail to understand what they have been told or to fully comply with therapy. Thus, a follow-up visit to ensure comprehension and compliance is an essential part of management.

The follow-up appointment

A follow-up appointment 6–8 weeks after the initial visit is important to ensure compliance with the instructions regarding diet and precipitating factors, and comprehension of the explanation and reassurance provided on the first visit. If the understanding is not complete, further discussion may be necessary. Continued bulking with bran should be encouraged if successful, and it may now be worked into the diet. If unsuccessful, the substitution of psyllium could be considered. In the unimproved patient, the environmental stresses to which the patient is subjected must be explored again and diagnostic alternatives considered. However, further investigation such as endoscopy, small bowel enema, intravenous pyelography, computerized tomography,

ERCP and ultrasound without specific indication should be avoided. These may have untoward effects. More importantly, such indecision and repeated testing undermines the patient's confidence in the diagnosis. An open mind must be kept about the irritable bowel sufferer since he or she is not immune to organic disease. However, a positive diagnosis may be made with confidence and seldom needs alteration.[29] If no new information surfaces at the second visit no new tests are required.

Although no drug can be recommended for all IBS patients, certain drugs may be useful in some situations. In the patient who has severe, predictable, post-prandial pain, anticholinergic drugs administered before meals may be effective.[64] It is impractical to attempt a 24-hour cholinergic blockade for symptoms that are intermittent and unpredictable.

In patients with the diarrhea-dominant IBS, loperamide seems to be effective.[65] Often those with diarrhea suffer incontinence and the resulting embarrassment may be the most significant disability. Loperamide increases anal sphincter tone, an action which might benefit such patients.[66] Loperamide does not pass the blood-brain barrier and thus lacks some of the undesirable central nervous system effects of other antidiarrheal drugs. Although on principle one should not take such a drug indefinitely it might be used selectively in a patient who anticipates a diarrheal attack at the time of a stressful event.

In the patient with severe abdominal pain who is unresponsive to other measures, amitriptyline may provide a remission. Such patients may not be obviously depressed, and amitriptyline may act by means other than as an antidepressant.

The smooth muscle relaxant effect of oil of peppermint has been demonstrated to be effective in two out of three short-term studies.[67-69] While the drug might be considered to be a harmless placebo, it should be noted that peppermint relaxes the lower esophageal sphincter, thus risking gastroesophageal reflux.[68,70]

In the diarrhea-dominant irritable bowel patient, cholestyramine has shown occasional benefit.[71] It may be that binding of bile salts by this anion exchange resin is sufficient to reverse the diarrhea. Some patients have idiopathic bile salt malabsorption.[72]

The IBS affects patients for long periods of their lives so no drug therapy is acceptable as a long-term solution. This is particularly applicable to psychoactive drugs such as diazepam. Such drugs do not primarily benefit the irritable bowel patient but may be useful in the management of short-term anxiety.

In all phases of management of the irritable bowel, encouragement and reassurance should be continued as the patient's need for these is great. Continuing medical care should be assured for the unimproved patient since such patients are particularly vulnerable to practitioners of alternative medicine, and all the hazards that their practices imply.[73]

Prognosis

The prognosis of the irritable bowel in terms of life expectancy is excellent, but for abolition of symptoms it is not so good. *Table 4* summarizes several studies which indicate that most adults with the irritable bowel are still symptomatic 1-10 years later.[29,35,74-76] In a very small study, half of a group of 34 children continued to have irritable bowel symptoms 30 years later.[75] Thus, there is evidence that the irritable bowel affects most sufferers for long periods of their lives. This reinforces the notion that drugs or diets which might have harmful affects should be avoided. In one study only 4 of 77 patients diagnosed to have the irritable bowel needed a change

Author	Year	Patients	Follow-up (years)	Result
Chaudhary and Truelove[35]	1962	126	1–10	63% still symptomatic
Waller and Misiewicz[74]	1969	50	1	Little change
Christensen and Mortensen[75]	1975	34 children with pain	30	16 (47%) have IBS
Holmes and Salter[29]	1982	77	6	57% symptomatic, 4 had alternative benign diagnoses
Harvey et al [76]	1987	104	5–8	74% had some symptoms, none changed diagnosis

Table 4 Prognosis in IBS.

in diagnosis 6 years later.[29] In another study, none of the patients said to have the IBS required a change in diagnosis 5–8 years later.[76] Thus, the diagnosis is a stable one and may be made with confidence.

There is another important side to the prognosis of the irritable bowel. Not only do such patients undergo much unnecessary investigation and treatment,[28] but they are particularly liable to surgery as well.[30,31,77] The study by Creed illustrates this point.[30] Of 119 patients who underwent appendectomy, a normal appendix was found in 63. Compared to the 56 who had inflamed appendices removed and 62 non-operated controls, those with normal appendices were more likely to have had an important life event within the previous 6 months, to be female, to have psychological symptoms and to be depressed. Furthermore, those who had normal appendices removed were more likely to have continued bowel symptoms 1 year later. The gut impact of the IBS sufferer's psychosocial environment cannot be ignored.

The unsatisfied patient

Few physicians are so successful in treating the IBS that all their patients are satisfied. The anxiety, depression and often hostility demonstrated by some unsatisfied patients challenge the physician's skill. At all stages it is important to continue emotional support and ensure continuity of care.

Many patients are convinced that they are sensitive to certain items in the diet. There is little to substantiate this and food allergy without extra gut symptoms is unusual and difficult to prove. One study at Cambridge, England appears to demonstrate sensitivity (not an allergy) to the products of wheat, poultry, milk and other food stuffs.[78] The Cambridge group have had great success through the use of elimination diets in diarrhea-prominent IBS patients. Unfortunately, these results have not been duplicated elsewhere.[79,80]

Should the doctor/patient relationship deteriorate, there are certain referral options. If the patient is obviously disturbed a psychiatric consultation may be useful. However, most IBS patients neither need nor profit from such referral. There are anecdotal reports of success with biofeedback but few centres have facilities for this.[81,82] One trial demonstrated that hypnosis was effective in resistant cases.[83] This study was not blinded and needs confirmation. During and beyond such referrals the physician should retain control of the patient's care.

It may be useful to refer the unsatisfied patient to a consultant. It is important for the physician to take the initiative here rather than let the patient seek help without guidance. The consultant, preferably in another medical centre, will likely reinforce the diagnosis, endorse the plan of management and return the patient to the original physician's care. His or her credibility thus restored, the first physician may find subsequent management easier.

Conclusions

Despite great technological advances in the study of intestinal function, the exact nature of the dysmotility responsible for the irritable bowel has not been identified, and symptoms have not been correlated with physiologic phenomena. As a result there is no diagnostic test for the irritable bowel and it must be defined by its symptoms. Nevertheless, it is possible to make a positive diagnosis of the irritable bowel with confidence, and this is crucial to successful management. Since most patients with this very common disorder do not see a physician it is necessary to establish on the first visit why the patient has come. This allows the physician to reassure the patient, explain the nature of the symptoms and prescribe an alteration of his or her diet through the use of increased fibre. Bran has at least a strong placebo effect. A follow-up visit is necessary to reinforce the reassurance and explanation. In the unimproved patient, diagnostic alternatives and the judicious use of drugs might be considered. If the patient seems to be losing confidence in his or her physician, a referral may have a salutary effect. The irritable bowel is a long-term disorder and some of its sufferers are liable to inappropriate investigations, treatments and even surgery. Thus, it is important for the physician to maintain control over the patient's care and at all times listen, explain and reassure.

References
1 Manning AP, Thompson WG, Heaton KW *et al.* Towards positive diagnosis of the irritable bowel. *Br Med J* 1978; **ii**: 653–4.
2 Kruis W, Thieme CH, Weinzierl M *et al.* A diagnostic score for the irritable bowel syndrome. *Gastroenterology* 1984; **87**: 1–7.
3 Kumar D, Wingate DL. The irritable bowel syndrome: a paroxysmal motor disorder. *Lancet* 1985; **ii**: 973–7.
4 Connell AM. The motility of the pelvic colon. II. Paradoxical motility in diarrhoea and constipation. *Gut* 1962; **3**: 342–8.
5 Snape WJ, Carlson GM, Cohen S. Colonic myoelectric activity in the irritable bowel syndrome. *Gastroenterology* 1976; **70**: 326–30.
6 Taylor I, Darby C, Hammond P. Comparison of rectosigmoid myoelectrical activity in the irritable colon syndrome during relapses and remissions. *Gut* 1978; **19**: 923–9.
7 Thompson WG. The irritable bowel: one disease, or several, or none? In: Read NW (ed). *Irritable Bowel*, Vol I. Grune & Stratton, 1985. pp 3–16.
8 Ford MJ. The irritable bowel syndrome. *J Psychosom Res* 1986; **30**: 399–410.
9 Swarbrick ET, Hegarty JE, Bat L *et al.* The site of pain from the irritable bowel. *Lancet* 1980; **ii**: 443–6.

10 Moriarty KJ, Dawson AM. Functional abdominal pain: further evidence that whole gut is affected. *Br Med J* 1982; **i**: 1670-2.

11 Kingham JGC, Dawson AM. Origin of chronic right upper quadrant pain. *Gut* 1985; **26**: 738-8.

12 Almy TP. The irritable bowel syndrome: back to square one? *Dig Dis Sci* 1980; **25**: 401-3.

13 Thompson WG. The irritable bowel syndrome: prevalence, prognosis and consequences. *Can Med Assoc J* 1986; **134**: 11-3.

14 Thompson WG, Heaton KW. Functional bowel disorders in apparently healthy people. *Gastroenterology* 1980; **79**: 283-8.

15 Drossman DA, Sandler RS, McKee DC et al. Bowel dysfunction among subjects not seeking health care. *Gastroenterology* 1982; **83**: 529-34.

16 Sandler RS, Drossman DA, Nathan HP et al. Symptom complaints and health care seeking behaviour in subjects with bowel dysfunction. *Gastroenterology* 1984; **87**: 314-8.

17 Whitehead WE, Winget C, Fedaravicius AS et al. Learned illness behaviour in patients with irritable bowel syndrome and peptic ulcer. *Dig Dis Sci* 1982; **27**: 202-8.

18 Greenbaum D, Abitz L, Van Ergeren L et al. Irritable bowel syndrome prevalence, rectosigmoid motility and psychometrics in symptomatic subjects not seeing physicians. *Gastroenterology* 1984; **86**: 1097 (abstr).

19 Bommelaer G, Rouch M, Dapoigny M et al. Epidemiologie des troubles fonctionnels dans une population apparement saine. *Gastro Clin Biol* 1986; **10**: 7-12.

20 Dent OF, Goulston KJ, Zubrzycki J et al. Bowel symptoms in an apparently well population. *Dis Colon Rectum* 1986; **29**: 243-7.

21 Fielding JF. A year in outpatients with the irritable bowel syndrome. *Irish J Med Sci* 1977; **146**: 162-5.

22 Sullivan SN. Management of the IBS: a personal view. *J Clin Gastroenterol* 1983; **5**: 499-502.

23 Switz DM. What the gastroenterologist does all day. *Gastroenterology* 1976; **70**: 1048-50.

24 Ferguson A, Sircus W, Eastwood MA. Frequency of "functional" gastrointestinal disorders. *Lancet* 1977; **ii**: 613-4.

25 Harvey RF, Salih SY, Read AE. Organic and functional disorders among 2,000 outpatients. *Lancet* 1983; **i**: 632-4.

26 Welch GW, Stace NH, Pomare EW. Specificity of psychological profiles on irritable bowel syndrome patients. *Aust NZ J Med* 1984; **14**: 101-4.

27 Drossman DA, McKee DC, Sandler RS et al. Psychosocial factors in the irritable bowel syndrome: a multivariate study of patients and nonpatients with IBS. (In press).

28 Thompson WG. A strategy for management of the irritable bowel. *Am J Gastroenterol* 1986; **81**: 95-100.

29 Holmes IM, Salter RH. Irritable bowel syndrome — a safe diagnosis. *Br Med J* 1982; **285**: 1533-4.

30 Creed F. Life events and appendectomy. *Lancet* 1981; **i**: 1381-5.

31 Fielding JF. Surgery and the irritable bowel syndrome: the singer as well as the song. *Ir Med J* 1983; **76**: 33-4.

32 Sox HC, Margulies I, Sox CH. Psychologically mediated effects of diagnostic tests. *Ann Intern Med* 1981; **95**: 680-5.

33 Hyams JS. Sorbitol intolerance: an unappreciated cause of functional gastrointestinal complaints. *Gastroenterology* 1983; **84**: 30-3.

34 Ravich WJ, Bayless TM, Thomas M. Incomplete intestinal absorption in humans. *Gastroenterology* 1983; **84**: 26-9.

35 Chaudhary NA, Truelove SC. The irritable colon syndrome. *Quart J Med* 1962; **31**: 307-23.

36 Svedlund J, Sjodin I, Ottosson JO et al. Controlled study of psychotherapy in irritable bowel syndrome. *Lancet* 1983; **ii**: 589-91.

37 Soltoft JI, Gudmand-Hoyer E, Krag B et al. A double blind trial of wheat bran on symptoms of irritable bowel syndrome. *Lancet* 1976; **i**: 270-2.

38 Manning AP, Heaton KW, Harvey RF et al. Wheat fibre and the irritable bowel syndrome. *Lancet* 1977; **ii**: 417-8.

39 Brodribb AJM. Treatment of symptomatic diverticular disease with a high fibre diet. *Lancet* 1977; **i**: 664-6.

40 Ornstein MH, Littlewood ER, Baird M et al. Are fibre supplements really necessary in diverticular disease of the colon? A controlled clinical trial. *Br Med J* 1981; **282**: 1053-6.

41 Weinreich J. The treatment of diverticular disease. *Scand J Gastroenterol* 1982 (suppl 79): 128-9.

42 Cann PA, Read NW, Holdsworth CD. What is the benefit of coarse wheat bran in patients with irritable bowel syndrome. *Gut* 1984; **25**: 168-73.

43 Lucey MR, Clark ML, Lowndes JO, Dawson AM. Is bran efficacious in irritable bowel syndrome? A double blind placebo controlled study. *Gut* 1987; **28**: 221-5.

44 Cowgill GR, Anderson WE. Laxative effects of bran and "washed bran" in healthy men. *JAMA* 1932; **98**: 1866-75.

45 Cleave TL. *The Saccharine Disease*. Bristol: John Wright & Sons 1974.

46 Burkitt DP, Walker ARP, Painter NS. Effect of dietary fibre on stools and transit times, and its role in the causation of disease. *Lancet* 1972; **ii**: 1408-12.

47 Thompson WG, Patel DG, Tao H *et al*. Does uncomplicated diverticular disease cause symptoms? *Dig Dis Sci* 1982; **67**: 605-8.

48 Hodgson WJ. The placebo effect: is it important in diverticular disease? *Am J Gastroenterol* 1977; **67**: 157-62.

49 Ritchie JA, Truelove SC. Treatment of irritable bowel syndrome with lorazepam butylbromide and isbaghula husk. *Br Med J* 1979; **i**: 376-8.

50 Ewerth S, Ahlberg J, Holmstorm B *et al*. Influence on symptoms and transit time of Vi Siblin R in diverticular disease. *Acta Chir Scand* 1980; **500** (suppl): 49-50.

51 Longstreth GF, Fox DD, Youkeles L *et al*. Psyllium therapy in the irritable bowel syndrome. *Ann Intern Med* 1981; **95**: 53-6.

52 Prior A, Akbar FA, Schroff NE *et al*. A double blind study of isbaghula in irritable bowel syndrome. *Gut* 1986; **27**: 625 (abstr).

53 Kumar A, Kumar N, Vij JC *et al*. Optimum dosage of isbaghula husk in patients with irritable bowel syndrome: correlation of symptom relief with whole gut transit time and stool weight. *Gut* 1987; **28**: 150-5.

54 Lichstein J, Mayer JD. Drug therapy of the unstable bowel (irritable colon). *J Chron Dis* 1959; **9**: 394-404.

55 Kasich AM, Fein HD, Miller JW. Comparative effect of phenaglycodol, meprobamate and a placebo on the irritable colon. *Am J Dig Dis* 1959; **4**: 229-34.

56 Wayne HH. A tranquillizer-anticholinergic preparation in functional gastrointestinal disorders – a double-blind evaluation. *Can Med Assoc J* 1969; **79**: 111-5.

57 Page JG, Dirnberger MS. Treatment of the irritable colon syndrome with Bentyl (dicyclomine hydrochloride). *J Clin Gastroenterol* 1981; **3**: 153-6.

58 Fielding JF. Domperidone treatment in the irritable bowel syndrome. *Digestion* 1982; **23**: 125-7.

59 Kruis W, Weinzierl M, Schussler P *et al*. Comparison of the therapeutic effect of wheat bran, mebeverine and placebo in patients with the irritable bowel syndrome. *Digestion* 1986; **34**: 196-201.

60 Brody H. The lie that heals: the ethics of giving placebos. *Ann Intern Med* 1982; **97**: 112-8.

61 Park LV, Covi L. Non blind placebo trial: an explanation of neurotic outpatients' response to placebo when its inert content is disclosed. *Arch Gen Psychiat* 1965; **12**: 336-45.

62 Wolff HG, DuBois EF, Cottell M *et al*. Conferences on therapy: the use of placebos in therapy. *NY State J Med* 1946; **46**: 1718-27.

63 Eghert LD, Battit GE, Welch CE *et al*. Reduction of postoperative pain by encouragement and instruction of patients. *N Engl J Med* 1964; **270**: 825-7.

64 Snape WJ Jr, Wright SH, Battle WM *et al*. The gastrocolonic response: evidence for a neural mechanism. *Gastroenterology* 1979; **77**: 1235-40.

65 Cann PA, Read NW, Holdsworth DP *et al*. Role of loperamide in management of irritable bowel syndrome. *Dig Dis Sci* 1984; **29**: 239-42.

66 Read MW, Read NW, Barber DC *et al*. Effects of loperamide on anal sphincter function in patients complaining of chronic diarrhea with fecal incontinence and urgency. *Dig Dis Sci* 1982; **27**: 807-13.

67 Rees WDW, Evans BK, Rhodes J. Treating irritable bowel syndrome with peppermint oil. *Br Med J* 1979; **ii**: 835-6.

68 Dew MJ, Evans BK, Rhodes J. Peppermint for the irritable bowel. *Br J Clin Pract* 1984; **38**: 394-8.

69 Nash P, Gould SR, Barnardo DE. Peppermint oil does not relieve the pain of irritable bowel syndrome. *Br J Clin Pract* 1986; **40**: 292–3.

70 Sigmund CJ, McNally EF. The action of a carminative on the lower esophageal sphincter. *Gastroenterology* 1969; **56**: 13–8.

71 Shapiro RH, Fleizer WD, Goldfinger JE *et al*. Cholestyramine responsive idiopathic diarrhea. *Gastroenterology* 1970; **58**: 993 (abstr).

72 Thaysen EH, Pedersen L. Idiopathic bile salt catharsis. *Gut* 1986; **17**: 965–70.

73 Smart HL, Mayberry JF, Atkinson M. Alternative medicine consultations and remedies in patients with the irritable bowel syndrome. *Gut* 1986; **27**: 826–8

74 Waller SL, Misiewicz JJ. Prognosis in the irritable bowel syndrome: a prospective study. *Lancet* 1969; **ii**: 753–6.

75 Christensen MF, Mortensen O. Long-term prognosis in children with recurrent abdominal pain. *Arch Dis Child* 1975; **50**: 110–4.

76 Harvey RF, Manod AC, Brown AM. Prognosis in the irritable bowel syndrome: a 5-year prospective study. *Lancet* 1987; **i**: 963–5.

77 Burns DG. The risk of abdominal surgery in irritable bowel syndrome. *South Afr Med J* 1986; **70**: 91.

78 Jones VA, McLaughlin P, Shorthouse M *et al*. Food intolerance: a major factor in the pathogenesis of the irritable bowel syndrome. *Lancet* 1982; **ii**: 1115–7.

79 Bentley SJ, Pearson DJ. Food hypersensitivity in irritable bowel syndrome. *Lancet* 1983; **ii**: 295–7.

80 Farah DA, Calder I, Benson L *et al*. Specific food interolance: its place as a cause of gastrointestinal symptoms. *Gut* 1985; **26**: 144–8.

81 Beuno-Miranda F, Cerulli M, Schuster MM. Operant conditioning of colonic motility in irritable bowel syndrome. *Gastroenterology* 1976; **70**: 867.

82 Engel BT, Nikoomanesh P, Schuster MM. Operant conditioning in the treatment of fecal incontinence. *N Engl J Med* 1974; **290**: 646–9.

83 Whorwell PJ, Prior A, Faragher EB. Controlled trial of hypnotherapy in the treatment of severe refractory irritable bowel syndrome. *Lancet* 1985; **i**: 1232–3.

Surgical management of lower gastrointestinal motility disorders

M R B Keighley

Investigation

Patients studied

Patients with long-standing functional bowel disorders deserve appropriate physiologic investigation. During the past 10 years, 82 patients have been referred for surgery at the Birmingham General Hospital, England, with chronic long-standing constipation with a normal barium enema; 16 patients were referred with constipation having radiologic evidence of megacolon or megarectum; 39 patients have been seen with a long-standing history of tenesmus, bleeding, diarrhea and intermittent constipation where endoscopic investigation confirmed the presence of a solitary rectal ulcer; 160 patients have been seen with a full thickness rectal prolapse; and 177 patients have been referred with fecal incontinence *(Table 1)*. The surgical management of these patients and their long-term outcome follow-up are described here.

For the purposes of this communication, all patients with Crohn's disease, ulcerative colitis, complicated diverticular disease, malignant disease of the large intestine and radiation proctocolitis have been excluded. Only patients with long-standing severe debilitating bowel disorders are subject to intensive physiologic assessment.

Manometry, electromyography, compliance and sensory assessment

Manometric assessment is made of the sigmoid colon, rectum and anal canal. Pressure measurements are obtained using a low pressure infusion pump and a four-channel recorder. Pressure measurements are obtained at rest, in the left lateral and seated position during maximum pelvic floor contraction and during attempted defecation.

The rectoanal inhibitory reflex is assessed after introducing incremental volumes into a rectal balloon. The rectoanal inhibitory reflex is defined as a 30% reduction in resting anal canal pressures after rectal distension.

Threshold anal sensation is evaluated in the upper, middle and lower zones of the high pressure zone of the anal canal using a constant current stimulator.

Rectal capacity is assessed and the following sensory parameters are recorded: threshold sensation, constant sensation and maximum tolerated volume. Rectal compliance is also evaluated by inflation of air into a rectal balloon and recording intra-balloon pressures using an air-filled transducer.[1-5]

Electromyography is then performed using a concentric needle electrode placed in the external sphincter and in the puborectalis. Resting action potentials are monitored and the degree of recruitment assessed during maximum pelvic floor contraction. Increased electrical activity is also assessed during attempted defecation. Sigmoid motility disorders are then evaluated using a continually perfused catheter placed in the sigmoid colon to measure resting motility index at 20 and 25 cm from

213

Condition (number of patients)	Surgical procedure	Outcome
Chronic constipation (82)		
36 Outlet obstruction alone	36 Anorectal myectomy	29 Normal bowel habit (7 constipated)
22 Outlet obstruction and slow transit constipation	22 Anorectal myectomy	7 Normal bowel habit (15 constipated)
	15 Subtotal colectomy later	13 Normal bowel habit (2 constipated)
24 Slow transit constipation alone	20 Subtotal colectomy	13 Normal bowel habit (4 stoma) (3 constipated)
Megacolon and megarectum (16)		
7 Megacolon alone	7 Subtotal colectomy	4 Normal bowel habit (3 constipated)
9 Megacolon and megarectum	5 Restorative proctocolectomy	5 Diarrhea
	4 Stoma	
Solitary rectal ulcer (39)		
10 Associated intussusception	7 Rectopexy	1 Normal bowel habit (6 tenesmus)
Rectal prolapse	6 Rectopexy	5 Normal bowel habit (1 constipated)

Continued

Rectal prolapse (160)

107 Incontinence and prolapse	71 Normal bowel habit (20 constipated) (16 incontinent)
53 Prolapse alone	37 Normal bowel habit (13 constipated)

Incontinence alone (177)

134 Pelvic floor neuropathy	37 Normal bowel habit (67 incontinent) (10 stoma)
43 Sphincter damage	32 Normal bowel habit (3 incontinent) (2 stoma)
7 Ectopic anus	6 Normal bowel habit (1 constipation:stoma)
8 Rectovaginal fistula	6 Normal bowel habit (1 persistent fistula)

In the Pelvic floor neuropathy row: 114 Post-anal repair. In the Sphincter damage row: 37 Sphincter repair. In the Ectopic anus row: 7 Rerouting procedures. In the Rectovaginal fistula row: 7 Repair.

Table 1 Patients with lower gastrointestinal motility disorders referred for surgical correction at the Birmingham General Hospital, England, over the past 10 years.

the anal verge. The influence of intrarectal bisacodyl is assessed using 5 mg of fresh bisacodyl. The response to a standard meal has also been evaluated in some patients.

Colonic transit is also assessed while patients are taking a normal diet with a mean daily fibre intake of 40 g/day when laxatives are withheld. Fifty radio-opaque granules are taken by mouth and a plain x-ray of the abdomen is obtained 5 days later so that the number of residual markers can be counted. Transit is recorded as percentage of radio-opaque markers passed within 5 days.[6,7]

Radiologic studies

Defecating proctograms have been performed more recently. A suspension of 120 g of cellulose with 'Barritop' is introduced into the rectal ampulla. The patient is then seated on a water-filled tire mounted on a lavatory pan. Screening of the pelvis is performed by lateral radiographs and the examination is recorded on video for subsequent playback. The perineum is marked with a radio-opaque tube and the symphysis pubis is also identified with a metal marker. The degree of perineal descent is assessed at rest in relation to the pubococcygeal line as well as the anorectal angle and length of the anal canal. Following maximum pelvic floor contraction, changes in the anorectal angle are assessed together with any elongation of the anal canal and upward displacement of the lower rectum. Screening is then conducted for 1 minute during attempted defecation to identify evidence of an incomplete intussusception, a full thickness rectal prolapse, a rectocele and the changes in the anorectal angle which occur during defecation. This examination also evaluates the degree of rectal emptying by measurement of the weight of contrast material passed during 1 minute. All patients undergo a barium enema examination in order to assess evidence of megacolon or megarectum and as a means of identifying underlying inflammatory bowel disease.[8-10]

Chronic constipation

Etiology

Severe chronic constipation may be secondary to a variety of factors. It is important for the clinician to exclude some of the more common causes such as drug therapy,[11,12] endocrine disorders,[13,14] poisons, congenital and acquired lesions affecting the cauda equina, Hirschsprung's disease,[15] megacolon and megarectum,[16] and operative damage to the pelvic autonomic plexus, a phenomenon that frequently complicates abdominal hysterectomy.

Once these predisposing abnormalities have been excluded there remains a group of patients who have long-standing severe chronic constipation. Some of these patients have a motility disorder that is associated with delayed transit through the colon,[17] but in others there may also be evidence of impaired rectal emptying associated with the increased electrical activity of the puborectalis during attempted defecation. This latter abnormality has been termed 'outlet obstruction'. In some patients outlet obstruction occurs alone while in others it may be associated with slow transit constipation.

Surgical management

During the past 10 years, 82 patients with idiopathic chronic constipation have been identified. Thirty-six of these patients had evidence of outlet obstruction alone, 22 had outlet obstruction in association with slow transit constipation, while 24 patients

had slow transit constipation alone. The initial approach to the management of patients with outlet obstruction alone or in combination with slow transit constipation has been an anorectal myectomy.

Anorectal myectomy: anorectal myectomy is performed under general anesthesia with the patient in the lithotomy position. A Parks anal retractor is inserted with the handles vertical. After infiltration of the submucosal and intersphincteric plane with adrenaline and saline (1:300,000), a transverse incision is made approximately 1 cm above the dentate line posteriorly. The mucosa is then separated from the internal sphincter and the rectal smooth muscle by scissor dissection. The mucosa is then retracted away from the internal sphincter using the third blade of the Parks retractor. In order to remove the entire length of the internal sphincter, the mucosa below the dentate line must be dissected off the smooth muscle until the lower limit of the muscle is reached. After further infiltration in the intersphincteric plane, the internal sphincter and rectal smooth muscle is then dissected from the posterior fibres of the external sphincter and puborectalis. A 1 cm width of smooth muscle is then excised over a length of 10 cm after marking the distal margin with a suture. After hemostasis, the mucosal incision is closed using a continuous catgut suture. A sponge is left inside the anal canal for 4 hours for tamponade. The excised specimen of smooth muscle and internal sphincter is subsequently examined histologically to exclude Hirschsprung's disease.

Thirty-six patients have had an anorectal myectomy performed for outlet obstruction alone. In six of these patients there was evidence of short segment Hirschsprung's disease upon histologic examination. Twenty-nine of 36 patients obtained complete resolution of symptoms following anorectal myectomy with return to normal bowel habit. None of the patients developed incontinence but bleeding was reported in 3 patients and 1 developed a submucous abscess postoperatively. All patients with short segment Hirschsprung's disease were improved by anorectal myectomy. Although 7 patients continued to require intermittent laxatives, all were improved by the operation. By contrast, in 22 patients undergoing an anorectal myectomy where there was evidence of both outlet obstruction and slow transit constipation, 7 achieved a satisfactory functional result while 15 obtained no benefit whatsoever and continued to require large doses of laxatives.

Physiologic studies in patients undergoing anorectal myectomy have revealed a significant reduction in resting anal canal pressures following this operation. There also appears to be a significant reduction in the pressures obtained in the anal canal during attempted defecation.[18]

Forty-six patients were shown to have evidence of slow transit constipation identified by low resting motility index in the sigmoid colon and failure to respond to bisacodyl; these patients also had impaired excretion of radio-opaque markers 5 days after their ingestion.

Subtotal colectomy and ileorectal anastomosis: 35 patients with slow transit constipation have been treated by subtotal colectomy and ileorectal anastomosis. The operation is performed through a mid-line incision with the patient prone and with a urethral catheter inserted immediately before operation. After a full laparotomy the omentum is preserved and the entire colon is removed. The ileum is transected just proximal to the ileocecal valve and the rectosigmoid junction is divided at the sacral promontory. An end-to-end anastomosis is performed without a covering ileostomy. Of the 35 patients who have undergone subtotal colectomy for slow transit constipation, 26 have an almost normal bowel habit. However, 5 patients have persistent constipation requiring laxatives and in 4 patients there has been complete failure to evacuate and all have subsequently required an ileostomy. Severe postoperative intestinal obstruction has been a feature in 7 of the 35 patients who underwent subtotal colectomy and ileorectal anastomosis. None of the patients has become incontinent following operation. However, bowel habit is often erratic and patients still complain of intermittent abdominal distension, nausea and lethargy.

Megacolon and megarectum

Sixteen patients have now been identified with chronic long-standing constipation where the diameter of the colon and rectum have been grossly abnormal following routine barium enema examination. Although identification of megacolon can be extremely difficult by radiology alone, all of the patients in this category had gross impairment of rectal sensation and were unable to appreciate volumes of more than 300 mL distending the rectal ampulla.

Seven patients with megacolon alone were treated by subtotal colectomy and ileorectal anastomosis but only 4 of these achieved normal bowel habit. Three patients with persistent constipation were later shown to have developed a megarectum. Nine patients initially demonstrated as having megacolon and megarectum either underwent restorative proctocolectomy or merely the raising of a stoma. Blind loop ileostomy was performed in 4 patients and this completely controlled symptoms. However, in 5 patients a stoma was refused and restorative proctocolectomy with ileopouch anal anastomosis was performed. One patient developed severe intestinal obstruction following restorative proctocolectomy but all patients now have good functional results and the mean frequency of defecation is 4/24 hours. None of the patients is incontinent and none has a history of soiling.

Solitary rectal ulcer

Etiology
Most patients with solitary rectal ulcer presented with rectal bleeding, mucus discharge and tenesmus. Abnormal bowel habit was common and 28 of the 39 patients with solitary rectal ulcer had a history of chronic long-standing constipation. Not all patients with a solitary rectal ulcer had an established ulcer and in some the only abnormality was an area of erythema with polypoidal projections on the anterior rectal wall.[19-22]

There are various theories as to the cause of the solitary rectal ulcer syndrome. Some series report a high proportion of patients with complete rectal prolapse. In some patients clinical evidence of a rectal prolapse is lacking but many of these patients have recently been shown to have an incomplete or an occult prolapse demonstrated on defecography.[23] It has been suggested that ulceration occurs at the apex of the intussusception as a result of ischemia. Another explanation for the causation of solitary rectal ulcer is based upon electromyographic studies which have shown that in some patients the puborectalis muscle becomes hyperactive during straining thereby traumatizing an area of the anterior rectal mucosa during defecation.[24]

Of the 39 patients with solitary rectal ulcer seen over the past 10 years, 10 were shown to have an incomplete intussusception on defecography. In addition, 6 patients with a full thickness rectal prolapse were identified clinically. Electromyographic studies indicated that only 6 patients had evidence of increased puborectalis activity during attempted defecation. Rectal sensation was impaired in some patients; in others, spikes of resting anal canal pressures indicated episodes of involuntary external sphincter activity. In others, involuntary external sphincter activity was only generated after balloon distension.

Treatment

Thirteen patients with a solitary rectal ulcer have now been treated by abdominal rectopexy. In 7 patients, rectopexy was merely performed for an incomplete intussusception identified by defecography. However, in only 1 of these patients was normal bowel habit subsequently achieved; the remaining 6 patients continue to have symptoms of tenesmus, mucous discharge and rectal bleeding with a persistent ulcer. By contrast, in the 6 patients who underwent rectopexy for full thickness rectal prolapse complicated by solitary rectal ulcer, 5 obtained excellent functional results and the ulcer appeared to heal. Only 1 patient had persistent constipation. These studies appear to indicate that the presence of an incomplete intussusception demonstrated during defecography in patients with a solitary rectal ulcer is of academic interest only. There appears to be no justification for surgical treatment in such patients since symptoms are rarely alleviated by rectopexy.

Rectal prolapse

Etiology

Rectal prolapse is often associated with incontinence and in approximately two-thirds of patients with a rectal prolapse, incomplete control of defecation is recorded in the history. Some younger patients with a rectal prolapse may have a history of prolonged constipation.

Rectal prolapse occurs almost exclusively in female patients. Males usually have some underlying abnormality such as rectal polyps, rectal bilharzia or long-standing chronic constipation. Recent radiologic studies have indicated that full thickness rectal prolapse is caused by an intussusception of the rectum through the pelvic floor.

As a result there is laxity of the lateral ligaments, attenuation of the mesorectum, a prolonged rectovaginal pouch and weakness of the pelvic floor.

Electromyographic studies of the puborectalis indicate evidence of partial denervation in many patients. Resting anal canal pressures are significantly lower in patients with rectal prolapse compared with age- and sex-matched controls and there is usually manometric evidence of impaired squeeze pressures in the anal canal of patients with rectal prolapse. By contrast, rectal sensation is normal although the anorectal angle at rest is generally obtuse.

It was found that the resting motility index in the sigmoid colon was normal in patients with a history of prolapse alone but was increased in patients with a history of incontinence in association with rectal prolapse. In many young patients with rectal prolapse, there is evidence of colonic inertia as indicated by delayed transit of radio-opaque markers through the colon.[25-28] Surprisingly, rectal prolapse is not confined to patients who are multiparous; 20% of the female patients have never had children.

Surgical treatment

There are various approaches to the surgical management of rectal prolapse. Use of the Thiersch wire is often unsuccessful in that the prolapse may not be contained or the wire is tied too tightly resulting in chronic constipation. More recently, the use of silastic rings around the anal canal and puborectalis has produced more encouraging results. Nevertheless, 17% of patients developed recurrent rectal prolapse.[29] Perineal procedures may be used for the repair of rectal prolapse and the Delormes operation has received recent interest.[30] Although this is a low morbidity operation, there is an 8–12% recurrence rate with this procedure.[31] Another approach in the management of rectal prolapse is to perform a perineal rectopexy together with a post-anal repair.[32] This is an interesting approach in the management of rectal prolapse but the follow-up for these operations is relatively short and already the recurrence rate is of the order of 8–10%.

Rectopexy: abdominal rectopexy is considered by many to be the operation of choice for rectal prolapse, particularly as radiologic studies indicate that the primary abnormality is one of intussusception. Use of the Ivalon sponge has been popular for many years and, although successful in 90% of patients, there is a risk of infection around the sponge; a number of patients referred after previous surgical repair of rectal prolapse have already had an Ivalon sponge which has been unsuccessful.

A simple posterior rectopexy has been developed at this institute using polypropylene mesh which is sutured to the sacrum in the mid-line and then to the divided lateral ligaments of the rectum after it has been fully mobilized posteriorly (*Figure 1*).

Abdominal rectopexy is performed with the patient in the supine position after catheterization. A lower mid-line incision is made. The sigmoid colon is held and the peritoneum on the lateral aspects of the upper two-thirds of the rectum is divided. No attempt is made to divide the anterior peritoneal reflection between the rectum and the vagina. The mesorectum is divided, preserving the superior hemorrhoidal

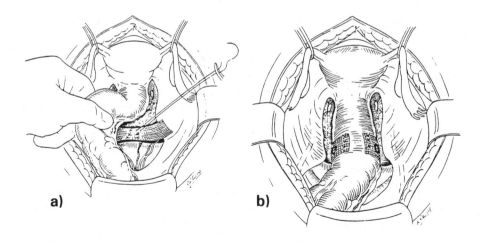

a)   b)

Figure 1   (a) Rectopexy using polypropylene mesh which is sutured to the sacrum. (b) Completed rectopexy. Reproduced with permission from Keighley MRB, Fielding JWL, Alexander-Williams J. Results of Marlex Mesh abdominal rectopexy for rectal prolapse in 100 consecutive patients. *Br J Surg* 1983; **70**: 229–31.

vessels without damaging the pelvic autonomic plexus or the pre-sacral veins. The rectum is mobilized down to the tip of the coccyx. The lateral ligaments are divided. A 2x3 cm rectangle of polypropylene mesh is prepared. Three sutures are placed through the periosteum of the sacral promontory just inside the pelvis which are sutured in the mid-line to the polypropylene mesh. The rectum is then thoroughly retracted in an upward direction and the lateral aspects of the polypropylene mesh are sutured to the divided lateral ligaments of the rectum. Two vacuum suction drains are placed in the pelvis and the abdomen is closed.

A total of 160 rectopexy procedures have been performed for patients with full thickness rectal prolapse. Thirty-two percent of the patients were over the age of 80; in 11% the operation was performed under spinal anesthesia because of anesthetic risk.

Of 107 patients having posterior rectopexy with a history of prolapse and incontinence, 23 had persistent troublesome incontinence requiring a subsequent post-anal repair. The results of secondary post-anal repair for persistent incontinence have been disappointing and only 7 of 23 patients have achieved full continence following post-anal repair. The operation of post-anal repair under these circumstances is often difficult because the retrorectal space has already been dissected during the abdominal rectopexy. Unfortunately there is no means at present of detecting those patients who are likely to have persistent incontinence after abdominal rectopexy. Therefore, combined rectopexy and post-anal repair cannot be justified since the risks of infection must be greater in patients having the dual operation. When the functional results of the 107 patients who underwent rectopexy for prolapse and incontinence were analyzed, 71 reported a normal bowel habit postoperatively, 20 had troublesome constipation often associated with a redundant sigmoid colon and 16 patients remained incontinent despite a previous post-anal repair.

The results of rectopexy in the 53 patients having rectal prolapse alone are also encouraging. Thirty-seven have a normal bowel habit although 13 patients have had troublesome constipation postoperatively.

Recurrent rectal prolapse has been reported in only 1 of 160 patients having abdominal rectopexy. There has been no operative mortality and morbidity has been low.

Abdominal rectopexy is therefore felt to be the operation of choice for patients with full thickness rectal prolapse and that post-anal repair should be reserved for patients with troublesome fecal incontinence despite correction of the rectal prolapse.

Fecal incontinence

Etiology

Fecal incontinence is a distressing symptom which is often associated with social isolation. The principal etiologic causes have been: obstetric trauma, idiopathic fecal incontinence, previous anal surgery and a variety of neurologic conditions.

Many patients with fecal incontinence have a history of a functional bowel disorder. Therefore, not only are resting anal canal and squeeze anal pressures significantly lower than age- and sex-matched controls, but in many of these patients there is increased motility in the sigmoid colon. Intestinal transit is generally normal but rectal and anal sensation is commonly impaired in patients with idiopathic fecal incontinence or in patients who have developed incontinence following obstetric trauma. A number of patients with fecal incontinence have abnormal perineal descent and almost all patients have electromyographic evidence of partial denervation to the pelvic floor.[33-37]

Surgical treatment

Surgical treatment of fecal incontinence is reported to be encouraging, and in the absence of central neurologic abnormalities, post-anal repair has been advised for patients with pelvic floor neuropathy and external sphincter reconstruction for those with deficiencies in the external anal sphincter.[76,38]

Post-anal repair: post-anal repair is performed with the patient in the lithotomy position with the buttocks placed well over the end of the operating table supported by a wedge to achieve adequate access to the skin over the tip of the coccyx. The patient is catheterized and draped. Preoperative antibiotics are given. A curved post-anal incision is made approximately 2 cm behind the anal canal (*Figure 2*). The anterior skin flap is raised towards the anus and the circular fibres of the external sphincter are identified. Dissection proceeds over the external sphincter and by retracting the external sphincter posteriorly the plane between the internal and external anal sphincter is opened. By gentle gauze dissection it is soon possible to insert a small curved Kocher's retractor anteriorly so that the lateral edges of the external sphincter and the inner fibres of the puborectalis sling can be retracted posteriorly (*Figure 2*). After this manoeuvre it is possible to introduce a wider Kocher's retractor anteriorly to facilitate access.

The crucial step in the operation is to divide Waldeyer's fascia transversely. This must be completely divided so that the veins on the posterior aspect of the rectum can be easily identified. Following this manoeuvre it is easy to sweep the rectum anteriorly off the entire sacrum to the level of the sacral promontory. A large curved Kocher's retractor is then inserted over the rectum to expose the pelvic floor muscles behind. The fibres of the puborectalis and pubococcygeus can be easily identified together with the ischiococcygeus on either side of the pelvis.

Although a two- or three-layer repair used to be applied, a single-layer mass closure technique has now been adopted by the author. By placing a series of interrupted Dexon sutures posteriorly, it is possible to creep forward apposing the puborectalis and pubococcygeus to the lateral extremities of the muscle fibres. These sutures must be ligated and not tied until all are in position. A curved Kocher's retractor is then withdrawn and curved cholecystectomy forceps inserted to prevent the anterior skin flap from obscuring the view. The sutures are then tied, two vacuum drains may be inserted in the retrorectal space and the skin is apposed with prolene.

Recent experience suggests that with long-term follow-up, the functional results of post-anal repair are much worse than has hitherto been reported in the literature.

Of 134 patients with pelvic floor neuropathy, 114 have now undergone post-anal repair. Follow-up has ranged from 1–11 years; however, only 37 of 114 patients have achieved normal bowel habit. Sixty-seven remain incontinent though many of these patients admit that symptoms are much better following surgical repair than they were beforehand. Ten of these patients have now eventually required an intestinal stoma. There is no doubt that patients with a functional bowel disorder in the sigmoid colon in association with fecal incontinence generally have a poor response to post-anal repair. However, it also appears that patients with gross electromyographic abnormalities in the puborectalis preoperatively do poorly. Hence, post-anal repair should be confined to those patients with mild incontinence and with reasonable muscle function as indicated by preoperative electromyographic studies.

Graciloplasty: all 10 patients who have undergone graciloplasty where post-anal repair has been unsuccessful have had uniformly disappointing results; in none of these patients has continence been restored.

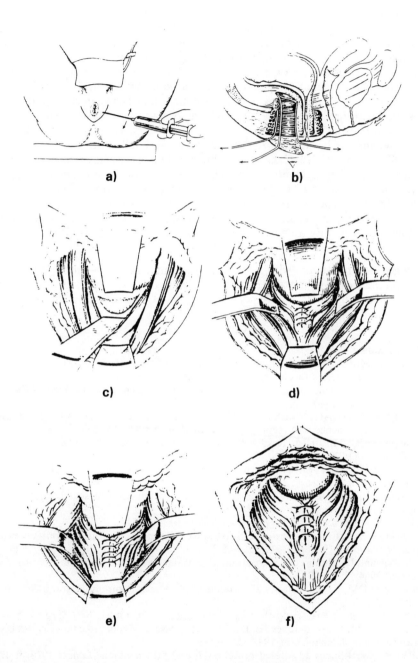

Figure 2 Intersphincteric post-anal repair: (a) incision after infiltration with adrenaline; (b) lateral view of the exposure; (c) pubococcygeus, puborectalis and ischiococcygeus displayed, Waldeyers fascia opened; (d) repair of ischiococcygeus; (e) repair of puborectalis; (f) repair of pubucoccygeus. Reproduced with permission from Keighley MRB, Fielding J. Management of faecal incontinence and results of surgical treatment. *Br J Surg* 1983; **70:** 463–8.

Sphincter repair: sphincter repair is performed in the lithotomy position if the defect is anterior but in the prone position if the defect is posterior. The anocutaneous junction is divided transversely over the site of the defect so that the mucosa can be dissected away from the scar tissue and preserved The lateral dissection defines healthy sphincter muscle on either side of the scar tissue. This is carefully dissected from the internal sphincter and a tape is placed under the healthy sphincter ring at a site lateral to the scar tissue. The scarred material of the external sphincter is then dissected with healthy muscle and divided. A flap-over Mayo repair is performed in two layers using the scar tissue to secure the sutures. The mucosa over the repaired sphincter muscle is then approximated to the perianal skin.

Of 43 patients with external anal sphincter damage, 37 have undergone sphincter repair using a flap-over procedure. Of these, 32 now have normal bowel habit, 3 remain incontinent and 2 eventually required an intestinal stoma. These results suggest that sphincter reconstruction provides excellent long-term results but the long-term results of post-anal repair are much worse than those reported earlier in patients followed-up for only a short period of time.

Others: seven patients with an ectopic anus have had a re-routing procedure and in 6 continence has been restored. Eight patients with a rectovaginal fistula were seen. Seven underwent repair; 6 have normal bowel habit, and only 1 patient has a persistent rectovaginal fistula.

References
1 Farthing MMLG, Lennard-Jones JE. Sensibility of the rectum to distension and the anorectal distension reflex in ulcerative colitis. *Gut* 1978; **19**: 64–9.
2 Ihre T. Studies on anal function in continent and incontinent patients. *Scand J Gastroenterol* 1974; Suppl **925**: 1–80.
3 Neil ME, Parks AG, Swash MH. Physiological studies of the anal sphincter musculature in faecal incontinence and rectal prolapse. *Br J Surg* 1981; **68**: 531–6.
4 Bartolo DCC, Jarratt JA, Read NW. The cutaneo-anal reflex: a useful index of neuropathy? *Br J Surg* 1983; **70**: 660–3.
5 Aaronson I, Nixon HH. A clinical evaluation of anorectal pressure studies in the diagnosis of Hirschsprung's disease. *Gut* 1972; **13**: 138–46.
6 Shouler P, Keighley MRB. Changes in colorectal function in severe idiopathic chronic constipation. *Gastroenterology* 1986; **90**: 414–20.
7 Poisson J, Devroede G. *Surg Clin Am* 1983; **63**: 197–217.
8 Patriquin H, Martelli H, Devroede G. Barium enema in chronic constipation: is it meaningful? *Gastroenterology* 1978; **75**: 619–22.
9 Wasserman IF. Puborectalis syndrome (rectal stenosis due to anorectal spasm). *Dis Colon Rectum* 1964; **7**: 87–97.
10 Preston DM, Lennard-Jones JE, Thomas BM. The balloon proctogram. *Br J Surg* 1984; **71**: 29–32.
11 Smith B, Grace RH, Todd IP. Organic constipation in adults. *Br J Surg* 1977; **64**: 313–4.
12 Present DM, Lennard-Jones JE. Does failure of bisacodyl-induced colonic peristalsis indicate intrinsic nerve damage? *Gut* 1982; **23**: A891.
13 Rees DW, Rhodes J. Altered bowel habit and menstruation. *Lancet* 1976; **i**: 475–80.
14 Preston DM, Lennard-Jones JE. Gynaecological disorders and hyperprolactinaemia in chronic constipation. *Gut* 1983; **24**: A480.
15 Nissan S, Bar-Maor JA, Levy A. Anorectal myomectomy in the treatment of short segment Hirschsprung's disease. *Ann Surg* 1969; **170**: 969–71.
16 Lane RHS, Todd IP. Idiopathic megacolon: a review of 42 cases. *Br J Surg* 1977; **64**: 305–10.
17 Watier A, Devroede G, Arhan P, Duguay C. Mechanisms of idiopathic inertia. A manifestation of systemic disease? *Dig Dis Sci* 1983; **28**: 1025–33.
18 Yoshioka K, Keighley MRB. Anorectal myectomy for outlet obstruction. *Br J Surg* (In press).

19 Kennedy DK, Hughes SR, Masterton JP. The natural history of benign ulcer of the rectum. *Surg Gynecol Obstet* 1977; **144**: 718–20.

20 Martin CJ, Parks TG, Biggart JD. Solitary rectal ulcer syndrome in Northern Ireland. 1971-1980: 51 cases in the whole of Northern Ireland. *Br J Surg* 1981; **681**: 744–7.

21 Rutter KRP, Riddell RH. The solitary ulcer syndrome of the rectum. *Clin Gastroenterol* 1975; **4**: 505–30.

22 Madigan MR, Morson BC. Solitary ulcer of the rectum. *Gut* 1969; **10**: 871–81.

23 White CM, Findlay JM, Proce JJ. The occult rectal prolapse syndrome. *Br J Surg* 1980; **67**: 528–30.

24 Rutter KRP. Electromyographic changes in certain pelvic floor abnormalities. *Proc R Soc Med* 1974; **67**: 53–6.

25 Keighley MRB. Anal function and faecal incontinence. In: Jerrell D, Lee E, eds. *Topics in Gastroenterology*. Oxford: Blackwell Scientific Publications, 1981; 305–23.

26 Keighley MRB, Fielding JWL, Alexander-Williams J. Results of Marlex Mesh abdominal rectopexy for rectal prolapse in 100 consecutive patients. *Br J Surg* 1983; **70**: 229–31.

27 Keighley MRB, Fielding J. Management of faecal incontinence and results of surgical treatment. *Br J Surg* 1983; **70**: 463–8.

28 Keighley MRB, Shouler P. Clinical and manometric features of the solitary rectal ulcer syndrome. *Dis Colon Rectum* 1984; **27**: 507–12.

29 Jackman FR, Francis JN, Hopkinson BR. Aspects of treatment. Silicone rubber band treatment of rectal prolapse. *Ann R Coll Surg Engl* 1980; **62**: 384–5.

30 Morson JRT, Jones NAG, Vowden P, Brennan TG. Delorme's operation: the first choice in complete rectal prolapse? *Ann R Coll Surg Engl* 1986; **68**: 143–5.

31 Christiansen J, Kirkegaard P. Delorme's operation for complete rectal prolapse. *Br J Surg* 1981; **68**: 537–8.

32 Wyatt AP. Perineal rectopexy for rectal prolapse. *Br J Surg* 1981; **68**: 717–9.

33 Duthie HL. Progress report on anal continence. *Gut* 1971; **21**: 844–52.

33 Read NW, Bartolo DCC, Read MG. Differences in anal function in patients with incontinence to solids and in patients with incontinence to liquids. *Br J Surg* 1984; **71**: 39–42.

34 Henry MM, Parks AG, Swash MH. The pelvic floor musculature in the descending perineum syndrome. *Br J Surg* 1982; **69**: 470–2.

35 Henry MM, Parks AG, Swash MH. The anal reflux in idiopathic faecal incontinence: an electrophysiological study. *Br J Surg* 1980; **68**: 531–6.

36 Read NW, Hanford NH, Schmuten AC. A clinical study of patients with faecal incontinence and diarrhoea. *Gastroenterology* 1979; **76**: 747–56.

37 Parks AG, Potter NH, Hardcastle J. The syndrome of the descending perineum. *Proc R Soc Med* 1966; **59**: 477–82.

38 Browning GGP, Parks AG. Postanal repair for neuropathic faecal incontinence: correlation of clinical results and anal canal pressures. *Br J Surg* 1983; **70**: 101–4.

Index